DEPARTMENT OF COMMUNITY MEDICINE

Recent Advances in
COMMUNITY MEDICINE

ALWYN SMITH PhD FRCP FRCGP FFCM

Professor of Epidemiology and Social Oncology,
University of Manchester, Manchester, UK

Recent Advances in
COMMUNITY MEDICINE

EDITED BY
ALWYN SMITH

NUMBER THREE

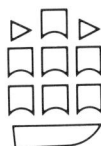

CHURCHILL LIVINGSTONE
EDINBURGH LONDON MELBOURNE AND NEW YORK 1985

CHURCHILL LIVINGSTONE
Medical Division of Longman Group Limited

Distributed in the United States of America by
Churchill Livingstone Inc., 1560 Broadway, New York,
N.Y. 10036, and by associated companies, branches
and representatives throughout the world.

First published 1985

ISBN 0 443 030219
ISSN 0144 1256

British Library Cataloguing in Publication Data
Recent advances in community medicine. – No. 3
  1. Community health services – Periodicals
  362.1′0425   RA425

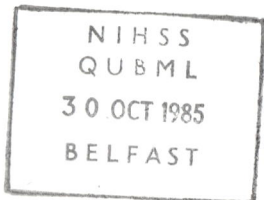

Printed in Great Britain at The Pitman Press, Bath

Contributors

SHEILA ADAM MD MFCM MRCP DCH
Specialist in Community Medicine, North West Thames Regional Health Authority

MICHAEL ALDERSON MD FFCM
Chief Medical Statistician, Office of Population Censuses and Surveys, London

JOHN R ASHTON MBBS MSc(Soc Med) MRCPsych MFCM
Senior Lecturer in Community Health, Liverpool University Medical School

ELIZABETH M BADLEY MSc DPhil
Deputy Director, Arthritis and Rheumatism Council Epidemiology Research Unit,
University of Manchester Medical School, Manchester

JOHN C. BELL BVSc MRCVS DVSM
Divisional Veterinary Officer, Ministry of Agriculture, Fisheries and Food

F. A. BODDY FRCP(Ed) FFCM
Director, Social Paediatric and Obstetric Research Unit, University of Glasgow

JOHN C. CATFORD MA MSc(Social Medicine) MRCP MFCM DCH
Specialist in Community Medicine, Wessex Regional Health Authority

DIANA K. CHISHOLM BA MB BChir(Cantab)
SHO, Department of Epidemiology and Community Medicine, University Hospital
of South Manchester

ANNE EARDLEY BA(Soc Sci) MSc MA(Econ)
Research Officer, Department of Epidemiology and Social Research, University
Hospital of South Manchester; Honorary Research Fellow in Epidemiology and
Social Research, Department of Oncology, University of Manchester

DIANA ELBOURNE BSc(Soc) Dip Stats, Msc(Stats)
Research Officer, National Perinatal Epidemiology Unit

ANDREA KNOPF ELKIND BSocSc MSc
Senior Research Officer, Department of Epidemiology and Social Research,
University Hospital of South Manchester; Honorary Research Fellow in
Epidemiology and Social Research in the Department of Oncology, University of
Manchester

TOM FRYERS MD PhD FFCM DRCOG DPH
Senior Lecturer in Community Medicine, University of Manchester; Specialist in
Community Medicine, North West Regional Health Authority; Director Psychiatric
and Mental Handicap Registers, Salford

N. S. GALBRAITH MB FRCP FFCM DPH
Director, Communicable Disease Surveillance Centre, Public Health Laboratory
Service, London

M. J. GOLDACRE MA MSc BM BCh FFCM
Specialist in Community Medicine, Oxford Regional Health Authority; Lecturer in
Social and Community Medicine, University of Oxford; Honorary Acting Director,
Unit of Clinical Epidemiology, University of Oxford, Oxford

J. A. MUIR GRAY MD MRCGP MRCP(Glas)
Specialist in Community Medicine, Oxfordshire Health Authority; Fellow of Green
College, Oxford

DAVE HARAN BSc MEd PhD
Senior Research Officer, Department of Epidemiology and Social Research,
University Hospital of South Manchester; Honorary Research Fellow in
Epidemiology and Social Research, Department of Oncology, University of
Manchester; Honorary Lecturer in Faculty of Education, University of Manchester

PATRICIA HOBBS MSc PhD
Deputy Head, Department of Epidemiology and Social Research, University Hospital
of South Manchester; Honorary Research Fellow in Epidemiology and Social
Research in Department of Oncology, University of Manchester

LESLEY MUTCH MB ChB
Research Officer, National Perinatal Epidemiology Unit

STEPHEN R. PALMER MA MB BChir MFCM
Consultant Epidemiologist, PHLS Communicable Disease Surveillance Centre
(Wales); Regional Public Health Laboratory, University Hospital of Wales, Cardiff

LAURA L. PENDLETON BSc MSc PhD
Research Officer, Department of Epidemiology and Social Research, University
Hospital of South Manchester; Honorary Research Fellow in Epidemiology and
Social Research, Department of Oncology, University of Manchester

P. O. D. PHAROAH MD MSc FFCM
Professor of Community Health, University of Liverpool

ALWYN SMITH PhD FRCP FRCGP FFCM
Professor of Epidemiology and Social Oncology, University of Manchester

BRENDA E. SPENCER BA MSc
Research Officer, Department of Epidemiology and Social Research, University
Hospital of South Manchester; Honorary Research Associate, Department of
Obstetrics and Gynaecology, University Hospital of South Manchester; Honorary
Research Fellow in Epidemiology and Social Research, Department of Oncology,
University of Manchester

D. R. R. WILLIAMS PhD MFCM
University Lecturer in Community Medicine, Cambridge University; Honorary
Specialist in Community Medicine, East Anglian Regional Health Authority

PHILIP H. N. WOOD MB FRCP FFCM
Director, Arthritis and Rheumatism Council Epidemiology Research Unit and
Professor of Community Medicine, University of Manchester Medical School;
Honorary Regional Specialist in Community Medicine

MARTIN C. WOOLAWAY MBBS MSc(Community Medicine)
Senior Registrar in Community Medicine, Wessex Regional Health Authority

Contents

1. The epidemiological basis of community medicine

Alwyn Smith

If there is such a person as the casual reader of a volume entitled Recent Advances in Community Medicine, that person might expect a catalogue of achievements rather than of aspirations. Nevertheless, it is important in a continually changing world to provide something more than a chronicle of immediate past history and advance in community medicine consists as much in the identification of opportunities as in their exploitation. An account of advances in most branches of medicine will be largely preoccupied with developments at the level of science rather than of practice since once an innovation is accomplished it becomes part of established tradition.

The principal science upon which the practice of community medicine is based is epidemiology whose concern is with the study of the health of human communities. A less than complimentary review of an earlier volume in this series expressed disapproval of the amount of attention devoted to what were dismissed as largely political questions and the lack of what the reviewer would have preferred and thought of as epidemiological topics. In presenting this latest volume one can only admit that a similarly inclined reviewer might have similar reservations. But it is important to consider not only whether the criticism is just but also whether the distinction is justified. In other words, how far is epidemiology the political study of health?

Much of the admitted confusion that has characterised some discussion of the nature and function of epidemiology arises from failure to resolve the question of whether epidemiology is a science or only a method. This requires some preliminary consensus concerning both the nature and function of *science* and the criteria that may be used in defining a science. Although the extensive literature of the philosophy of science is characterised by considerable controversy, there is general agreement that science has two main preoccupations:

(a) the disciplined recording of observations, with all that that implies in terms of the development of observational technique, experimental design, and analysis, and

(b) the use of the accruing data to construct a systematic interpretation of our experience of the universe which both provides a satisfactory explanation of data, and leads to constructive conjectures which may be tested against further data.

What is less completely agreed is that science has an implicit purpose which is to permit us to *improve* our experience of the universe. The distinction between scientific explanations and theological ones might be summarised, at least in Western culture, by the observation that while religion helps us to endure our predicament, science helps us to change it.

Science is discernibly, if not quite categorically, divided into *sciences*. Although superficially they differ from one another most obviously in their investigational techniques there are more profound considerations that distinguish the different sciences. First, sciences differ from one another in their domains of enquiry, the particular aspects of the universe to which they address themselves. Second, they differ in the kinds of models (theories) they use to interpret their domains. This is partly because different domains may require different theoretical models (e.g., astronomy and geology) but sometimes it is the theoretical difference that distinguishes two sciences with similar domains (e.g., physics and chemistry; sociology and psychology). Third, the nature of the domain and the structure of the theory may prescribe a characteristic set of investigational methods, which thus follow from rather than dictate the subject matter and theoretical structure of the science. Finally, some sciences arise quite explicity from an intended field of practical application as do the sciences (as distinct from the technical practices) of engineering, agriculture and medicine.

Although the uses of science depend very much on the users, what is generally intended by scientists to be useful is their results. These are not simply the data recorded by scientific research but the systematic explanatory models (theories) that scientists construct from their data. Theory is the intended useful end-product of scientific activity. Nevertheless, the investigational methods of science may also be found useful in day-to-day technical practice. This has been particularly the case in medicine where techniques originally developed for purposes of scientific enquiry often turn out to be useful tools for investigating practical problems.

EPIDEMIOLOGY AS A SCIENCE

We can now examine epidemiology in terms of the criteria by which it may be distinguished both as *science* and as *a science* and consider in turn its methods, its domain of enquiry, its theoretical structure and its applications.

Methods
These need not detain us long. Most of the investigational methods used by epidemiologists have been eclectically borrowed from other population sciences. A good knowledge of them could be acquired by the average science-trained student in a week-end. Essentially, epidemiology proceeds by observing or estimating the incidence of health events or the prevalence of health states among characterisable sub-groups of the community identifiably experiencing particular vicissitudes. Standard sampling techniques are used when total population data are difficult or inconvenient to assemble. There is room for considerable improvement in the detailed techniques used for obtaining and analysing data but for the most part such improvement would involve little more than raising epidemiological standards to the levels generally prevailing in other population sciences.

Domain of enquiry
The term *epidemiology* is derived from Greek words implying the study of events happening to communities. Historically, epidemiology began with the study of *epidemics* which were episodes in which the observable occurrence of illness became

locally and transiently increased. Diseases which did not display such epidemicity were thought of as either sporadic, endemic or absent from the community under consideration As the available observational techniques become more effective it became clear that most illnesses display spatial and temporal as well as other interesting variations in different communities and epidemiology has consequently extended its range of concern to all illnesses and indeed to variations in levels of health. Many definitions of epidemiology have been proposed; the writer's own is 'that branch of medical science that is concerned to interpret the health experience of human communities'.

As with most very brief definitions, much depends on the precise meaning to be attached to some of the words that are used. However, if the preliminary observations on the nature and function of science and sciences are accepted, the main residual problems concern what is to be understood by the terms 'health' and 'community'.

The issue of health poses no particular problem if we agree that it has to be quite widely understood. The writer defines health as representing 'a level of physiological function and anatomical completeness sufficient to permit an individual to perform an acceptable social role'. Thus an individual's health may be as much a function of the community's social development as of the individual's body, and ill-health is as much a social as a physiological phenomenon. If we define disease as the absence of health it follows that health is the absence of disease and such concepts as 'positive health' are seen to have no useful meaning. A community is a much more complex notion; it is clearly more than a category of persons or even a population. A community may be defined (for these purposes) as 'an aggregation of individuals sharing a concern for the quality and duration of their individual and collective survival'. Thus a climbing team, a work force, a city or nation, or the population of the world may in different contexts, represent communities. Such a category as the individuals listed on a particular page of the telephone directory would not normally constitute a community unless the page were missing and they banded together to remedy the situation. The important issue is that if human individuals did not live in communities epidemiology would be largely pointless since its findings could not be usefully applied.

The essential function of a human community is to protect the interests of its members. Epidemics of sickness seem to have been identified as an important threat at a very early stage in human history and avertive rituals or other procedures were developed to deal with them. Most such action is necessarily based on at least an implicit explanation of how, or why, the threat arises. Such explanations, in common with other explanations of human experience, became scientific in a recognisably modern sense during the very earliest periods for which we still have records, and over the last two or three thousand years these explanations have become elaborated and articulated. An historical account of these developments shows that they represent a coherent and continuous development of a distinct intellectual tradition.

Not everyone uses the term epidemiology to describe this intellectual tradition. Some writers have sought to limit the use of the term to describe an arbitrary selection of methods used in epidemiological enquiry. Nevertheless, the clear development of public health as a branch of human social activity and the evident and, indeed, necessary development of an underlying explanatory system upon which it could be based, is more or less universally acknowledged. The terms that have been used to describe this explanatory system have, however, been numerous and diverse. Public health theory, social medicine, state medicine, health science, population medicine, and medical ecology, have all had their proponents. But 'epidemiology' seems to commend itself on both historical and etymological grounds.

Theoretical structure
A problem that is encountered in any survey of modern epidemiology is its relative absence of distinctive theory. This has led some epidemiologists to see their science as no more than a method and has resulted in the literature of the subject coming to resemble a vast stock-pile of almost surgically clean data untouched by human thought. Such research hypotheses as are explicit (or more often implicit) seem to derive mainly from the theory of other disciplines. Indeed, much recent British work published as epidemiological might more reasonably be viewed as the work of investigators from other disciplines employing methods derived from epidemiology to pursue their own concerns.

This bias towards empiricism has not always been a feature of epidemiology. Indeed, from the time of Hippocrates until the eighteenth century the discipline was almost wholly theoretical since no appropriate investigational methods were available for empirical enquiry. We owe the origin of modern epidemiological method to John Graunt who developed techniques for collecting and analysing data on attributed causes of death and on the personal characteristics of the deceased individuals. His innovation ushered in a period of theoretical and methodological development which culminated in the work of nineteenth century epidemiology in the field of communicable disease. But the eventual declining relevance of the infection model to the newer problems of twentieth century epidemiology was associated with an increasing predominance of methodological over theoretical concerns. In the present century, advances in the technology of data processing and in the power of statistical methods have further tilted the balance towards empiricism.

Another probable influence that has emphasised this trend has been the progressive isolation of epidemiology and epidemiologists from the practitioners of practical public health. The reasons for this isolation have been relatively unexplored, but, in Britain, it is clear that by the time university Chairs began to be created in what was often called Social Medicine, individuals with professional experience in public health were generally considered inappropriate or ineligible to occupy them. One important historical reason for this was that medical officers of health had, since the early years of the century, largely forsaken their consultative role as community physicians in order to assume responsibility for the day-to-day direction of the extensive personal health and other services which they had brought into being to solve public health problems left largely neglected by the clinicians of the day. Having relinquished the community physician's role in favour of that of manager, their need to command and to pursue a scientific explanation of the health experience of human communities declined. That science, deprived of contact with practical problems, grew ever more esoteric and empirical. For it is a paradox that when a science is closely engaged in informing a branch of practice it requires a stronger theoretical base than when allowed to escape from everyday reality. Practitioners require principles; mere data are scarcely ever useful since they can rarely be accumulated sufficiently quickly for the purposes of practical decision-making and data isolated from the interpretive context of theory are frequently equivocal if not actually meaningless.

The isolation of epidemiology from public health had the further effect of fostering a closer association between epidemiologists and clinical scientists. The possibility of using methods borrowed from epidemiology for the examination of hypotheses arising in these other sciences and the paucity of theory capable of generating genuinely epidemiological hypotheses, promoted an opportunistic eclecticism in much so-called epidemiological research.

Another circumstance which has hindered the development of a central body of coherent epidemiological theory has been the increasing concern of a large number of other scientific disciplines, and fields of professional practice, with the health of human communities. Many factors other than the practice of public health or medicine have contributed to health change and many other scientific disciplines have explored these issues. Any comprehensive body of epidemiological theory would need to accommodate elements of the theory of other disciplines but the education of most epidemiologists has tended to limit their awareness of, or concern for, disciplines outside medicine. Since the contribution of clinical disciplines to epidemiological understanding is inevitably somewhat fragmentary, epidemiological theory has become relatively impoverished.

However, a historical view of the development of epidemiology does permit the identification of a theoretical framework for the subject. Isolated writings in the last few decades have contributed to the delineation of a current and future theoretical development. In considering the development of epidemiological theory for the present and future, it is convenient to distinguish four principal theoretical perspectives which are now considered under the headings of the clinical perspective, the ecological perspective, the demographic perspective, and the socio-political perspective.

The clinical perspective
The earliest epidemiologists seem to have been physicians (or licensed healers) who used the data of their clinical experience to generate and support conjectures about the causes and consequences of disease. Hippocrates and Galen are commonly regarded as early epidemiologists although it is uncertain how far their conjectures were intended to lead to practical policies. Clearly, study of the distribution and determinants of disease prevalence requires data on disease occurrences and physicians were in the best position to acquire suitable data. Later physicians who used their clinically acquired data in an epidemiological way included Sydenham, Percival and Heberden and in our own century the fashion has become re-established.

Two major problems in the use of clinical data for epidemiological purposes are the difficulty of identifying the communities or populations to which the experience relates and the selective presentation of a community's experience of illness to any individual physician. These difficulties seriously inhibited the development of clinical epidemiology until it became possible to pool the collective experience of the physicians serving a defined community and this remains a major problem when large volumes of data are required. The Royal College of General Practitioners has pioneered such collaborative studies in this country on a major scale.

A more serious limitation of clinically based epidemiology is the general lack of interest among clinicians in the causes or consequences of illness and the intense preoccupation of medical science and teaching with the mechanisms of disease. Much of this derives from the relative lack of access to relevant data; the majority of clinicians with sufficient opportunity for research pursue their work in institutional environments which insulate them from their patient's experience of domestic and working life. The problem is compounded by a prevalent ideology among clinicians which limits their role to counsellor of individual patients and makes them reluctant to engage in the political arena where issues relevant to the public health inevitably need to be discussed.

In spite of this, clinicians undoubtedly made important contributions to the body of empirical data on which epidemiologists may draw and have occasionally contributed to epidemiological science. An acknowledgement by more doctors of the truth of Virchow's assertion that 'should medicine ever fulfill its great ends it must enter into the larger political and social life of our time . . .' would greatly enhance the relevance of the clinical contribution. Meanwhile one must particularly acknowledge the major contributions made to epidemiology by clinicians working in the specialties of general practice, psychiatry, geriatrics, trauma surgery, occupational medicine and obstetrics — all fields in which consciousness of the need to develop services for communities is as important as the capacity to respond to the needs of individuals.

The ecological perspective
The dependence of human health on the relationship of man to his habitat and to other creatures that share it, is the longest established tradition of epidemiological thought. It is evident in the writings of Hippocrates and it was the main theme of eighteenth and nineteenth century epidemiology. Beginning in the late eighteenth century, with the observations of Percival and others that health and sickness was associated with housing and working conditions as well as with season and climate, epidemiologists continued throughout the nineteenth century to specify in detail those aspects of habitat that were unhealthy. The identification of pathogenic micro-organisms and the demonstration that their transmission depended on the contamination of air, water and food, was an important achievement which made possible the new sciences of medical microbiology and immunology.

In the late nineteenth and early twentieth centuries recognition of the role of intermediate hosts and vector species and the concept of both inherited and acquired immunity permitted an elaboration of the ecological perspective and led, in respect of communicable disease, to productive theoretical models. The concept that disease outbreaks represented a disturbance of a symbiotic equilibrium between human hosts, parasitic infective agents, and the environment which influenced their interdependence, informed the researches of such epidemiologists as Ross, Greenwood and Frost.

More recently, the ecological perspective has embraced epidemiological studies of accidental and other trauma, and of diseases arising from the dissemination of toxic products of human and other activity. This has, so far, been most effective in the environment involved in studies of occupational disease and injury, but has begun to be fruitful in a wider context in relation to such issues as atmospheric and other pollution.

An aspect of the ecological perspective, so far relatively neglected, is the significance of the interaction between habitat and human genetic structure: the possibility that changes in habitat and consequent changes in life-style disrupt the adaptive relationship that has developed between human experience and human genotype. For example, lipid storage capability, possibly arising from the human species' long experience of under-nutrition, may be disadvantageous for humans with an over-abundant food supply. The application of ecological genetics to problems of human health represents a potentially productive extension of the ecological perspective in epidemiology.

The demographic perspective

The relationship between human health and the structure and growth of human populations has been curiously neglected by modern epidemiologists, with the notable exception of McKeown, although it was a major feature of epidemiology in the nineteenth century. The average duration of human life has approximately doubled for the world as a whole and trebled for the more favoured parts of the world during the last two hundred years, having probably remained almost constant for some two million years before that. Although the consequent rapid increase in human numbers is the most dramatically obvious result of this change in life expectation, many other important demographic changes have flowed from it which are of great significance in relation to human health. The changed age structure of human populations and the enormous growth of human migration are significant examples where the demographic perspective might be expected to enrich epidemiological enquiry.

There are also areas where the ecological and the demographic perspective overlap. The environmental implications of human population growth are obvious enough. The profound disturbance in human genetic structure which may be expected from changes in the size and structure of populations remains so far largely unconsidered, still less, explored.

The socio-political perspective

The socio-political perspective originated in the recognition by the nineteenth century public health practitioners that implementation of policies deriving from epidemiological study called frequently for skill and persistence in the political arena. This was particularly true of the development of clean water supplies and safe sewage disposal and has continued to be important in the present century in relation to atmospheric pollution and other industrial hazards and more recently to the issues of cigarette smoking and diet. Public health depends crucially on public policy and a comprehensive understanding of the determinants of a community's health must embrace political analysis.

Considerable attention has been devoted to issues related to what may be summarised as the social causes and consequences of changes in the mortality and morbidity experience of human communities. However, it is possible to be critical of the extent to which attempts have been made to explore the meaning of the simple social categories frequently employed in such researches. Demonstrations of mortality and morbidity differentials among categories defined in terms of sex, marital status, and social class, have frequently been accepted as the outcome rather than the point of departure for epidemiological enquiry.

More recently, the socio-political perspective has involved studies of the functioning of health and medical services, and of their utilisation by the communities they have been established to serve. That such studies contribute also to the development of the theory of other disciplines does not invalidate them as epidemiological studies. The nature and functioning of services and their accessibility and utilisation are major determinants of the prevalent levels of health in human communities.

The socio-political perspective has increased in importance because of the changing pattern of prevalent types of illness. Chronic illnesses have replaced acute as the dominant type. Chronic illness differs from acute not simply in its time scale but most significantly in its age-distribution and aetiology. Whereas the acute illnesses which have seemed most significant for most of man's history occurred throughout the age-span and derived largely from identifiable single causes in the external physical environment, chronic illnesses are more often multifactorial and associated to a much greater extent with human behaviour and the 'normal' processes of ageing. They are therefore less amenable both to prevention and to cure and must be dealt with to a much greater extent by adjustment of the social environment. Any understanding of the health of the elderly is impossible if social issues are neglected.

Applications
The science so far described has three evident functions:

1. It is one of the sciences of man and therefore makes a contribution to human biology and to the human sciences.
2. It is one of the sciences of health and therefore makes a contribution to medical science which in turn provides a rational basis for all medical practice.
3. Most specifically it is the scientific basis for the practice of community medicine which may be defined as the branch of medical practice that is concerned to improve the health experience of human communities.

Community medicine is the name now given in Britain to the branch of medical practice that is still known in most other countries as public health. It is distinguished from the clinical specialties which may be defined as being concerned in their various ways with promoting the health of human individuals. Community medicine, as practised in Britain differs from the activity known as public health in the USA in being much more the province of doctors. It has therefore been much more sharply distinguished than its US counterpart from the simple administration and management of the health services. Community medicine is not primarily an administrative activity but a branch of the practice of medicine.

Medical practice of every kind consists essentially of the provision of advice delivered to an appropriate client and directed towards helping in the solution of the client's health problems. The clinician's client is usually an individual, occasionally a family; the community physician's client is a community. The community physician's advice is usually directed to agencies of the community that are concerned with policies that may affect health and, most importantly, the agencies that make decisions on the structure and function of the services that deliver health and medical care. If advice is to be professional it must be based on disciplined investigation of the circumstances of the problem which must be interpreted against a background of relevant theory.

Epidemiology is central to the practice of community medicine but it is less generally realised that a viable epidemiology depends on a healthy practice of community medicine. Although the formally recognised practice of this specialty did not exist before the fifth decade of the nineteenth century when 'medical officers of health' became the first full-time community physicians, the function has a somewhat longer history. Doctors have advised their communities on matters of public policy relevant to health for almost as long as they have advised their individual patients. The significant developments in Britain were initiated when Percival urged the formation of the Manchester Board of Health in the late eighteenth century and laid down two principles which have guided the subsequent developments of the distinctively British practice of public health. These principles were (1) that a community's health depends on the community and its agencies specifically pursuing policies designed to promote health and (2) that such policies require to be based on a rigorously scientific examination of the determinants of community health. The subsequent formal arrangements made by communities to retain and consult public health doctors gave an impetus to the required scientific researches which were largely initiated and carried out by these early full-time community physicians.

The recent relative decline of epidemiology as the scientific basis of practice in community medicine and as a force in medical science resulted partly from the increasing preoccupation of community physicians with service management but also from the separation of academic epidemiology from practical community medicine. This latter trend has had the effect that epidemiological science has weakened its theoretical basis and predictably failed to find an adequate substitute in eclectic borrowing from the theory of the clinical and laboratory sciences.

A further damaging trend has been the search for an apolitical epidemiology. It is difficult to understand how a science whose basic function is to provide a rational basis for public *policy* could be *apolitical*. It is only in the English language which uses the synonyms *policy* and *politics* in slightly different contexts that such a notion could arise. The public health movement is inescapably political and generally progressive, hence the particular victimisation of public health doctors in right-wing dictatorships.

Health depends not only on medical technology but increasingly on public policy in the fields of trade, agriculture and taxation as well as on political decisions concerning the arrangements made for providing and controlling health and related services. The machinery for constructing and operating these health-related policies is complex, but the discipline of community medicine is involved in providing the professional advice for the policy-making process.

Advising the community's decision-makers on health issues is not an exclusive province of professional community physicians. To some extent all physicians function in a community medicine mode in that they have a responsibility to the community as well as to individuals. But community physicians are the principal channel of that advice and the scientific context in which such advice has necessarily to be interpreted is an epidemiological one. If all physicians are to function to some extent as community physicians then all medical science must embrace an epidemiological dimension. The responsibility for ensuring this is essentially vested in those who are employed primarily in the academic or service practice of community medicine.

If epidemiology is the science on which medicine in general, and community medicine in particular, bases its counsel relevant to health aspects of public policy, then it must embrace the issues that are relevant to health maintenance and improvement and develop a theoretical foundation capable of providing the rational basis for health promotive strategies. The first requirement is a recognition of the essentially political nature of the salient issues. Most initiatives for better health require recognition of the structure and function of human society and the need to mobilise and deploy resources in a purposeful way. A useful epidemiology needs to establish its theoretical framework in social and political as well as in biological terms. An epidemiology which seeks to limit itself to the excercise of an arbitrary array of elementary statistical procedures, applied eclectically to whatever ends are dictated by current fashion, will not only fail to honour its traditional devotion to the pursuit of the public health, it will also bore its practitioners out of their minds.

2. The origins of ill-health

An appraisal of strategy for health for all and its implications

Philip H. N. Wood   Elizabeth M. Badley

A new era dawned when, in May 1977, the thirtieth World Health Assembly adopted the aim of 'attainment by all citizens of the world by the year 2000 of a level of health that will permit them to lead a socially and economically productive life' (WHO, 1977). This aspiration is commonly referred to as HFA 2000. Its unique quality is collective espousal of what is acknowledged as a fundamentally social goal.

A seven-year period having elapsed since the key resolution was adopted, it is opportune to consider what underlies this aim and what the implications may be. The exercise is the more topical because a preliminary formulation of objectives or targets in support of the global strategy has been issued by the Regional Committee for Europe of the World Health Organization (EURO) only within the last year (WHO, 1983). Similar developments have been taking place on the other side of the Atlantic Ocean, culminating in the issue of implementation plans for attaining the objectives of the nation in the United States (PHS, 1983).

ASPIRATIONS FOR HEALTH

Health is generally regarded as a fundamental human right. WHO defines it as a state of complete well-being mentally, physically, and socially. More practically, WHO acknowledges that health is also an extremely valuable resource, healthy people can realise their full potential, and healthy societies can achieve maximum social and economic development. These are the precepts that influenced member states in undertaking commitment for the next two decades.

The nature of health

The notion of health represents an ideal. Ideals are both important and necessary, inspiring dedication to challenging tasks. Nevertheless, whilst recognising their value it is also essential to appreciate their limitations. The latter are illuminated by George Bernard Shaw's response to an invitation to address the Ancoats Brethren; he rejected the suggested title, 'realisable ideals', saying that no ideal worth a damn was realisable. Health would certainly have satisfied him in this respect since, as Dubos (1965) has indicated, 'the concept of perfect and positive health cannot become a reality because man will never be so perfectly adapted to his environment that his life will not involve struggles, failures, and sufferings.'

It is a tautology to describe health as a sense or feeling of wholeness because both terms derive from the same root, as does the word holy. Nevertheless, the significance of this formulation rests on the fact that it draws attention to perceptions of experience, rather than to any more objective status of the individual. The sense or feeling is approximated by role fulfilment, including the discharge of obligations that others expect of us. This is what is good of itself, and the intactness or perfection of the organism or its bodily shell is only instrumentally good and not necessarily critical to realisation of this existential end.

Against this background it is instructive to examine the EURO objectives for what they reveal about influences that determine health. All told there are 82 targets and, as they have not so far had wide currency, we have summarised them in a series of tables. Where appropriate the latter include an indication of current British performance in relation to each objective. This has been done not from lack of concern with what is happening elsewhere, but because the targets are intended for integration into a national strategy. It is therefore more coherent and illuminating to regard British experience as an illustrative case study.

We have not been able to incorporate the American objectives into the tables since they were formulated in too different a style. This is a pity because, although the target areas are similar, instructive differences in emphasis are apparent. Readers will also find it helpful to consult the PHS report (1983) for its identification of antecedent biomedical problems, such as control of blood pressure levels, reduction in sodium ingestion, fertility control, immunisation, and the like.

Health for all

Under the title of 'adding years to life', Table 2.1 shows the more conventional measures of 'health' status. These include overall life expectancy and mortality rates in infants, mothers, young and older children, young adults, and the middle aged. Specific causes are also identified — ischaemic and rheumatic heart disease and stroke; cancer of the lung and uterine cervix; motor vehicle, home, and occupational accidents; and suicide. We have distinguished between experience in England and Wales and that in Scotland, to indicate the range of variation that may be encountered.

Great Britain had a head start in industrialisation, and therefore also in the improvement in living standards to which this usually gives rise. There is thus little cause for congratulation in the fact that current British rates are generally quite close to what we have termed augmented targets (i.e. those appropriate for countries that have already achieved the main, lower level, objectives), and even less grounds for satisfaction in regard to, say, lung cancer, where the basic standard does not yet apply in the UK.

Beneath the neutered experience indicated in Table 2.1 is appreciable variation on 'the scale of life's chances' (Morris, 1975). The most readily retrievable information relates to sex, and indicates that death rates at various ages differ considerably between men and women. Similar differences in magnitude are seen in relation to social class, and to area of residence (Table 2.2).

WHO acknowledges that there is room for improvement in these directions by inclusion of supplementary targets, elimination of differences in rates between localities, socioeconomic strata, and the sexes. This is a more intractable problem, to which the Black Report (DHSS, 1980) testified. Some aspects will be considered elsewhere in this volume, but it is worth identifying the general challenge for an enquiring mind, what are the determinants of differential experience? Simple explanations related to 'absolute' factors such as material poverty have been shown to

Table 2.1 WHO targets concerned with adding years to life

No.	Target in support of WHO European Regional Strategy for HFA 2000 (WHO, 1983)*	Current British rate† E & W	Scotland
1	Life expectancy of 70 (75+) years; halve differences between AG&S	74	72
2	Infant mortality <30 (<15) per 1000 live births; if <15, eliminate A&G	11	11
3	Maternal mortality <20 (<10) per 100 000 live births; if <10, eliminate A&G	9	10
4	Death rate <70 (<50) per 100 000 at ages 1–4	46	47
	Death rate <35 (<25) at ages 5–14; if better, eliminate A&G	23	25
5	Death rate <95 (<80) per 100 000 at ages 15–34	64	79
	Death rate <675 (<570) at ages 35–64; if better, reduce AG&S	634	807
6	Ischaemic heart disease DR <200 (20% less) per 100 000 at ages 35–64; if better, reduce AG&S >1/3	190	262
7	Stroke deaths reduced 50% at ages 35–64	37	63
8	Rheumatic heart disease death rate <1 per 100 000 at ages <65	2	3
9	Lung cancer DR <55 (<30) per 100 000 at ages 35–64; if better, eliminate A&G	66	85
10	Cervical cancer death rate reduced >25% in women at ages 35–64	10	10
11	Motor vehicle accident DR <25 (<15) per 100 000; if better, reduce G	11	14
12	Fatal home accidents rate reduced >30%, & home accidents >15%	10	14
13	Reduce rate of fatal accidents at work >50%	2 } (GB)	
	Reduce rate of occupational accidents >25%	1890 } (GB)	
14	Death rate from suicide <20 per 100 000	9	10
	Death rate from attempted suicide <100; if better, reduce suicide by >25%	343 (Edin)	

* In most instances the full formulation of a target generally begins with 'By the year 2000 no country or group within a country will have', or words to that effect; for brevity the specification has often been inverted – e.g. presented as less than (<) when the original stated 'not more than'.
Targets levels specified in parentheses (augmented targets) apply to countries that have already attained the basic objective.
DR = death rate; differences between: areas (A) = geographical areas; groups (G) = socioeconomic groups; S = sexes; GB = British rate; Edin = data from Edinburgh only.
† Expressed in terms (i.e. units) corresponding to those of the relevant target; where denominator for target not specified, this is per 100 000 in the relevant age group.

Table 2.2 Current English performance on conventional measures of 'health' status according to between-group differences*

Target No.†	Rates in age groups to which target relates‡ In sexes Male	Female	In social classes SC 1	SC V	In localities Highest	Lowest
1	71	77	72	69	na	na
2	25	18	12	31	13	10
3	—	16	9	23	18	5
4: 1–4	52	41	46	119	60	40
5–14	27	18	23	51	25	20
5: 15–34	86	42	39	93	70	57
35–64	797	475	562	950	809	550
6	303	80	149	268	285	158
7	43	30	27	66	89	50
8	1.6	3.2	(6)	(13)	7	1
9	96	36	31	126	88	19
10	—	11	4	25	8	5
11	15	6	15	37	15	11
12	8	11	na	na	na	na
13	na	na	na	na	na	na
14 (suicide)	11	6	13	22	9	6

* Data on social class older, mainly from 1972 occupational mortality experience and confined to males of working age; offered mainly for illustration.
† Corresponding to those identified in Table 2.1
‡ Expressed in terms (i.e. units) corresponding to those of the relevant target; rates shown in parentheses to emphasise that magnitude has changed appreciably since period from which data derived.
— = Not applicable; na = not available.

be inadequate. The operation of more subtle and relative influences, assimilating individual and group frames of reference, have to be sought.

Turning to the buzz phrases, 'adding health to life' and 'adding life to years' (Table 2.3), most of the objectives are less precise. Performance under these heads throughout the European region is too disparate for WHO to be able to set more exact targets. This unfortunately leaves ample room for dissembling, with the danger of erosion of the determination to accomplish what is feasible. For example, experience

Table 2.3 Other WHO targets directly concerned with health for all

No.	Target in support of WHO European Regional Strategy for HFA 2000 (WHO, 1983)*	Current British rate†
	A Adding health to life	
15	Eliminate indigenous measles, [rates shown: per 1000 at all ages]	2
	poliomyelitis,	0
	neonatal tetanus,	0
	congenital rubella,	0.09
	diphtheria,	0
	congenital syphilis	0.003
	& indigenous malaria [rate shown = imported cases]	0.03
16	Average years free from major diseases and disabilities >65,	na
	>80% without permanent disability by 65 yrs (rate shown = in those 65–74)	49%
17	Eliminate thalassaemia [rates shown: per 1000 live births]	na
	& rhesus incompatibility in the newborn;	3
	reduce incidence of Down's syndrome, [trisomy 21 = 1.5]	2
	neural tube defects,	8 E&W 11 Sc
	haemophilia, } by >80%	na
	Duchenne muscular dystrophy, (males)	0.3
	& fragile x-linked mental retardation	2
	reduce consequences of phenylketonuria	0.07
	& congenital hypothyroidism	na
18	Substantially reduce disability [rates shown: per 1000 adult population]	28 imp
	due to diseases of musculoskeletal system & connective tissue	5 dis
19	Substantially reduce mental disease and disability	101 imp
	[mental retardation & mental illness combined]	12 dis
20	Reduce occupational diseases & occupational exposure to chemical, physical, & biological health risks	
21	DMF † <4.5 (<3) in 12-year-old children,	3.2
	and <4 (<2) missing teeth at ages 35–44; if better, eliminate G	9
	B Adding life to years	
22	4 out of 5 people to perceive their health as being good	3 in 5
23	Better financial means, physical accessibility to public facilities, & social opportunities to lead active life according to their own choice for all old people	?
24	Physical, social, & economic opportunities to exploit to the full their capacities for a socially & economically productive life for all disabled persons, so as to be fully contributing members of society to extent allowed by those capacities & their own choice	?

* See corresponding footnote to Table 2.1; E & W = England & Wales; Sc = Scotland; imp = impairment (all degrees); dis = severe disability.
† Expressed in terms (i.e. units) corresponding to those of the relevant target; where denominator for target not specified, this is per 100 000 in the relevant age group.
‡ DMF = decayed, missing, or filled teeth.

Table 2.4 WHO targets concerned with the prerequisites for health*

No.	Target in support of WHO European Regional Strategy for HFA 2000 (WHO, 1983)†
25	By 1990 Europe will be free from the fear of war
26	Reduce present differences in health status between countries by at least half [see Table 2.1]
27	Reduce present differences in health status between socioeconomic and social groups by at least half [see Table 2.2]; absolute poverty as a cause of ill-health will be removed
28	By 1990 all people will have access to and be able to afford the foods necessary for adequate nutrition [28% live on or below poverty margin]
29	By 1990 all people will have the opportunity of obtaining an adequate basic education; + adult literacy rate >90% [estimated as 94% in Britain]
30	By 1990 everyone will have adequate and safe drinking-water and sanitation
31	By 1990 everybody will be housed in accommodation meeting at least minimum health standards for human habitations [6% of dwellings classified as unfit, & 5% lack 1 or more amenities; 21% lack sole use of 4 indoor amenities — flush WC, sink/basin + cold water, fixed bath or shower, & gas or electric cooker]
32	By 1995 all people, including the disabled and the handicapped, will have an opportunity of engaging in a useful occupation and playing a socially significant role [unemployment in the nondisabled of order of 12%]

* Where possible, current British ratings shown in square brackets.
† See corresponding footnote to Table 2.1.

in the United States offers a stark contrast to unsatisfactory British efforts at controlling measles and rubella. To compensate for these limitations it will be necessary to formulate well-defined national objectives for the open-ended dimensions; the current British ratings included in the tables contribute to this endeavour by clarifying the order of each problem as it is today.

Prerequisites for health

Table 2.4 enumerates conditions without which health cannot be attained. Target 25 indicates that WHO does not share the British Medical Association's diffidence in acknowledging the health relevance of peace and the threat posed by nuclear proliferation. Differential health experience is featured again, emphasising what a thorny dilemma this is. Then come the traditional public health concerns of nutrition, drinking water and sanitation, and housing, coupled with education as another contributor to wholeness. Finally there is role opportunity, a sore challenge in the face of mounting structural unemployment.

Table 2.5 is concerned with health promotion, a subject discussed elsewhere in this book. The topic is considered by WHO in relation to life styles. Of itself that is unexceptionable, although certain assumptions are commonly associated with this approach; we shall scrutinise these suppositions in the later parts of our commentary.

Table 2.6 focuses on health protection by identifying extraneous hazards. Control of these problems by containment is related to environmental and occupational health, but social and political dimensions are hinted at in target 56. Further remarks on current British performance are probably redundant; the ratings really speak for themselves.

Table 2.5   WHO targets concerned with lifestyles conducive to health*

No. Target in support of WHO European Regional Strategy for HFA 2000 (WHO, 1983)†

A General

33   By 1990 public policy will make healthy lifestyles the easier lifestyles to choose
34   By 1987 all countries will have ensured effective community participation at all levels of policy-making concerned with developments relating to lifestyles and their implementation
35   By 1990 all people will be better able to make mature decisions regarding their own choice of lifestyle
36   By 1990 >90% of individuals of all groups and communities will be well aware of the health implications of their lifestyles, be motivated to protect their health, and regard unhealthy behaviour as socially less acceptable
37   By 1990 each country will have developed measures to strengthen family and other social networks so as to enable people to choose, want, and maintain healthy lifestyles
38   By 1995 >90% of people will have healthy eating habits; <5% will be affected by obesity [16% of those aged 15–65 are 20% or more overweight]
39   By 1990 >90% of people will have the opportunity and the motivation to spend the amount of time on physical activity needed for good health
40   By 1995 >90% of people, particularly vulnerable groups (such as the elderly, the disabled, the widowed, youth, and migrant workers) will have the opportunity and resources to participate in social life at a level which provides a sense of identity, self-esteem, and general wellbeing
41   By 1995 >80% of people, including vulnerable groups such as those in institutions, the disabled, the elderly, etc, will have an opportunity of leading an emotionally satisfying sexual life in harmony with the needs, beliefs, and values of the individual and society

B Specific

42   By 1990 reduce tobacco consumption >50% [average cigarettes/wk: m 148, f 98] >80% of population will be non-smokers [currently 62% of men & 67% of women are non-smokers]
43   By 1990 no group will have a consumption of pure alcohol per person aged 15+ years >15 (>10) litres per year [currently 15% of population consume >10 litres per annum] if better, further reduce by >20% & eliminate significant S
44   By 1995 (substantially) reduce use of illicit psychoactive drugs [registered addicts: 12.9 m & 4.9 f per 100 000]
45   By 1995 >95% of all drivers will be safe and considerate [8% of drivers commit indictable offences during course of a year]

* Where possible, current British ratings shown in square brackets.
† See corresponding footnote to Table 2.1; target levels specified in parentheses (augmented targets) apply to countries that have already attained the basic objective; S = socioeconomic group differences.

The desirable properties of systems of health care are highlighted in Table 2.7. We have introduced subheadings, which made it necessary to alter the order of presentation of targets (viz. 68–71). Perhaps all that is needed at this juncture is to sound a warning against a complacent British predilection to equate primary health care (PHC) with primary medical care of the type to which we are accustomed from general practitioners. PHC in fact has rather different connotations.

The aim of PHC is to close the gap between 'haves' and 'have nots' in regard to health resources. The basis of the approach is enunciated in the Declaration of Alma Ata (WHO, 1978). The point we are wishing to stress is in Article 4, which states that 'the people have the right and duty to participate individually and collectively in the planning and implementation of their health care'.

To a considerable extent PHC can therefore be regarded as a renegotiation of power. Expressed more analytically, it is concerned with restoration of autonomy to

Table 2.6 WHO targets concerned with a healthy environment*

No.	Target in support of WHO European Regional Strategy for HFA 2000 (WHO, 1983)†
46	By 1990 all people will have a better chance of living in housing and in urban and rural environments that will protect them against health hazards and enable them to live a healthy life
47	Reduce exposure to occupational hazards to such an extent that incidence of occupational diseases from known hazards reduced 50%
48	By 1995 (significantly) reduce human health risks from water sources
49	By 1995 (substantially) reduce health risks from air pollution in both outdoor & closed environments, & adopt internationally binding agreements to curb air pollution across frontiers
50	By 1995 eliminate major known health risks from waste generated in homes & in industry
51	By 1995 protect all people effectively against unnecessary exposure to radiation
52	By 1995 (significantly) reduce risk of direct and indirect human exposure to potentially toxic chemicals
53	By 1990 (significantly) reduce health risks from food contamination [rate for food poisoning per 100 000: 2.3] and potentially harmful additives [20 (approx. 4% of total) of the EEC-accepted food additives (coded by E designations) are recognised as being toxic]
54	By 1995 (significantly) reduce the environmental risks of accidents
55	By 1995 (significantly) reduce environmental risks of exposure to pathogenic microorganisms and parasites
56	By 1990 people aged 15+ years will be aware of the major categories of environmental health hazards and their consequences, and local communities as well as the producers of such risks will be motivated and mobilised to reduce them
57	By 1990 have multisectoral and well-coordinated national environmental health systems that include proper machinery for risk assessment, planning and management, and effective international agreements to curb environmental pollution affecting more than one country

* Where possible, current British ratings shown in square brackets.
† See corresponding footnote to Table 2.1.

those from whom it has been expropriated. Many conventions have developed as medical healing has become more professionalised, particularly relating to how patients and their problems are regarded. Some of these customs cannot be viewed as amounting to anything other than restrictive practices, and PHC challenges their continuance.

Basis for attaining health

It is a truism that these various objectives are unlikely to be attained unless their interdependence is recognised. This means that a strategy is required, together with an infrastructure of legislation, resources, education, management, and information and evaluation systems (Table 2.8). Once again we have found it necessary to alter the order of presentation, though this time by a complete table.

Two aspects excite comment. First, performance indicators will be necessary to monitor progress. Unfortunately those currently being applied in the UK are scarcely likely to contribute to this process, being concerned solely with economic housekeeping — and mainly in the context of occult attempts at cost cutting. The same is true of their nearest analogues in the United States, diagnosis related groups or DRGs (Editorial, 1983); these in fact are more Procrustean, because hospitals get reimbursed not for costs actually incurred with particular patients but only according to average

Table 2.7   WHO targets concerned with appropriate care*

No. Target in support of WHO European Regional Strategy for HFA 2000 (WHO, 1983)†

A Priorities, distribution, and integration

58   By 1990 have health systems based on primary care and effectively supported by secondary and tertiary care, and ensure a proper balance between health promotion, prevention, cure, care, and rehabilitation

59   By 1990 ensure all sectors whose services influence health (water, agriculture, education, industry, etc) acknowledge that safeguarding the population's health must be an overriding concern in their activities as well, and that such sectors cooperate closely with the health sector in this endeavour

60   By 1985 ensure effective and representative community participation at all levels of health care organisation and development

61   By 1995 secure distribution of resources according to need, while ensuring the physical, economic, and cultural availability, accessibility, and acceptability of services to the local population and providing for good functional integration between units at different levels

68   By 1990 achieve the necessary coverage of essential secondary services, providing specialised care to patients as well as advice and support to the primary health care level, and conducting personpower training and research

69   By 2000 achieve the necessary coverage of tertiary services, giving the most specialised care to patients referred from the primary or secondary levels, offering advice and support to such levels, and conducting specialised training and a broad range of research

70   By 1987 have a clear national policy and a formal mechanism for systematic assessment of the quality of care, so that by 1990 all new and existing promotive, preventive, diagnostic, treatment, rehabilitative, and care technologies will be adequately assessed and be applied to patients who really need them, with their informed consent

71   By 1995 (substantially) reduce the abuse, improper use, and overuse of licit drugs

B Primary health care

62   By 1990 ensure the primary health care system provides effective health promotive and preventive services to all individuals and population groups in need — including services for genetic counselling, family planning, immunisation [ratings: diphtheria, tetanus, & poliomyelitis 83% pertussis & measles 53%], selective screening [cervical smear rate in females: 12 per 100 000], maternal and child welfare, occupational and school health, counselling on matters related to lifestyles and health, together with epidemiological surveillance of disease

63   By 1990 ensure the primary health care system offers the provision of appropriate diagnostic, treatment, and rehabilitative services to the whole population

64   By 1990 ensure the primary health care system provides the elderly, the disabled, and other groups in special need with a full range of services, including health promotion, prevention, counselling, treatment, rehabilitation, home care, institutional care, & outreach services

65   By 1987 ensure the organisation of health personnel at primary level is community-based and coordinated, so as to facilitate teamwork, promote broad understanding of the patient's life situation, foster a family-oriented form of health care delivery, and actively involve the personnel in research and teaching

66   By 1987 recognise the importance of health care given by individuals, families, and self-help groups, which is supportive of as well as being supported by the care given by health professionals

67   By 1995 evaluate health care given by providers operating outside the formal health care system, so that support may be given to alternative health care practices that have been shown to be safe and effective

* Where possible, current British ratings shown in square brackets.
† See corresponding footnote to Table 2.1.

durations of stay and associated investigations, etc, for typical patients in the relevant diagnostic class.

Performance indicators are concerned with quality control, and initiatives in general practice (Buckley, 1983; Irvine, 1983) offer a much more constructive approach to this particular task at the level of the individual practitioner. As far as the system is concerned, WHO has issued a series of seven booklets clarifying various

Table 2.8   WHO targets concerned with support measures

No.	Target in support of WHO European Regional Strategy for HFA 2000 (WHO, 1983)*
75	By 1986 develop a national strategy to attain health for all and adopt the necessary legislation to make its implementation possible and its application effective
76	By 1984 establish a managerial process geared to the attainment of HFA 2000, actively involving communities and other sectors in the development, implementation, and evaluation of the national strategy for reaching that goal
77	By 1986 establish national policy and machinery for systematic assessment of health technology, so that by 1990 all major new and already existing health technology will have been evaluated in terms of its effectiveness, efficiency, safety, and acceptability, & from the point of view of national health policy & economic constraints
78	By 1987 spend at least 5% of the gross national product on health, ensuring preferential allocation of resources to implement the national strategy so as to attain health for all by the year 2000
79	By 1988 adapt the planning, production, and management of health personpower more closely to national health needs and health-for-all policies, with more emphasis on primary health care, promotion, prevention, & rehabilitation, as well as appropriate use of diagnostic & therapeutic methods
80	By 1988 have strong health education programmes drawing on a wide range of public and private resources, ensuring balanced & mutually reinforcing support to basic HFA policies and programmes
81	By 1988 ensure that education of personnel for sectors other than health will provide adequate information on HFA principles, and training in the practical implications of the national HFA policy and programmes as applied to their own sector
82	By 1985 establish health information systems capable of supporting managerial processes for national health development, assessing progress towards health for all, disseminating relevant scientific information, and providing the public with appropriate information

* See corresponding footnote to Table 2.1.

aspects of the HFA strategy. The one on indicators for monitoring progress (WHO, 1981) offers guidance that takes account of four types of measure:

— indicators of health policy (e.g. proportion of resources devoted to particular goals);
— social and economic indicators related to health;
— indicators of provision of health care (see next paragraph);
— indicators of health status and quality of life.

The second point to be made is that the initiatives of the Körner committee (1982) may contribute to target 82, at least if they are implemented. Much though they are to be welcomed, however, they cannot help but exhibit some limitations in the HFA context in the absence of an explicit health-related goal for the National Health Service (NHS) and a strategy for how this might be attained. Supermarket management philosophies (DHSS, 1983), and the covert upheaval of the NHS which they aspire to accomplish, are disturbingly more irrelevant for the same reasons, even though superficially they might appear to allow Britain to reach target 76 by the specified deadline.

One other component is acknowledged, the need for investment in research to make good deficiencies in knowledge (Table 2.9). Despite the initiatives of Zuckerman (1961), which led to the allocation of research budgets to ministerial departments concerned with services, such as the Department of Health and Social Security (DHSS), and those of Rothschild (1971), directed at the social relevance of research and the means of its application, Britain has a long way to go to reach target 72. In fact

Table 2.9 WHO targets concerned with research

No.	Target in support of WHO European Regional Strategy for HFA 2000 (WHO, 1983)*
72	By 1985 have machinery for systematically analysing the research support required for health-for-all development, for the effective application of new knowledge from research in health policy and programme formulation, and for making academies of science, universities, and other research bodies active partners in health-for-all development
73	By 1988 have a national research plan based on the country's own health-for-all development priorities, one which will make national academies of science/health research councils, universities, and other research bodies and institutions active contributors to planned and coordinated health-for-all research
74	By 1990 devote a (substantial) amount of total health expenditure to financing the national health-for-all research plan

* See corresponding footnote to Table 2.1.

the whole notion of mission-oriented endeavours of this type tends to be somewhat alien for the biomedical research community, engendering a diffidence in assuming such obligations that can be detected in, for example, the deliberations of WHO's European Advisory Committee for Medical Research (WHO, 1982).

HOW ILL-HEALTH ARISES

Is there a conceptual model underlying WHO's formulations, or those of the Department of Health and Human Services in the United States (PHS, 1983)? Or do the recommendations represent just an eclectic shopping basket of randomly associated ideas, i.e. a wholly empirical exercise? We cannot presume to answer that question, although we agree with McKeown (1983) in his echoing of Kuhn (1970), that the old paradigm is changing but the new one (to provide a basis for health strategies) is not yet clearly defined.

As a contribution to this challenge, we have been seeking a framework to encompass the various circumstances that give rise to ill-health. We have approached this by attempting to project back to the origins of disease from our work on the nature of experiences associated with its consequences (Wood & Badley, 1978, 1981); the latter formed the basis for the *International Classification of Impairments, Disabilities, and Handicaps* (WHO, 1980). Before describing our framework, however, we need first to dissect the basis for present understanding.

Evolution and history
It is necessary to start by appreciating that individuals of the human species, and their health, are in a dynamic and yet vulnerable state (Dubos, 1965). In other words, the species is part of an ecosystem in which the balance of nature can be altered. One reflection of this is the manner in which disease experience has changed at different stages of evolution and history.

Paraphrasing McKeown's (1976) analysis, the major problems for hunter-gatherers appear to have been trauma and undernutrition. The means of abating the latter became available with improved food production following the neolithic revolution, even if the potential was not realised because of the associated rise in fertility. However, the resultant aggregation in villages promoted increased passage of epidemics so that infections also became a major scourge. Both of these features were enhanced, respectively, by the much later agricultural and industrial revolutions. Following not long after, the sanitary revolution was associated with reduction in the toll of infection and, coupled with declining birth rates, this allowed so-called 'degenerative' conditions and mental ill-health to emerge to the forefront.

Turning our gaze momentarily towards the future, we can do no better than quote McKeown (1983) at some length

'In discussions of the changing pattern of disease it is generally assumed that the infections were the diseases of the past and that the non-communicable diseases which have partially replaced them are the problems of the indefinite future. Except in relation to conditions determined before birth this assumption is questionable; it is unlikely that the infections were predominant before the historical period and in time the roles may again be reversed. . . . Man's long term relation to his parasites is a much more open question. Where it is possible to prevent contact with them, as in the case of organisms spread by water and food, there is no reason to doubt that control will continue to be effective. We cannot have the same confidence about diseases caused by organisms normally found in the body or conveyed by vectors such as the mosquito, tick, or snail. . . . The disappearance of an infectious disease provides no certainty that it has gone forever. Smallpox, for example, is said to have been eradicated, but we can hardly believe that the virus, or others capable of evolving into it, has disappeared forever from the animal reservoirs from which it presumably initially emerged. Predictions about future health trends are notoriously unreliable, but my own guess is that 100 years from now it is more likely that . . . environmental hazards will be strictly controlled . . . than that diseases such as influenza, malaria, and the common cold will have been eradicated.'

From the perspective just established it should be clear that the sources of influence on health lie both within the individual and externally in the society in which he or she lives. Such influences may be health-promoting or deleterious, though few exhibit direct and immediate one-to-one relationships. The heart of the problem lies in the nature of these relationships, appreciation of which is coloured by our assumptions about causality. The latter must therefore be submitted to fairly rigorous scrutiny.

Causal relationships

An outline developed by Bradford Hill (1965) is most helpful, even though it by no means resolves all the difficulties. He offered nine criteria for consideration before deciding that causation was the most likely interpretation of an observed association between two variables, one that was 'perfectly clear-cut and beyond what we would care to attribute to the play of chance'. These criteria are reproduced in Table 2.10, although for purposes of illustration we shall discuss them in a slightly different order so as to sustain a historical perspective.

It seems likely that one of the first perceptions of cause and effect relationships developed in regard to physical injury. The contingent connection between slipping on the proverbial banana skin and fracture must have been inescapable, however much such occurrences may have been attributed to divinely instigated nemesis or whatever. Of the causality criteria in Table 2.10, temporality was the key to recognising the relationship.

Before proceeding further it is worth expanding a little on a distinct aspect of temporality, what might be designated as proximity. This concerns the time for an occurrence to become manifest. The connection between events distributed over short time spans is not too difficult to appreciate. In marked contrast are delayed manifestations, such as occur with rheumatic fever and hepatitis, and chronic exposure, as with silicosis, radiation, and hypersensitivity. Perceiving relationships of this type is much more taxing, and the difficulties are heightened when it is possible for exposure to be sustained (e.g. tobacco) or relatively brief (asbestos).

Table 2.10   Criteria for evaluation of whether an observed association might be interpreted as being indicative of causation*
(from Hill, 1965)

1   *Strength* of the association (in statistical terms)
2   *Consistency* (replication)
3   *Specificity* (criteria of necessity and sufficiency)
4   *Temporality* (which is the cart and which the horse?)
5   *Biological gradient* (dose-response relationship)
6   *Plausibility* (biologically†)
7   *Coherence* (triangulation)
8   *Experiment* (e.g. animal studies)
9   *Analogy*

* Not forgetting the three causal fallacies: post hoc ergo propter hoc; confusion of cause and effect; deception of common cause.
† Recall the advice of Sherlock Holmes: having eliminated the impossible, whatever remains, however improbable, must be the truth.

What is noteworthy is that, collectively, we tend to take a different view of these various occurrences. For example, high concentrations of a toxic gas are regarded as causing injury, whereas chronic low exposure leads to 'disease'. Similarly, a big mechanical force applied to the spine is viewed as trauma but repeated small doses give rise to 'disc degeneration'. Our comprehension of the phenomena of ageing is rendered similarly uncertain for related reasons (Wood, 1976). What complicates matters is that different social valuations are attached to these various conceptions; these are evident in eligibility for compensation.

Returning to our theme, the next step is usually attributed to Hippocrates (1849), when he counselled that 'whoever wishes to investigate medicine properly, should proceed thus . . . consider the seasons of the year, . . . the winds, . . . qualities of the waters, . . . the ground, . . . the mode in which the inhabitants live and what are their pursuits'. We can appreciate that this guidance is wise, but it does not really resolve whether the associations indicated are causal.

Some help can be derived from what might be regarded as internal consistency, which Bradford Hill (1965) accords separate status as the property of biological gradient. The classical example of this is observing that a given association also exhibits a dose-response relationship; for example, that not only do smokers carry a greater risk of lung cancer than nonsmokers, but that the degree of risk is related to how heavily the individual smokes. Whether this provides independent evidence is debatable because some, such as Fisher (1959), regard gradient as only a reiteration of the main association to be explained. Nevertheless, failure to find a dose-response relationship does constitute a challenge to accepting that an association may have causal significance.

Further progress could not really be made until particular maladies had been identified. This depended on a cluster concept in regard to disease, associating together various disparate clinical features to yield a unique entity that could be subjected to speculation (Feinstein, 1967; Wood, 1982). Given this establishment of specificity, space-time interaction could then be detected, with appreciation of contagion and other communicable experiences. The criteria underpinning this latter development were strength and consistency.

It is interesting to realise that 'proof' of these phenomena was not possible until the remaining criteria had been satisfied, plausibility, coherence, experiment, and analogy. What ultimately emerged, of course, was the germ theory and its later refinement with acknowledgement of the role of vectors; the latter represented a remarkably developed appreciation of the complexities of events. Fulfilment of the criteria of plausibility and coherence owed a great deal to acquisition of the capacity to expand dimensions; this was provided by development of the microscope. Haddon (1980) has argued cogently that lack of a similar facility in regard to time retarded appraisal of the dynamics of accidents, until means such as high-speed cameras, accelerometers, and radiation detectors had become available.

Aetiological appreciations

The more general significance of these advances was that they encouraged a notion of unifactorial determination, a single factor appearing to be both necessary and sufficient to account for the occurrence of these forms of ill-health. Industrial intoxications, such as with beryllium (although really no more than a subclass of accidents), together with vitamin deficiencies and certain other nutritional disturbances, also conform to this pattern. Single gene defects such as the inborn errors of metabolism can also be accommodated within this scheme of things, even if at times necessitating invocation of constructs such as incomplete penetrance to explain why observations don't correspond to predicted patterns.

The important limitation to be acknowledged is that the conditions just mentioned exemplify the only model for disease aetiology that we really comprehend at present. Hence the temptation to try to fit other disorders into a similar mould, as with the idea that cancer may be due to a 'virus'. At the same time the externality of agents conceived of in this way reinforces excusal from blame, one of the attributes constituting part of the sick role.

What we have depicted so far could be regarded as an essentially clinical outlook on disease experience. Epidemiology had its formal roots in these developments, but it has evolved an independent and complementary perspective. This has included recognition that the occurrence of conditions can rarely be explained adequately just by the operation of a single agent; in other words, an appreciable part of the variance is not accounted for in this way, so that the agent cannot be a sufficient cause.

Tuberculosis illustrates some of these characteristics. Familial influences were identified, as well as links with poverty, and some of these attributes could be manipulated until effective treatment rendered such initiatives less pressing. Thus the simple framework of *cause (a)→result (a)* had to be admitted as being only quasi-unifactorial. The epidemiological response was to attempt to be more comprehensive by advancing a model loosely referred to as multifactorial, one which took account of the host (persons), the agent, and the environment (time and place of affection, etc.).

However, designation as multifactorial actually tends to obscure as much as it reveals because one has to differentiate between pleiotropy, composite aetiology, and heterogeneity; this has been explored by Murphy (1972), and has been illustrated by one of us (Wood, 1978).

To some degree matters were advanced when Lalonde (1975) developed his new perspective on the health of Canadians. This took account of biological and genetic factors, environmental hazards, life style and behaviour, health care, and the organisation of that care and regionalisation. The horizons of many engaged in the field were probably enlarged by this work, and certainly it is since then that there have been reasonable attempts to integrate both sociocultural factors, including stress (McQueen & Siegrist, 1982), and a so-called ecological perspective (e.g. Catalano, 1979) with more conventional biomedical concepts.

A different emphasis is evident in McKeown's (1983) consideration of the basis for health strategies. In this he develops an apparently uncomplicated taxonomy of disease, those determined before birth, those due to deficiencies and hazards, and those due to maladaptation. Much though we endorse a large part of his thesis, the appraisal nevertheless still tends to be too rooted in a single-factor type of approach. Perhaps this is why he found intellectual contortions necessary to achieve the simplicity; the latter became possible only by subsuming both predators and parasites into the same category of food shortage as that affecting humans.

The potential for confusion and even conflict on these matters is epitomised by pellagra. Here is a specific vitamin deficiency, therefore exemplifying unifactorial determination; and yet at the same time it occurred in persons of a particular social status in the southern United States, with associated inadequacies in diet, so suggesting a more complex or multifactorial aetiology. These contrasting outlooks stemmed not from the so-called facts, but from what observations happened to be made and from the interpretations that were then attached to such findings. At root the differences are fundamentally both epistemological and philosophical in nature.

Methodological implications

This controversial aspect of the medical paradigm derives from what Kuhn (1970) referred to as the conventions of a discipline, the presuppositions adopted to facilitate experimentation and communication. Their kernel consists of postulates about the sources of knowledge, from which is developed the basis for methodology, the modes of description (such as quantitative or qualitative), the setting (be it in the field or the laboratory), and the level of analysis (individual or aggregate).

For the investigator there is, of course, a profound disincentive to adopting more complex models of aetiology. Not only are such appreciations likely to be more taxing to the intellect for assimilation, but they also have unhappy methodological implications. The single factor model is very precise, allowing of 'definitive' testing. What can compare, for example, with the exactness of prediction of ratios of occurrence for Mendelian traits? More complex models tend to be analytically messy; the danger of confounding is increased, and derivative estimates (such as relative risk, or heritability) are generally rather crude.

The easiest way of dealing with such difficulties might appear to be to ignore them. Presumably this is why Collingwood (1940), in his remarks on empiricism and phenomenalism, stated: 'In the lowest type of low-grade thinking we are unaware that every thought we find ourselves thinking is the answer to a question. We are wholly unaware that the question arises from a presupposition.' A similar notion was conveyed in John F. Kennedy's remark that the greatest enemy of truth is not the lie but the myth.

The myth often serves as the foundation for the walls of a prison within which investigators operate, but not all the barriers are insurmountable. Some are even self-imposed. One is created by our jargon (Bross, 1964), which itself is constrained by our appreciation of the world. For instance, descriptive observations are often cloaked under the guise of 'risk factors'. The justification for this nomenclature is that the attributes are found to have predictive power, and they are frequently expressed in 'sophisticated' terms (e.g. population attributable risk or etiologic fraction — Rothman, 1976). Nevertheless, almost unawares, loose usage can encourage a sleight of intellect whereby simple prediction is transformed into causal significance, yet without rigorous scrutiny of this attribution.

Another obstacle is related to the means by which scientists make decisions, tending to be cautious because a large loss is attached to erroneous conclusion. Others are perhaps less immediately tractable, being founded on methodological difficulties including those related to what we discussed earlier, proximity. But the taken-for-granted presupposition still tends to be the cornerstone. A simple example concerns acceptance of the reality of a 'phenomenon', for which the cause has then to be sought. For instance, it has recently been argued that the so-called placebo response may well be no such thing, representing little more than regression to the mean (McDonald et al, 1983).

Perhaps in like vein is a challenge to the idea that Britain is experiencing an epidemic of coronary heart disease (Bartley, 1983). We have not had the opportunity to review all the evidence, but Bartley's suggestion that the conventional appraisal has gained credibility because of the social and political roles such ideas play in different periods does introduce another perspective on how the data should be regarded.

Somewhat complementary is the possibility that, having become so accustomed to thinking of ill-health in relation to specific diseases, we may be neglecting other types of experience. The relatively 'nonspecific' increases in morbidity and mortality associated with bereavement, retirement, and unemployment cannot be dismissed simply because no particular ailments can be implicated. As Marmot (1976) has suggested, there may be profit in diverting attention to states of vulnerability as the entities of concern.

Yet other barriers are potentially more sinister, because of opportunities for what can amount to inadvertent collusion. One concerns the fact that useful new observations can always have the capacity to disturb the established order, with political and economic consequences that are generally likely to be unwelcome. At the same time it is the corresponding establishment that will most often be approached for the funding of such studies.

Another is that the timidity of orthodoxy can reinforce the barriers, to neglect of an important aspect of the scientist's relationship with society. The Nobel laureate, Salvador Luria, gave succinct expression to this aspect: 'The scientist, after all, is a person for whom the present knowledge is not adequate. Therefore he should also be a person for whom the present society is not adequate. If you are not resigned to the present state of knowledge, you should not be resigned to the present state of organisation.'

Tacit assumptions

A rather different aspect of 'methodology' concerns the practical application of any insights gained. In essence one can identify two types of response to problems — that of the revolutionary who, following the principle of the Etruscan phalanx, concentrates all his force on what Mao Zedong termed the principal contradiction; and that of the evolutionary, who is sensitive to intricacy and appreciates that there are limits to the scale of intrusion in a democratic society, and who therefore seeks multiple interventions directed at as many points as possible of the web of complexity.

Single factor models obviously lend themselves to the first of these tactics, encouraging what is almost a paradox; that orthodox attitudes tend to favour the revolutionary thrust. This is reflected in statements such as 'a programme for intervention is, however, unlikely to be effective unless the illnesses can be defined and attributed to single factors or groups of factors that act synergistically and are amenable to intervention' (Doll, 1983). The point we wish to bring out is that such claims are coloured by unacknowledged views of the world and its organisation. As we have suggested, these views are often of the nature of myths, and unfortunately they may obscure from our vision the possibility of alternative prescriptions for action.

Although it leads us on to dangerous ground, this part of our thesis may not be very persuasive unless we offer examples. One is provided by a critique of work linking 'social structure' to the aetiology of depression in women (Williams, 1982). On the face of it a comprehensive causal analysis of sociopsychological factors had been developed. However, as Williams notes, the methodological primacy accorded to cause over motive, and to context over agency, and failure to examine the dialectical relationship between these dimensions, are incompatible with (and therefore negate) the political implications claimed for this work.

Other theoretical contradictions are evident in the stressful life events approach. Mestrovic & Glassner (1983) cite an instance when they criticise the common assumption that health is natural, as if it represented some sort of homeostasis, rather than acknowledging Durkheim's view that, as far as behaviour is concerned, 'disease no less than health is inherent in the nature of living things. The two states are not contraries'. Before dismissing these difficulties as what might be expected of psychosocial enquiry, however, it is salutary to remember that many biomedical attributes tend to lack any theoretical foundation; this subject is explored by McQueen & Siegrist (1982).

For our other example we would confront studies directed at the identification of more material environmental influences. For example, an extremely detailed enquiry has recently concluded that on present evidence it seems unlikely that the total effect of all types of pollution, other than in the workplace, can cause more than 1 per cent of all fatal cancers (Doll, 1983). Even occupational factors appeared to be responsible for only 4% of malignancies.

Certainly this could appear as a convenient exoneration of the American way of life, and so to what extent can it be accepted at face value? We admire the elegance and rigour of Doll & Peto's (1981) study, and we appreciate how they tried to head off the simplest levels of misunderstanding with their perceptive concept of avoidability. Very fundamental difficulties nevertheless remain. What is problematic in interpretations of this type is how the environment and the workplace are regarded, how 'pollution' is characterised, and how meaningful links are sought.

Interpreting evidence

The dilemma can be illustrated by a brief consideration of mortality in coalminers. Standardised mortality ratios (SMRs) are increased markedly, and the straightforward approach is to relate this to their occupation. However, somewhat similarly elevated SMRs are also recorded in their spouses, who do not work underground. This means one has to entertain at least two other types of possibility. One is that there might be quite wide dissemination of undetected material pollutants in the locality. The other, even more general, is that there may be some unappreciated lethal quality to the culture of mining communities, for which what might be regarded as the correlates of relative poverty appear to be a strong candidate.

Such an appreciation might not appear to be immediately productive, because of its generality; nevertheless it is not of itself unscientific in Popperian terms (Popper, 1959), since it could be submitted to falsification—providing one devised the appropriate study to test the ideas. Our purpose is to draw attention once again to the context in which observations are located. The appropriateness of study designs is customarily adjudged by rather technical standards. However, so narrow an outlook on the terrain is not really warranted because there is a theoretical minefield, the existence of which seems too often to be ignored.

Midgley (1979) describes the problem

'What counts as a fact depends on the concepts you use, on the questions you ask. . . . There is no neutral terminology. So there are no wholly neutral facts. All describing is classifying according to some conceptual scheme or other. We need concepts in order to pick out what matters for our present purpose from the jumble of experience, and to relate it to the other things that matter in the world. There is no single set of all-purpose "scientific" concepts which can be used for every job. Different enquiries make different selections from the world. So they need different concepts.'

To drive the point home, as Joris (1980) has done, 'every scientific discourse is based on a set of culture and ideology-bound *metaphors*, and has therefore to be read as metaphor, and not as an 'objective' transparent language that would stand in a one-to-one relationship with an immutable, absolute reality.'

Investigation has derived great power from William of Occam and his razor, what now tends to be enunciated as the principle of parsimony; hence part of the attraction of single factor models. The approach is sometimes castigated as 'reductionism', but this tends to neglect the point we have just made, from Midgley (1979). Nevertheless there is an inescapable hazard that reduction may deform, if not even violate, reality. Protection may be secured by paying particular attention to two of Bradford Hill's criteria, coherence and specificity, which we shall now consider a little further.

The coherence of an association can be examined by what amounts to triangulation, seeking other means of acquiring information that has a bearing on the question. For example, a concept of 'unnecessary untimely mortality' has been suggested (Rutstein et al, 1980), and has been exploited by Charlton and his colleagues (1983). A fairly widely appreciated method of examining coherence is to make comparisons of experience in the sexes, the excess of mortality in males presenting ready opportunities for study. We have been pursuing this to see whether removal of what may be 'untimely' makes the sexes as similar as it should. Miller & Gerstein (1983) have attempted a somewhat similar exercise in relation to the influence of smoking, and conclude the latter is the overwhelming 'cause' for the male–female nontraumatic longevity difference.

Both Fisher's early (1959) and Burch's persisting (1984) doubts about the causal role of tobacco stemmed from problems with coherence. The former was concerned by the incongruous findings on inhaling and neglect of urban–rural differences that were independent of smoking [which Doll & Peto (1981) have endeavoured to cope with], and the latter because trends in lung cancer mortality over time did not show synchrony with changes in tobacco consumption.

Underlying these difficulties is a human propensity encapsulated by the German poet Christian Morganstern:

> 'And thus in his considered view
> What did not suit, could not be true.'

Hamilton's (1974) advice to always concentrate on failures (i.e. what doesn't fit) offers a means of countering this vulnerability. In fact it is important to go out of one's way to seek evidence with a potential to challenge conclusions, as Popper (1959) has demonstrated.

Herein lies part of our concern over exoneration of 'pollutants' from a role in causing cancer. Surely a pollutant is no more than something that has been shown to have an unwanted effect, rather on a par with dirt being defined as matter in the wrong place. Doll & Peto (1981) remark that quite minor variations in both diet and living conditions can determine tumour development. Once identified, the responsible factors would thereafter merit designation as pollutants, and yet, as Doll & Peto note, these influences generally tend to be dismissed by investigators as just a potential nuisance. Such narrow views are then compounded by logic dangerously reminiscent of the claim that all swans are white, i.e. asserting that there are no non-white swans.

However, that is by no means the only source of difficulty. Doll & Peto stress that, with a few notable exceptions, there are no general epidemic increases in malignant disease. It is, perhaps, a pity that they did not bring out more clearly the limited time period being considered. Of course there can be no means of determining when our present cancer burden developed. On the other hand, it has been over the last two centuries (roughly, the period of industrialisation) that some of the greatest alterations in ways of life have occurred. This perspective suggests that it may be in precisely those 'nuisance' influences where the key factors could be located.

We have other misgivings as well. One centres on the third of Fisher's (1958) requirements for a correct statement of probability, which is that no relevant sub-set can be recognised; surely the distinctions made between initiators and promoters constitute just such heterogeneity? Once again we come back to which aspect of a situation is selected for examination. This is pertinent to Doll & Peto's unease, which we share, at being constrained by a narrow conventional view of occupation — the oversimplification of social variables to which epidemiological research has been prone (McQueen & Siegrist, 1982).

As is so often the case, an important contributory difficulty involves the criterion of specificity, with its attendant questions relating to necessity and sufficiency. In regard to the latter, is one seeking a sufficient cause (i.e. a single factor), or does one recognise that the situation is more complex and that components of a sufficient cause should be considered (Rothman, 1976)? Whilst not taking issue with the apparently dominant effect of smoking (because blocking the role of but one necessary component of a sufficient cause renders the joint action of the other components insufficient), we cannot help wondering how much other forces may be concealed under this influence.

Prescribing action
Fisher (1959) drew attention to a moral dilemma in regard to the engendering of fear in others. His own view was that the 'yellow peril' of modern times was the organised creation of states of frantic alarm, particularly by those who feel strongly on issues and demand that the hazards be brought home by means such as publicity.

We have chosen to echo these remarks because many of today's 'health' campaigns seem to be similarly vulnerable to the propensity of the species to prescribe how its fellows should live, an indulgence that is not infrequently associated with tunnel vision. What concerns us is the unsatisfactory and frequently ominous nature of the evidence on which these initiatives are based. For example, a recent television programme on heart disease was so concerned with the dangers of greasy junk foods, potato chips and the like so beloved of children, that it appeared to advocate confectionery as a substitute. What had happened to concern with dental caries?

We are reminded of a story of Kafka's about a country doctor, in which he said 'to write prescriptions is easy, but to come to an understanding with people is hard'. The comprehension that is currently exploited depends on a particular view of the species and its relationship with its surroundings. Expressed more explicitly, a narrow focus on aetiology too readily leads to polarisation between the individual and the environment. This is where it becomes so critical how these elements are regarded.

In his authoritative review of the prospects for prevention Doll (1983) concludes that the greatest opportunities lie with the modification of personal habits, especially smoking and (more speculatively) diet. It was not within his remit to confront the determination of these habits. However, if one wishes to act on his appraisal this becomes the nub of the situation. Let us start, therefore, with a fairly prevalent view which is reflected by the definition that life style is the set of behaviours adopted by personal choice (Lambert et al, 1982).

That may be true to some degree as far as the middle class is concerned, and most physicians and health promoters tend to have such comfortable backgrounds. However, to project such liberty in determining one's pattern of life to the majority is but another example of what George Bernard Shaw described, speaking of independence, as middle class blasphemy. One has also to appreciate that Judaeo-Christian values, which have influenced the development of most western societies, are very individualistic in their emphasis. Before knowing where one is, therefore, the notion of personal choice soon leads to victim-blaming, which too readily implies that collective action is not even appropriate.

McKeown (1983) acknowledges that the conditions of interest should be regarded as diseases of maladaptation. His appraisal is as follows.

'The most important medical advance in the nineteenth century was the discovery that infectious diseases were largely attributable to environmental conditions and could often be prevented by control of the influences which led to them; the most significant advance in the twentieth century is the recognition that the same is true of many non-communicable diseases.'

It is evident that WHO shares this view of the 'external' influences on life style (Table 2.5), and our purpose is just to question whether everyone committed to this endeavour has assimilated the point fully, with all its political implications.

INFLUENCES ON HEALTH

Having prepared the ground with an examination of intellectual obstacles to be overcome before a more sensitive appreciation can be developed, we can now take up further aspects of the tension between individual and 'environmental' influences on health.

Susceptibility and exposure

It is helpful to focus on the morbid end of these considerations, because health is difficult to think about in concrete terms other than by reference to its antitheses, disequilibria on the mental, physical, and social planes (Wood, 1972). The latter include deprivation, malnutrition and disease, and poverty, with a considerable degree of intercorrelation between these. The prime target of medical activity may be disease itself but, if one is to avoid securing the stable after its occupant has bolted, it is liability to disease that should be our major concern in the context of HFA.

As we shall be using superficially similar terms, it is necessary that we clarify their meanings.

Susceptibility is the most straightforward; it identifies innate tendencies as distinct from external circumstances. For example, in the case of an infectious disease the individual's susceptibility depends on his or her immunological defences which, in turn, are largely although not exclusively determined by inherited qualities (i.e. genetic constitution or, in Hippocratic nomenclature, diathesis). Predisposition is often used as a synonym for susceptibility, as in the designation 'predisposition frequency' for the ratio of affected family members (Penrose, 1953).

Liability represents not only the individual's innate tendency to develop or contract the disease (i.e. his susceptibility in the usual sense), but also the whole combination of external circumstances that makes him or her more or less likely to develop the disease. In this we are following Falconer (1965) and, as he goes on to illustrate for an infectious disease, liability includes the degree of exposure to the infective agent.

Liability (L) can thus be regarded as the resultant of (inherent) susceptibility (S) and (extrinsic) exposure (E). This relationship is depicted in Figure 2.1, where it can be seen that L may be the consequence of high S and low E, or vice versa, or of intermediate combinations. For his purpose (the computation of heritability), Falconer (1965) supposed that liability had a Gaussian distribution; as he claimed, this is not unwarranted assumption about its real nature.

The plot in Figure 2.1 portrays a linear pattern for L, which would be observed if both S and E were distributed in Gaussian fashion; i.e. if both are graded attributes, rather than being dichotomous (present/absent) characters. This point has not been

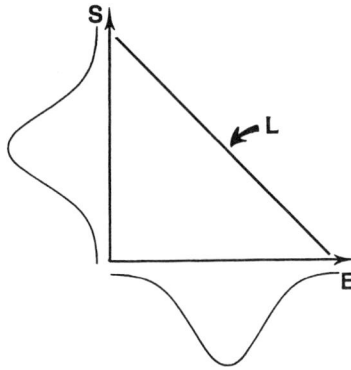

Fig. 2.1   Distribution of liability, depicting the interplay of susceptibility and exposure.

established, although it is a plausible assumption for further exploration and some work [e.g. on pneumoconiosis, Lindars & Davies (1967)] certainly supports such a view. However, we must acknowledge that other evidence is not in accord, at least superficially; e.g. the reported threshold influence (i.e. lack of a dose-response relationship) of physical exercise on ischaemic heart disease (Morris et al, 1973).

Obviously the relative contributions of S and E vary between different diseases; this is exemplified by portrayal of conditions on a spectrum extending from nature to nurture (e.g. Wood, 1978). Such variation would alter the slope of L. An estimate of the contributions can be derived by computing the heritability of liability, the maximum extent to which a genetic hypothesis could account for the observed distribution of disease in relatives; this is represented as h^2 and is expressed as a percentage. A minimum estimate for non-familial influences, E, would then be $(100-h^2)$ per cent although, as we shall show later on, this should not simply be equated with the environment conceived of in material terms.

Spectrum of determinants

We have just indicated that both susceptibility and exposure are likely to be appreciably more problematic than is currently acknowledged. This now needs to be taken a little further, in an endeavour to escape a simple dualism of intrinsic and extrinsic determinants of health. The circumstances that bear on health may be conceptualised in broad terms on a spectrum that extends from the insensible to the material. Figure 2.2 seeks to portray the range of 'topics' to be borne in mind, although no attempt has been made to indicate pathways in an exhaustive manner; to

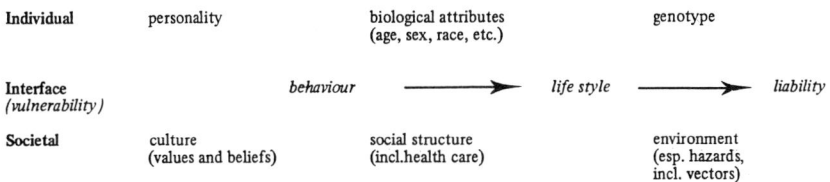

Individual	personality	biological attributes (age, sex, race, etc.)	genotype
Interface (vulnerability)		behaviour ⟶	life style ⟶ liability
Societal	culture (values and beliefs)	social structure (incl. health care)	environment (esp. hazards, incl. vectors)

Fig. 2.2   Internal (individual) and external (societal) sources of influence on health (extending on a spectrum from the insensible to the material: see text for explanation).

have done this would have produced a lattice of arrow shafts obscuring more than it revealed. Our main purpose is to suggest the direction of flow.

The bulk of this essay has been concerned to display the insecure foundation for succumbing to the temptation to equate susceptibility with genotype and exposure with the material environment; for that reason neither S nor E feature in Figure 2.2. Reverting to our earlier example of an infectious disease, immunological defences (S) are going to be influenced not only by the germ plasm but also by biological attributes such as age and ethnicity (whether the disease is endemic or an importation), by the vulnerability of the personality to stress (Rogers et al, 1980), and by the availability of nutrients, the latter being affected both by taboos operative in the culture and by economic and related factors determined by social structure.

Equally, exposure is influenced by age and sex (for example, in patterns of play), by cultural practices (including the location of habitations) and social structure (such as leads to social class differences), and by personality as mediated by behaviour and life style. The latter, of course, are also shaped by biology and culture (gender expectations, etc) and by social factors [most notably the availability of noxious agents such as alcohol, analgesics, and automobiles, Hetzel (1971)].

One value in exploring the interrelationships between the various factors represented in Figure 2.2 relates to the possibility of distinguishing between aetiologically distinct sub-sets, what may be regarded as underlying influences on the one hand and expressions that derive from them on the other. This leads us to make a further distinction.

Vulnerability is a term we have introduced for this purpose, with its accepted meaning of 'being open to attack'. Our intention is to restrict the concept of liability to established 'causes' of disease, and to speak of vulnerability when influences are of less certain or specific aetiological status (such as applies to many so-called risk factors).

We submit that behaviour and life style can be regarded only as derivative attributes, which is why we have depicted their location on the interfaces representing vulnerability, implying that they occupy a position further down the chain of causal circumstances than the factors that contribute to their determination. This is little more than a graphic representation of the situation Marx was describing when he said that men make their own history, but not under circumstances of their own choosing.

Two important implications stem from this appreciation. First, if one is to act on the conventional wisdom that prevention is better than cure, then it is on what we have referred to as the underlying influences that intervention should preferentially be brought to bear. Moreover, it is evident that the potential for intervention lies almost entirely with what have been designated as societal influences in Figure 2.2; the individual properties (age, sex, etc) are largely immutable.

Secondly, the amenability of vulnerability attributes to individual choice is much more limited than is commonly acknowledged, for reasons that we hope are by now apparent. This poses a serious challenge to Morris's Calvinistic assertion, one which is admittedly very acceptable to the established order, that 'the emergent principle of modern public health [is] that individual behaviour and *personal responsibility* are becoming crucial to further advance' (Morris & Heady, 1955; we have added the emphasis).

One other point that is worth remarking is the correspondence of what we have been categorising as the underlying determinants with accepted disciplines of enquiry—psychology, biological sciences, and genetics as far as the individual influences are concerned, and anthropology, the various social science sciences (including social administration and economics), and environmental sciences, such as geography, in regard to the societal influences. The significance of the fact that the activities of behaviourists and counsellors, who direct their energies to the vulnerability interfaces, have not so far been accorded the dignity of disciplinary status remains to be determined.

Options for intervention

It is time now to make more explicit some of the implications of our appraisal for intervention strategies. First, though, it may be helpful if we introduce a grid that we have found useful in ordering our own thoughts (Table 2.11). This endeavours to

Table 2.11 A grid for appraising options for intervention (extended from Wood, 1983 — after Leavell & Clark, 1965 & Haddon, 1980)

| | | Options for intervention | | |
| | | Communal | | |
Level of control	Individual	Access (*)	Physical surroundings	Social milieu
Primary (to prevent) a) Health promotion b) Protection (hazard containment)				
Secondary (to arrest) a) Reaction i Prompt response ii Screening b) Stabilisation i Cure ii Amelioration				
Tertiary (to repair) a) Restoration (control of disability) i Reconstruction ii Rehabilitation b) Maintenance (control of handicap) i Continuing care ii Enablement iii Support				

* Access relates to an intermediary, such as a vehicle or vector, or to the availability of a commodity (e.g. alcohol).

integrate an expanded Haddon (1980) matrix with Leavell's (Leavell & Clark, 1965) levels. We originally worked on this in the context of controlling disability (Wood, 1983) but we have now generalised the scheme. At the same time we have tried to break with the careless convention that speaks of secondary and tertiary 'prevention'—how can one prevent after the event has happened, and yet secondary and tertiary initiatives are, by definition, post hoc?

The idea of the grid is that it should be used as a checklist when considering options for the control of any health problem. Although it may not be possible to make an entry in every cell, the exercise should reduce the likelihood of neglecting fruitful possibilities. Readers may care to consult Haddon (1980) or Wood (1983) for specific examples of the use of more modest versions of this grid.

It can be seen in Table 2.11 that, whereas we have allowed a single column for options relating to individuals, communal initiatives have been differentiated into access, physical surroundings, and social milieu. The two latter probably need no further clarification, but our use of the term access may not be so transparent. We are thinking of two things under this head, the conventional vehicle or vector (be it an arthropod or a loose floorboard) and the availability of agents that are also commodities in human transactions (tobacco or alcohol, for example).

Our approach presents a stark contrast to the single factor interventions with which we have been taking issue earlier in this chapter. Moreover, as we hope the grid helps to make clear, most options for control depend on social policy initiatives. Even as far as the individual is concerned this still to a large extent applies; most secondary and tertiary interventions involve the availability of services, be these voluntary, insurance based, or provided by the state, and many primary control measures are equally influenced by forces outside the individual.

Turning now to health problems, their heterogeneity has to be acknowledged. Almost paradoxically, the desire for a general perspective has to take account of this. Again an evolutionary outlook is helpful. As long as the force of mortality was experienced in the perinatal period and childhood, the dominant influences of nutrition, development, and hygiene were paramount. Once this 'milestone' has been passed the diverse origins of ill-health become more obtrusive. Between one condition and another the balance of factors and the subtle influences of culture are likely to differ.

It is unlikely, therefore, that a universal prescription will be possible; the principal contradiction is probably located in the foundations of current social organisation and, unless this is to be confronted, initiatives will have to be taken on many fronts. By seeking a universal solution we would become vulnerable to an unscientific view, assaulting the most difficult problems while neglecting specific and potentially more rewarding challenges.

We would here introduce another consideration. Doll & Peto (1981) enunciate the sound maxim that, given two agents which account for a similar proportion of deaths, the one more amenable to control is of greater public health significance. To complement this view, if a particular measure appears in the grid (Table 2.11) for more than one condition (and dietary modification is one of the best current examples), then one would be tempted to attach higher priority to further evaluation of that measure.

There are three other lesser points we should like to make. The first is that thus far we have been principally concerned with what can be characterised as 'professional' appraisals of the phenomena associated with ill-health, be these biomedical or sociocultural in their orientation. Harking back to the principle of primary health care (PHC) that we discussed, regarding communal participation, it will also be necessary to take cognisance of so-called lay systems of belief (Blaxter, 1983; Williams, 1984), since these cannot help but reflect public perceptions of the genesis of ill-health and influence what might be done to change matters.

Secondly, the importance of context that we have stressed more than once applies equally to many laboratory findings. For example, current evidence indicates that an excessive sodium intake is potentially harmful. But is it the actual sodium load that matters, or is it some other property such as the sodium/potassium balance (MacGregor, 1983)? The public health interest in this is that it could extend our options — while trying to reduce the use of sodium in food processing, we could also promote potassium-rich foods such as citrus fruits. The principle is sound, even if the example may prove to be faulty; in fact existing social class differences in fruit consumption (much related to price) might indicate that such an initiative would only be likely to increase the social morbidity differentials even more.

Finally, we would sound a note of caution. Many interventions appear to have a potential for harm as well as benefit. For example, what may be good for your cholesterol may also increase a hazard of malignancy (Taylor, 1983). This is analogous to what the economists refer to as opportunity costs; we prefer the words of Socrates: 'If you marry, or if you do not, you will live to regret it'. Our conclusion, then, is to paraphrase Berger (1978): we need to be bold in our thinking and prudent in our prescriptions.

ACKNOWLEDGEMENT

We are indebted to our colleagues Orin Smith and Catherine Turtle for their work on the derivation of current British performance in relation to the WHO targets. Footnotes to the tables would have become unmanageable had the sources for all estimates been shown; however, we have prepared an appendix that lists this information and copies will be provided on request.

REFERENCES

Bartley M 1983 Coronary heart disease — a disease of affluence or a disease of industry? Bulletin of the Society for Social History of Medicine 33: 50–51
Berger P 1978 Facing up to modernity. Penguin Books, Harmondsworth
Blaxter M 1983 The causes of disease — women talking. Social Science and Medicine 17: 59–69
Bross I D J 1964 Prisoners of jargon. American Journal of Public Health 54: 918–927
Buckley E G 1983 Quality and the College. Journal of the Royal College of General Practitioners 33: 761
Burch P R J 1984 The Surgeon General's 'epidemiologic criteria for causality' — reply to Lilienfeld. Journal of Chronic Diseases 37: 148–156
Catalano R 1979 Health, behaviour and the community — an ecological perspective. Pergamon Press, New York
Charlton J R H, Hartley R M, Silver, R, Holland W W 1983 Geographical variation in mortality from conditions amenable to medical intervention in England and Wales. Lancet 1: 691–696
Collingwood R G 1940 Essay on metaphysics. Clarendon Press, London, p 35
Department of Health and Social Security (DHSS) 1980 Working group on inequalities in health (the Black Report). HMSO, London
DHSS 1983 NHS Management Inquiry, report (the Griffiths Report). HMSO, London
Doll R 1983 Occasional review — prospects for prevention. British Medical Journal 286: 445–453
Doll R, Peto R 1981 The causes of cancer — quantitative estimates of avoidable risks of cancer in the United States today. Journal of the National Cancer Institute 66: 1193–1308
Dubos R 1965 Man adapting. Yale University Press, New Haven
Editorial 1983 Payment by diagnosis. Lancet 2: 1403–1404
Falconer D S 1965 The inheritance of liability to certain diseases estimated from the incidence among relatives. Annals of Human Genetics 29: 51–76

Feinstein A R 1967 Clinical judgement. Williams & Wilkins, Baltimore
Fisher R A 1958 The nature of probability. Centennial Review 2: 261–274 [also reproduced in Fisher 1959]
Fisher R A 1959 Smoking — the cancer controversy; some attempts to assess the evidence. Oliver & Boyd, Edinburgh
Haddon W Jr 1980 Landmarks in American epidemiology — advances in the epidemiology of injuries as a basis for public policy. Public Health Reports 95: 411–421
Hamilton M 1974 Lectures on the methodology of clinical research, 2nd ed. Churchill Livingstone, Edinburgh
Hetzel B 1971 Life and health in Australia — The Boyer lectures, 1971. Australian Broadcasting Commission, Sydney
Hill A B 1965 The environment and disease — association or causation? Proceedings of the Royal Society of Medicine 5: 295–300
Hippocrates 1849 The genuine works of Hippocrates, Adams F (trans). Sydenham Society, London, vol 1, pp 179–222 [also reproduced in Barkhuus Arne medical survey from Hippocrates to the world travellers. Ciba Symposium 6, 1986 (1945)]
Irvine D 1983 Quality of care in general practice — our outstanding problem. Journal of the Royal College of General Practitioners 33: 521–523
Joris P 1980 In a discussion of Lacan's Ecole Freudienne de Paris. New Statesman 16 May p 750
Körner E 1982 Steering group on health services information — first report to the Secretary of State on the collection and use of information about hospital clinical activity in the National Health Service (the Körner report). HMSO, London
Kuhn T S 1970 The structure of scientific revolutions, 2nd ed. International Encyclopedia of Unified Science, vol 2, no 2. University of Chicago Press, Chicago
Lalonde M 1975 A new perspective on the health of Canadians, a working document. Information Canada, Ottawa
Lambert C A, Netherton D R, Finison L J, Hyde J N, Spaight S J 1982 Risk factors and life style — a statewide health-interview survey. New England Journal of Medicine 306: 1048–1051
Leavell H R, Clark E G 1965 Preventive medicine for the doctor in his community — an epidemiologic approach, 3rd ed. Blakiston Division, McGraw-Hill Book Co, New York
Lindars D C, Davies D 1967 Rheumatoid pneumoconiosis — a study in colliery populations in the East Midlands coalfield. Thorax 22: 525–532
McDonald G J, Mazzuca S A, McCabe G P Jr 1983 How much of the placebo 'effect' is really statistical regression? Statistics in Medicine 2: 417–427
MacGregor G A 1983 Nutrition: the changing scene — dietary sodium and potassium intake and blood pressure. Lancet 1: 750–752
McKeown T 1976 The modern rise of population. Edward Arnold, London
McKeown T 1983 A basis for health strategies — a classification of disease. British Medical Journal 287: 594–596
McQueen D V, Siegrist J 1982 Social factors in the etiology of chronic disease — an overview. Social Science and Medicine 16: 353–367
Marmot M 1976 Facts, opinions and affaires du coeur. American Journal of Epidemiology 103: 519–526
Mestrovic S, Glassner B 1983 A Durkheimian hypothesis on stress. Social Science and Medicine 17: 1315–1327
Midgley M 1979 Beast and man, the roots of human nature. Methuen, London, p 5
Miller G H, Gerstein D R 1983 The life expectancy of nonsmoking men and women. Public Health Reports 98: 343–349
Morris J N 1975 Uses of epidemiology, 3rd ed. Churchill Livingstone, Edinburgh
Morris J N, Heady J A 1955 Social and biological factors in infant mortality: v. mortality in relation to the father's occupation 1911–1950. Lancet 1: 554–559
Morris J N, Adam C, Chave S P W, Sirey C, Epstein L 1973 Vigorous exercise in leisure time and the incidence of coronary heart disease. Lancet 1: 333–339
Murphy E A 1972 The application of genetics to epidemiology. In: Stewart G T (ed) Trends in epidemiology — application to health service research and training. C C Thomas, Springfield, ch 3, p 102–138
Penrose L S 1953 The genetical background of common diseases. Acta Genetica 4: 257–265
Popper K R 1959 The logic of scientific discovery. Hutchinson, London
Public Health Service (PHS) 1983 Promoting health/preventing disease — implementation plans for attaining the objectives of the nation. Public Health Reports 98 suppl: 1–178
Rogers M P, Trentham D E, McCune W J et al 1980 Effects of psychological stress on the induction of arthritis in rats. Arthritis and Rheumatism 23: 1337–1342
Rothman K J 1976 Reviews and commentary — causes. American Journal of Epidemiology 104: 587–592
Rothschild Lord 1971 The organization and management of government R and D. In: A framework for government research and development. HMSO, London

Rutstein D D, Berenberg W, Chalmers T C et al 1980 Measuring the quality of medical care — second revision of tables of indexes. New England Journal of Medicine 302: 1146

Taylor K G 1983 Leading article — hypocholesterolaemia and cancer? British Medical Journal 286: 1598–1959

Williams G H 1982 Causality, morality, and radicalism — a sociological examination of the work of George Brown and his colleagues. Sociology 16: 67–84

Williams G H 1984 Lay beliefs about the causes of rheumatoid arthritis — implications for rehabilitation. International Rehabilitation Medicine 6: in press

Wood P H N 1972 Conceptual fallacies in health planning. Paper prepared for Third International Conference on Social Science and Medicine, Elsinore

Wood P H N 1976 Osteoarthrosis in the community. In: Wright V (ed) Osteoarthrosis. Clinics in Rheumatic Diseases 2: 495–507

Wood P H N 1978 Epidemiology of rheumatic disorders. In: Scott J T (ed) Copeman's textbook of the rheumatic diseases, 5th ed. Churchill Livingstone, Edinburgh, ch 3, Fig 3.4, p 32, and Fig 3.3, p 28

Wood P H N 1982 Advances in the classification of disease. In: Smith A (ed) Recent advances in community medicine — 2. Churchill Livingstone, Edinburgh, ch 13, p 169–183

Wood P H N, Badley E M 1978 An epidemiological appraisal of disablement. In: Bennett A E (ed) Recent advances in community medicine — 1. Churchill Livingstone, Edinburgh, ch 9, p 149–173

Wood P H N, Badley E M 1981 People with disabilities: toward acquiring information which reflects more sensitively their problems and needs. International exchange of information in rehabilitation monograph no. 12. World Rehabilitation Fund, New York

World Health Organisation (WHO) 1977 Resolution WHA 30.43. WHO, Geneva

WHO 1978 Primary health care — report of the international conference on primary health care, Alma Ata, USSR, September 1978. WHO, Geneva

WHO 1980 The international classification of impairments, disabilities, and handicaps — a manual of classification relating to the consequences of disease. WHO, Geneva

WHO 1981 Development of indicators for monitoring progress towards health for all by the year 2000. Health For All series, No 4. WHO, Geneva

WHO 1982 Report on the eighth session of the European Advisory Committee for Medical Research (document EUR/RC32/4). Regional Committee for Europe, WHO, Copenhagen

WHO 1983 Targets in support of the regional strategy for HFA 2000 (document EUR/RC33/9). Regional Committee for Europe, WHO, Copenhagen

Zuckerman S 1961 The management and control of research and development. Office of the Minister for Science. HMSO, London

3. The scope for prevention

John R. Ashton

Preventive medicine is once again a fashionable activity. For a time in the 1950s and 1960s it was assumed that the decline of infectious diseases meant that we could turn our attention to the use of modern technology to treat the diseases that remained and prevention became a Cinderella subject. There followed a slowly growing disenchantment with this approach and a return to a preoccupation with prevention. New expectations have now been raised and failures to take prevention seriously are beginning to have political consequences — consequences which in the Britain of the 80's cannot be ignored (DHSS, 1975; HMSO, 1977; Lalonde, 1974; USDHEW, 1979; WHO, 1981a). Already questions are beginning to be asked by Health Authority members about slow progress towards prevention goals and it is not infrequent to hear officers saying that 'we must be seen to be doing something about prevention . . .'. Of such beginnings are major changes made.

THE BACKGROUND

The population of England and Wales in 1086 was of the order of 1.25 million as estimated from the Domesday Book (Cartwright, 1977). For the next 600 years there was slow overall growth interrupted by occasional dramatic declines — for example as a consequence of the plague which may have reduced the population by anything up to a half in 1338 to 1349 (Waters, 1977). By 1695 the population stood at about 5.5 million. Accurate figures are available from the decennial census since 1801 when the population was nearly 9 million (Fig. 3.1). The population doubled in the first half of the nineteenth century and nearly doubled again in the second half. Since 1901 the increase has slowed down and has now stopped. McKeown has argued that the main reason for the population increase was a reduction in the death rate and a consequent increase in the expectation of life at birth; this change was largely due to a decline in mortality from infectious disease which in turn was attributable to improvements in nutrition and environmental conditions (McKeown, 1976).

McKeown's analysis is striking for its conclusion that with the exception of vaccination against smallpox, which was associated with 1.6% of the decline in the death rate from 1848 to 1971, it is unlikely that immunisation or therapy had a significant effect on mortality from infectious disease before the twentieth century. In particular, most of the reduction in mortality from tuberculosis, bronchitis, pneumonia and influenza, whooping cough and the food-and-water-borne disease had already occurred before effective immunisations or treatments were available.

Between 1900 and 1935 some specific measures contributed to the reduction in mortality from infections. These included immunisation against diphtheria, surgery in appendicitis, peritonitis and ear infections, salvarsan in syphilis, intravenous therapy

population (millions)

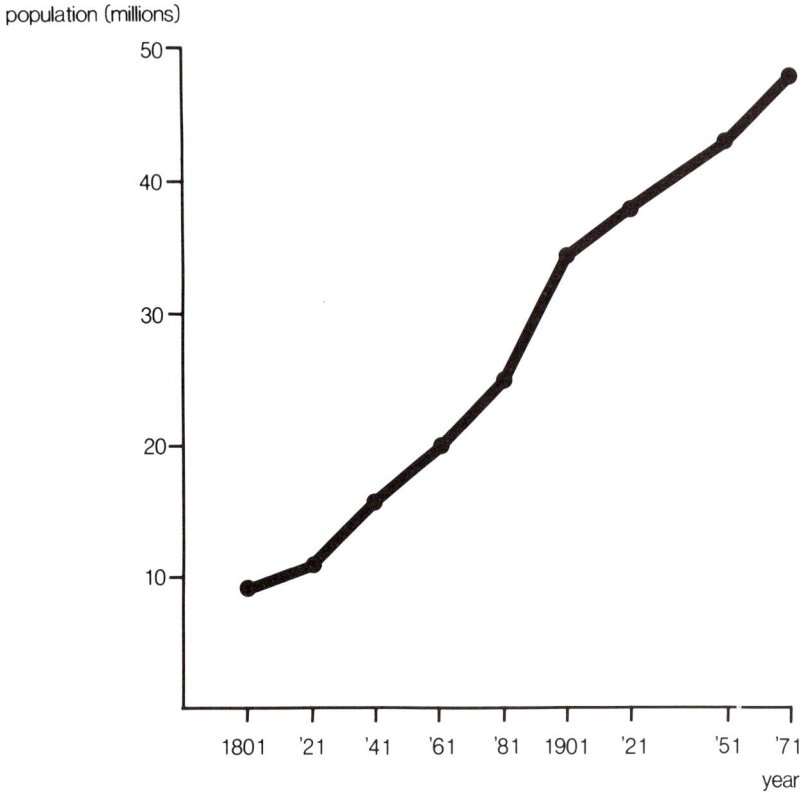

Fig. 3.1   Population of England and Wales at the time of the decennial census 1801 to 1971.

in diarrhoeal disease, passive immunisation against tetanus and improved obstetric care. However the total contribution of medical and surgical interventions to reductions of mortality has been small compared with the effect of environmental, 'public health' measures.

It is clear from McKeown's work that in the past the impact of medicine has been more on morbidity than on mortality and that the important determinants of health have been those which minimised the consequences of disturbances in the ecology in which human beings evolved. There appear to be biologically determined limits to the expectation of life and the efficient functioning of the organ systems of any individual. This has become particularly pertinent now that non-communicable diseases have superseded the communicable diseases in importance. The rational approach would appear to be to tackle those environmental factors which determine health and disease in the twentieth century with the same determination and vigour that was applied to their predecessors in the nineteenth.

THE NATURE OF CONTEMPORARY HEALTH PROBLEMS

In 1980 there were 656 000 live births in England and Wales and the infant mortality rate was 12.0 per 1000 live births (DHSS, 1982). The expectation of life for males surviving to their first birthday is about 70 years and for females about 76 years (DHSS, 1980).

Although much still needs to be done in ensuring that the conditions of pregnancy and neonatal life are optimal for the production of healthy surviving infants, not least with respect to inequalities between the social classes, in historical terms most of the attainable improvement has already been achieved. Infant mortality rates today are one-tenth of those at the turn of the century. A large part of this residual mortality is accounted for by death from congenital disorders in the first weeks of life for which there are no immediate prospects of prevention. However, the mortality during the first 12 months is still higher than in any other year until after the age of 50.

One consequence of the changes which have occurred over the last 100 years is that the age distribution of the population has altered and we now have a much higher proportion of elderly people in the population (Fig. 3.2, Table 3.1). It is increasingly

Table 3.1   The change in population distribution 1871 to 1981 in England and Wales

Year	Percentage aged over 65 years
1871	4.6
1901	4.6
1931	7.4
1971	13.0
1981	15.2

(Morris, 1975; OPCS, 1984.)

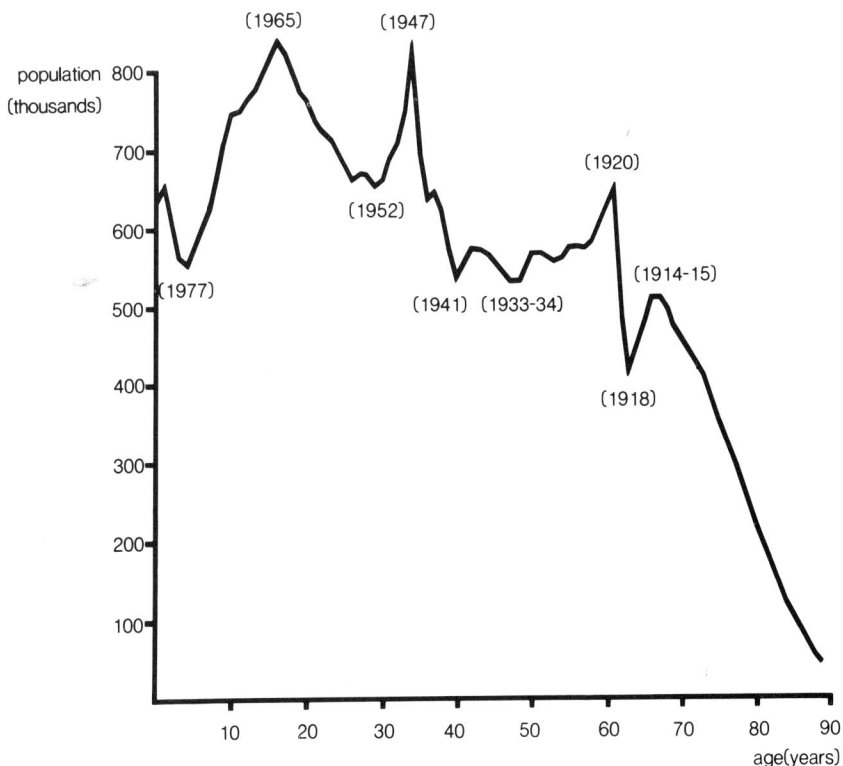

Fig. 3.2   Total population of England and Wales 1981. Source: Provisional mid-1981 population estimates for England and Wales and health areas. Ref. PPI 82/3 OPCS. Year of birth peak and trough cohorts in parentheses.

regarded as abnormal for people to die before they reach old age and the diseases to which death is attributed are to a large extent determined by initial genetic endowment and accumulated environmental insults over 60 or 70 years (Table 3.2) (WHO, 1980; WHO, 1982). A useful way of looking at the effects of mortality is in terms of the years lost as a result of premature death; this method of representation allows some weight to be attached to causes of death which affect the young (Table 3.3). Overall it is apparent that lifestyle and behaviour play an increasingly important part and morbidity before death has become an important consideration. It is clear too that a large proportion of premature deaths have preventable causes.

Table 3.2 Principal causes of death in England and Wales 1980

Rank	ICD number	Cause of death	Male	Female	Main age groups involved
1	390–459	Circulatory system	143 079	147 316	40+
2	140–239	Neoplasms	69 529	61 038	40+
3	460–519	Respiratory system	42 334	41 071	50+
4	800–999	Injury & poisoning	11 757	8 539	15–24, 65+
5	520–579	Digestive system	7 176	8 964	65+
6	580–629	Genitourinary system	3 734	4 001	65+
7	320–389	Central nervous system	3 117	3 366	65+
8	240–279	Metabolic disorders	2 597	3 843	55+
9	760–779	Perinatal conditions	1 865	1 283	Perinatal
10	746–759	Congenital anomalies	1 769	1 635	Under 1 year
11	001–139	Infectious/parasitic	1 229	1 010	65+
12	290–319	Mental disorders	1 126	2 182	70
13	780–799	Ill-defined conditions	1 042	1 465	75+
14	710–739	Musculoskeletal	742	2 362	65+
15	280–289	Blood disorders	654	1 018	65+
16	680–709	Skin disorders	120	353	65+
17	630–676	Pregnancy/childbirth	—	70	20–40

Source: Table 2 DH2 No. 7 Mortality Statistics 1980 OPCS.

Table 3.3 Priority conditions causing premature death in Mersey Region. Causes of years of life lost before the age of 70 years in 1980

Rank	Cause of death	Years of life lost	Percentage years lost
1	Heart disease	34 309	20.6
2	Perinatal causes	12 279	7.7
3	Cancer of respiratory system and lungs	10 218	6.4
4	Stroke	8 911	5.6
5	Road accidents	8 354	5.3
6	Congenital abnormalities	8 173	5.1
7	Pneumonia	5 960	3.8
8	Other external causes	5 203	3.3
9	Cancer of breast	5 159	3.2
10	Chronic lung disease	4 095	2.6
11	Brain and nerve diseases	3 951	2.5
12	Suicide	3 631	2.3
13	Blood cancers	3 394	2.1
14	Ill-defined conditions	2 939	1.9
15	Homicide and undetermined injury	2 653	1.7
16	Cancer of bowel	2 201	1.4
17	Cancer of stomach	1 871	1.2
18	Infectious diseases	1 822	1.1

Source: D. Pinder, Personal communication.

The actual perception of health problems and the priority attached to any particular one is influenced by a number of factors including the age-specificity of particular problems in relation to the demographic structure and variables such as the extent to which many people are involved in simultaneous afflictions (as in an aeroplane crash) or the extent to which an external agent can be held responsible (Ashton, 1983). Although death is the final common pathway for all of us and increasingly tends to occur in an institutional setting under medical surveillance, the extent of morbidity in the community depends to a large extent on how hard one looks; most disease occurs outside the medical context (Fig. 3.3).

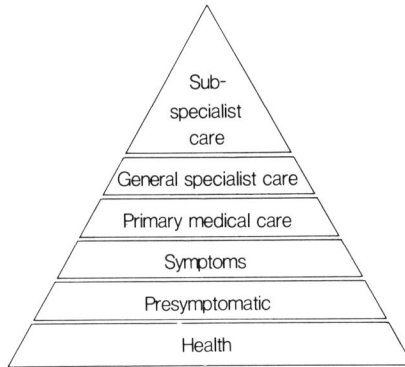

Fig. 3.3 The pyramid of health and disease.

Primary medical care marks the point at which ailments acquire medical labels and at which one assumes that some threshold of anxiety of interference with every day living has been crossed. The majority of general practice consultations are for self-limiting conditions where a wider level of education and understanding among the general public is essential if the population as a whole is to be able to make full use of health services when they are needed and be in a better position to deal with minor ailments without recourse to professional help (Table 3.4).

The use of general practice consultation as a measure of community morbidity is convenient but misleading. It depends on political and administrative factors such as access and on cultural factors such as the perception of illness and the tolerance of discomfort inconvenience and pain. In the survey which provided the baseline for the pre-war Peckham experiment only 9% of the people studied were free of disorder and disease (Table 3.5). More recent surveys have found that only 10% of a population studied could be classified as completely healthy in accordance with the WHO definition (Fry, 1979).

As so much 'disease' is transient, an alternative approach has been to employ diaries and to collect symptom data in the general population over a defined period. Dunnell & Cartwright (1972) found the incidence of a variety of symptoms in a random survey of British adults to be as high as 40% over a two week period.

Taken together the evidence suggests that much of what we know as ill-health is preventable by changes of life-style, behaviour and environmental influences and a great deal of that which is not preventable is self-limiting or amenable to self-care.

Table 3.4   Persons consulting in a year in a British General Practice of 2500 persons

Conditions		Persons consulting per 2500
1. Minor		
General:		
Upper respiratory infections		500
Emotional disorders		300
Gastrointestinal infections and upsets		250
Skin disorders		225
Specific:		
Acute tonsillitis		100
Acute otitis media		75
Cerumen		50
Acute urinary infections		50
Migraine		30
Hay fever		25
2. Major (new cases)		
Acute bronchitis and pneumonia		50
Myocardial infarction		7
Acute appendicitis		5
Strokes		5
All cancers		5
Severe depression		12
Suicide attempt		3
Suicide	(every 4 years)	1
3. Chronic		
Chronic rheumatism		100
Chronic mental illness		55
Chronic bronchitis		50
Chronic heart failure and angina		45
High blood pressure		25
Asthma		25
Peptic ulcer		25
Old strokes		15
Epilepsy		10
Diabetes		10
Parkinsonism		3
Multiple sclerosis		2
Chronic pyelonephritis	less than	1
4. Social pathology		
Poverty		100
Aged over 75 years		100
Severe physical handicap		70
Broken home		50
Chronic alcoholism		30
Deafness		25
Blindness		7
Severe mental handicap		10
Divorce		3
Illegitimate birth		3
Committed to prison		2

Source: Fry, 1979.

Table 3.5   Health: The relationship of disorder
to disease

	Percentage
Disorder with disease	31.6
Disorder without disease	59.0
Neither disorder nor disease	9.4

Source: Scott Williamson & Pearse, 1938; Ashton, 1977.

INEQUALITIES IN HEALTH

Superimposed on the situation so far described is the added dimension of inequalities in the experience of health and disease and of the availability of services to those in need (Townsend & Davidson, 1982). When the National Health Service was established in 1948 there were very few explicit objectives other than the broad goal that medical care should be equally available to all with equal need irrespective of the ability to pay.

The creation of the Health Service was but one part of a programme of social legislation introduced by the post-war Labour Government to implement the recommendations of the Beveridge Report, published in 1942. These recommendations were intended to rebuild the social fabric after the devastation of the 1930s depression and the Second World War and were meant to tackle Beveridge's five giant evils of 'Want, Disease, Ignorance, Idleness and Squalor' (Beveridge, 1942).

It was then the contemporary wisdom that an expenditure on health services would subsequently reduce after the initial backlog of disease had been worked off. That wisdom has changed and it is now usual to think not of a backlog but rather of an iceberg or of layers of an onion. We have come to have a much more realistic understanding of the relative nature of medical and social need and an appreciation that the thresholds which determine the tolerance of discomfort and distress are flexible in accordance with levels of material, psychological and social expectation.

One of the consequences of the imbalance towards emphasis on hospital care in the past 30 years has been that until recently there has been very little concern to evaluate the extent to which the total package of health and related services, both institutional and community-based were delivering the goods in terms of measurable outcome measures of the public health. Rather there was a tendency to assume complacently that as we had a National Health Service equity must automatically follow and this has been reinforced by a widespread and touching belief that medicine and the practice of medicine is automatically 'a good thing' irrespective of any evaluation. McKeown's work challenged this view and Tudor-Hart and Townsend argued convincingly that there were inversions in the provision of health services and that in effect those people who most need good quality accessible medical services are least likely to have them (Tudor-Hart, 1971; Townsend, 1974). The accumulating concern over health inequalities resulted in the Black Report on Inequalities in Health which has documented inequalities of mortality experience between men and women, the different social classes, between different parts of the country and between different racial groups. It shows clearly that major differences exist in the environmental factors which impinge on health, in the personal risk factors relating to lifestyle and in access to and use of preventive and treatment services. Above all the report singled out the concentration of severe inequalities in ten health districts as being the least favoured places in which to live (Table 3.6). The identification of these towns in this way is strongly reminiscent of a similar form of identification involving some of the same towns in Chadwick's report on the sanitary condition of the labouring population of Great Britain in 1842 (Chadwick, 1842). Chadwick's report resulted in the Public Health Act in 1848.

Table 3.6   The unhealthy districts

Salford
Tameside
Gateshead
Liverpool
South Tyneside
Tower Hamlets
Durham
Bolton
Wirral
North Tyneside

Townsend & Davidson, 1982.

THE PROBLEM AND THE TASK

The problem is becoming clearer. In his Harveian oration Sir Richard Doll comprehensively reviewed the field and concluded that modification of lifestyle, protection against trauma, control of infection and pollution, the screening of populations and the use of prophylactic medication are the areas of interest (Doll, 1983). He estimated that the avoidance of smoking alone would reduce the mortality from all cancer by about a third, would almost eliminate chronic obstructive lung disease and the complications of peripheral vascular disease, would reduce the age-specific mortality from aortic aneurysm by at least three-quarters and the mortality from myocardial infarction by about a quarter and would probably lead to a small reduction in perinatal mortality in the poorer socio-economic groups. Modifications of diet including the intake of alcohol and the control of obesity and the encouragement of physical exercise are now widely regarded as desirable public health goals. The realisation that preventive medicine must now be central to any health strategy has begun to influence the Political Parties in their policy formulation. The statement that our health centres should more accurately be described as sickness centres may be true at present but may not be so for much longer even though few health centres yet promote health through community activity as pioneered in the Peckham Health Centre (Fig. 3.4) (Horder, 1983; Ashton, 1977).

The message has been taken up by the World Health Organisation and linked to the concept of developing broad based Primary Health Care. The Global Strategy for attaining Health For All By The Year 2000 grew from the Alma-Ata conference on Primary Health Care in the USSR in 1978 (WHO, 1978; WHO, 1981a). The Alma-Ata Declaration which was signed by all member states reaffirmed the Organisation's commitment to the goal of obtaining Health For All as a fundamental human right. Primary Health Care was seen as the necessary cornerstone for the attainment of a level of Health For All By The Year 2000 which would permit everybody to lead socially and economically productive lives. The strategy consists of

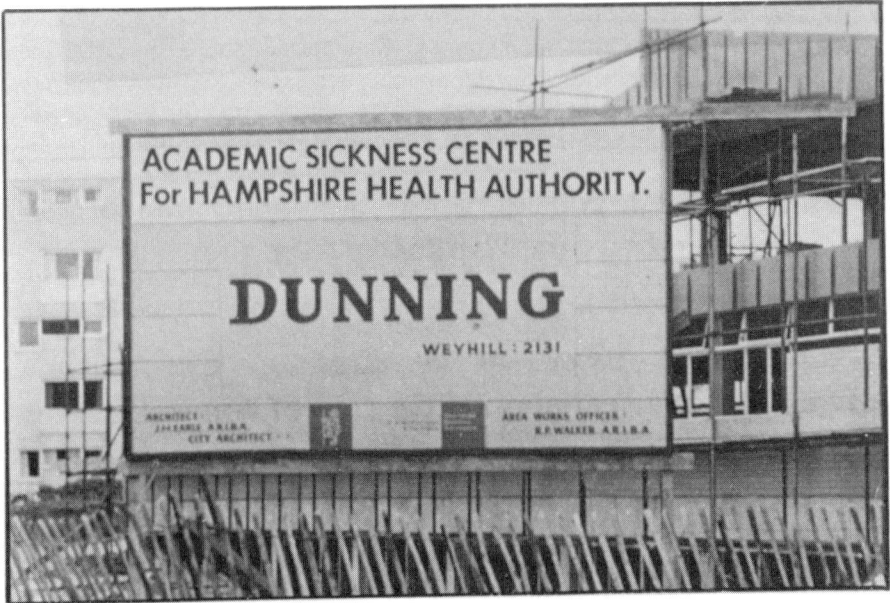

Fig. 3.4 Health centres or sickness centres?

three main elements: the promotion of lifestyles conducive to health, the reduction of preventable conditions and the provision of care which is adequate, accessible and acceptable to all.

The Health For All Strategy was adopted as a policy as resolution WHA 32.30 in the Thirty-second World Health Assembly in 1979. As a result each Region of WHO has produced its own strategy document and a large number of countries in all regions have since formulated national strategies, a notable exception being the United Kingdom which has a tradition of assuming that WHO is an organisation which helps countries in Africa and the Far East and to which we offer expertise (Horder, 1983; WHO, 1981a).

The key perspectives of the strategy are that it is aimed at the elimination of inequalities and is based on a broad public health concept of primary care; that is to say that defined populations are covered by defined primary health care personnel. This concept which has recently been well described by Tudor-Hart and by Kark offers an opportunity to synthesise the public health or population approach together with that of the personal physician (Tudor-Hart, 1981; Kark, 1981). The potential for this approach in the United Kingdom is considerable given the level of development of general practice training and organisation and the existence of a denominator in the form of a practice list. However the lack of training in field epidemiology and team work for primary health workers are currently major constraints and attempts to improve the state of some general practices in inner city areas revealed by various recent reports will probably require legislation to change the conditions of service of doctors and other health workers and ensure that Primary Health Care is adequately funded. Norway and Finland are two examples of countries which have faced up to this problem and passed a Primary Health Care Act.

In the Health For All Strategy it is intended that programmes for health promotion, disease prevention, therapy and rehabilitation should be developed and each signatory of Alma-Ata commits itself to developing the necessary education and research programmes to support the implementation of the strategy; decentralised control and active participation by the people themselves in their own health underpin the bottom-up approach to the development of programmes for health promotion (Fig. 3.5). The key is working with people not on them. Global and Regional indicators have been developed and it is intended that appropriate national and local indicators should be (Tables 3.7 and 3.8). In addition each country is expected to produce a biennial report on the progress made towards attaining the strategy goals.

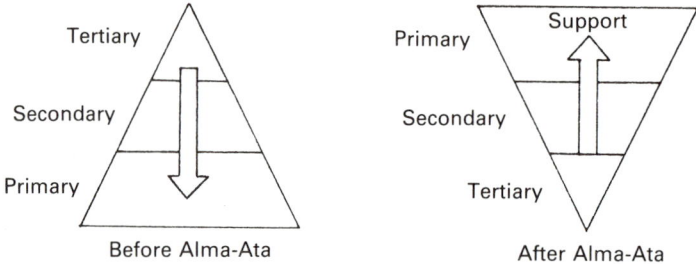

Fig. 3.5 Bottom-up not top-down in health for all by the year 2000. Reproduced with the permission of Professor H. Vuori.

There is great emphasis in the strategy documents on the need for intersectoral collaboration where the health interest is affected by the interests and activities of other sectors of society and other government departments. This need for inter-sectoral collaboration was also identified in the Black Report which made two specific recommendations to facilitate it:

1. The setting up of two government committees, a ministerial committee and an officials committee, as Fora for the integration of policy.
2. The setting up of an independent Health Development Council to play a key role in social planning.

Table 3.7 Global indicators

The number of countries in which:

1 Health for all has received endorsement as policy at the highest official level.
2 Mechanisms for involving people in the implementation of strategies have been formed or strengthened, and are actually functioning.
3 At least 5% of the gross national product is spent on health.
4 A reasonable percentage of the national health expenditure is devoted to local health care.
5 Resources are equitably distributed.
6 The number of developing countries with well-defined strategies for health for all, accompanied by explicit resource allocations, whose needs for external resources are receiving sustained support from more affluent countries.
7 Primary health care is available to the whole population.
8 The nutritional status of children is adequate.
9 The infant mortality rate for all identifiable subgroups is below 50 per 1000 live-births.
10 Life expectancy at birth is over 60 years.
11 The adult literacy rate for both men and women exceeds 70%.
12 The gross national product per head exceeds US$500.

Source: Global Strategy for Health for all by the Year 2000 WHO Geneva 1981. 'Health For All Series' No. 3.

Table 3.8   Regional indicators. List of suggested indicators of progress towards achieving health for all by the year 2000

Indicators of the attainment of health for all

Indicators of survival
1 Life expectancy at birth — by sex*
2 Infant mortality*
3 Perinatal mortality*
4 Comparative mortality in given ages among selected socio-economic and occupation groups
5 Specific mortality rates for selected causes (accidents, suicides)*

Indicators of lifestyle
1 Alcohol consumption per capita*
2 Tobacco consumption per capita*
3 Percentage of nonsmokers by age, sex and social class*
4 Drug abuse in adolescents and young adults*
5 Percentage of pregnancies before 15*
6 Incidence of sexually transmitted diseases*
7 Number of people in sports associations—by age

Indicators of 'quality of life'
1 Proportion of persons disabled as a result of permanent impairment — in selected age groups*
2 Incidence of waterborne diseases*
3 Percentage of population in households with an adequate water supply of safe water*
4 Percentage of population in households with an adequate waste disposal system*
5 Percentage of population exposed to given levels of selected pollutants*
6 Percentage of children below a given nutrititional state — by age
7 Birthweight in selected groups*
8 Absenteeism from work
9 Absenteeism from school
10 Criminality rates*
11 Levels of education in various age groups*
12 Percentage of population satisfied with their own level of health
13 Percentage of people over 70 years with low dependency status

Socio-economic indicators
1 Gross national product per capita*
2 Health expenditure as a proportion of gross national product*
3 Income distribution
4 Percentage of health expenditures financed by:
   — government (central and local)
   — social security (compulsory insurance)
   — private insurance
   — private direct payment
   — other
5 Percentage of population at 'poverty level'
6 Proportion of active population seeking employment

Indicators of progress at national level
   Indicators of progress towards primary health care
1 Percentage of population entering the health system through primary health care*
2 Percentage of first contact with specialists arising out of referral from primary health care
3 Number of doctors working alone in primary care practice and number of teams of 2, 3, 4, . . . partners
4 Number of persons working in primary care teams, other than doctors — by category (nurses, pharmacists, dentists, occupation therapists, social workers, etc.)
5 Percentage of nurses working in hospital and in the community*
6 Percentage of contacts in primary health care which do not involve curative services — by category:
   — family planning
   — surveillance
   — health education/promotion, etc.
7 Percentage of primary care teams with an established mechanism for community participation
8 Percentage of cost of health services devoted to primary care — of which, percentage devoted to pharmaceuticals*

Table 3.8 *cont'd*

Availability of services
  1 Classical resource-to-population ratios (physician, nurse, health post, hospital bed, etc.)*
  2 Average daily time of availability of primary health care services

Accessibility of services
  1 Average delay between occurrence of an emergency (accident, heart attack) and appropriate care
  2 Percentage of population with access to a source of primary health care within 15, 30, 60 minutes, or longer*
  3 Indicators of shortfall (number of people on waiting lists)

Utilisation of services
  1 Attendance rates — by type of service
  2 Proportion of children immunised against specific diseases*
  3 Duration of stay in hospital
  4 Cost per unit of service

Acceptability of services
  1 Percentage of general population not willing, or reluctant, to use a given type of service
  2 Percentage of users satisfied with the ways the services are provided

* Figures considered of particular relevance for the Regional Strategy.
Source: Regional Strategy for Attaining Health For All By The Year 2000 WHO for Europe EUR/RC30/8 Rev.1
27 February 1981.

THE TEAM APPROACH

Contemporary health problems are almost all multifactorial and have their roots as much in society as in biology. In general it is possible to identify three social levels at which action is necessary if a systematic approach is adopted. Such an approach should also take full account of the relative contributions of primary, secondary and tertiary prevention (Table 3.9) (Ashton, 1982).

If the style necessary for health promotion and preventive medicine in the twentieth century is participatory it must also be multidisciplinary. Dennis and colleagues have made a strong case for the need for multidisciplinary teams to work in partnership with each other and with the general public (Dennis et al, 1979). In their analysis they argue that one person alone in the tradition of the medical officer of health is no longer sufficient for the broadly based approach which is necessary today. Several English Regional Health Authorities have now set up Regional Health Promotion Teams (Ashton, 1982).

How such teams should be structured and run to achieve their greatest impact remains as yet an open question and there are arguments emerging about their fundamental philosophy. At present the teams which are in existence seem to have

Table 3.9 A framework for constructing prevention programmes

Level of action	Level of prevention		
	Primary	Secondary	Tertiary
Government			
Institutional			
Personal			

Ashton, 1982.

been functioning very much from the top down and operating in comparative isolation from the operational levels of primary care, health district and the active groups within the community. Neither have they developed appropriate health indicators to demonstrate the usefulness of what they do although this may soon be rectified (Catford, 1983).

For these teams to be able to fulfil their promise and become the effective catalysts of a modern locally based public health movement involving the general population, a clearly defined approach incorporating the following principles is necessary (Ashton, 1982):

1. Activity on health promotion and disease prevention should be carried out at the most decentralised level that is compatible with effective action.
2. There should be a team approach.
3. Participation by the community should be an over-riding principle.
4. Health promotion teams should have security of employment and independence of action.
5. A central strategic prevention plan for the promotion of health should be produced which is informed by the priorities and objectives decided at the periphery.
6. Health Promotion Teams should produce annual reports based on the development of appropriate indicators that can be used to assess progress and revise objectives.

THE WAY AHEAD AND A CAVEAT

The agenda for the new public health movement and many of its ingredients can be defined. The importance of appropriate information in the form of relevant or field epidemiology as the basis for regular reports must now be picked up and acted on. Unfortunately the Korner Committee failed to provide the guidelines for the information we need although the WHO indicators are a useful starting point (Korner, 1983; WHO, 1981a, b). Routinely available information and newly designed information systems will need to be supplemented by ad hoc surveys of the 'dipstick' variety such as those which were used to monitor the progress of the Karelia Heart Disease Prevention Project (Puska et al, 1981). At a local level such surveys may well be carried out as part of job creation schemes in conjunction with departments of community medicine, general practices, health districts, schools and occupational and community groups. For the epidemiological approach to become fully integrated into clinical practice and into the practice of other relevant sectors will require the development of appropriate training programmes for health care and other personnel (WHO, 1981c).

The development of approaches such as these will need to take place in close association with the community itself and have as their aim the provision of all three types of health education as described by Griffiths et al (1982). Initiatives along these lines which avoid victim blaming are now beginning to be described (Smith, 1982; Allen & Purkis, 1983).

A systematic approach must underline the new public health but our methods should not be constrained by any particular narrow model. The use of razzmattaz can be important but should not be seen as a substitute for systematic education and working with people rather than on them must be a key.

One important caveat must be borne in mind; the danger of setting up a false dichotomy between treatment and prevention (Morris, 1980). At the end of the day there are still many conditions which we do not know how to prevent and these will become more important in an aging population. High technology treatments should not be automatically decried for they offer great hope and relief to many people and in the future it is probable that they will acquire even more importance.

REFERENCES

Allen R, Purkis A 1982 Health in the round voluntary action and antenatal services. National Council for Voluntary Organisations, London

Ashton J R 1977 The Peckham Pioneer Health Centre: a reappraisal. Community Health 8: 132–137

Ashton J R 1982 Towards prevention — an outline plan for the development of health promotion teams. Community Medicine 4: 231–237

Ashton J R 1983 Editorial. Risk Assessment. British Medical Journal 286.

Beveridge W 1942 Social Insurance and allied services. Cmnd. 6404 2 volumes. HMSO, London

Cartwright F F 1977 A social history of medicine. Longmans, London

Catford J C 1983 Positive health indicators — towards a new information base for health promotion. Community Medicine 5: 125–132

Chadwick E 1842 Report on the sanitary condition of the labouring population of Great Britain. Edited by M W Flinn for Edinburgh University Press 1965

Dennis J, Draper P, Griffiths J et al 1979 Rethinking Community Medicine (A report from a study group). Guys Hospital London Unit for the Study of Health Policy.

DHSS 1975 Prevention and Health: Everybodys business. HMSO, London

DHSS 1980 On the state of the public health for the year 1978. HMSO, London

DHSS 1982 On the state of the public health for the year 1980. HMSO, London

Doll R 1983 Prospectus for prevention. British Medical Journal 286

Dunnell K, Cartwright A 1972 Medicine takers, prescribers and hoarders. Routledge and Kegan Paul, London

Fry J 1979 Common diseases: Their nature incidence and care. MTP, Lancaster

Griffiths J, Dennis J, Droper P 1982 Prevention and the community physician. In: Smith A (ed) Recent Advances in Community Medicine. Churchill Livingstone, Edinburgh

HMSO 1977 First report from the Expenditure Committee. Preventive Medicine, London

Horder J 1983 General Practice in 2000. Alma Ata declaration. British Medical Journal 286: 191–194

Kark S L 1981 The practice of community oriented primary health care. Appleton-Century-Crofts, New York

Korner E 1983 Steering Group on Health Services Information. A report from Working Group D. Community Health Services DHSS

Lalonde M 1974 A new perspective in the health of Canadians. Minister of Supply and Services, Canada

McKeown T 1976 The role of medicine. Nuffield Provincial Hospitals Trust, London

Morris J N 1975 The uses of epidemiology. Churchill Livingstone, Edinburgh

Morris J N 1980 Are health services important to the people's health? British Medical Journal 280: 167–168

OPCS 1980 Mortality Statistics Table 2 DH2 No. 7. HMSO, London

OPCS 1982 Provisional mid-1981 population estimates for England and Wales and health areas. PP1 82/3 HMSO, London

OPCS (1984) PP1–84/3

Pinder D 1982 Personal communication

Puska P et al 1981 Community control of cardiovascular diseases. The North Karelia Project. WHO ISBN 92 890 1006 1, Copenhagen

Scott Williamson G and Pearse I H 1938 Biologists in search of material. Faber and Faber, London

Smith C 1982 Community based health initiatives: a handbook for voluntary groups. National Council for Voluntary Organisation, London

Townsend P 1974 Inequality and the health service. Lancet 1179–1190

Townsend P and Davidson N 1982 Inequalities in health — The Black Report. Penguin Books, Harmondsworth

Tudor-Hart J 1971 The inverse care law. Lancet 405–412

Tudor-Hart J 1981 A new kind of doctor. Journal of the Royal Society of Medicine 74: 871–883

United States Department of Health, Education and Welfare 1979 Healthy people. The Surgeon General's report on Health Promotion and Disease Prevention. Background Papers. Bethesda Maryland US DHEW

Waters W E 1977 Matters of life and death. Inaugural lecture. University of Southampton

WHO 1978 Alma-Ata 1978. Primary Health Care. WHO, Geneva

WHO 1980 Prevention and control of chronic noncommunicable disease—Report on a WHO working group. ICP/CUD 020(2)

WHO 1981a Global strategy for health for all by the year 2000. WHO, Geneva

WHO 1981b Regional strategy for health for all by the year 2000. Health For All Series No. 3 EUR/RC 3018 WHO, Copenhagen

WHO 1981c Continuing education for primary health care. Report on a seminar. ICP/MPM019 WHO, Copenhagen

WHO 1982 Epidemiological studies on social and medical conditions of the elderly. Euro Reports and Studies 62. WHO, Copenhagen

4. Poverty and health services

F. A. Boddy

INTRODUCTION

By the middle of this century most European countries had adopted programmes of social legislation which had the alleviation of poverty as one of their purposes. The collective financing and supply of health services was generally a part of these schemes; there was an expectation that medical and related services would contribute to the reduction of illness and thus diminish observed inequalities in the health of different social groups (Titmuss, 1958). In the United Kingdom, the Beveridge Report (1942) included Disease as one of the 'five Giants' to be attacked on the road to reconstruction and assumed 'the establishment of comprehensive health and rehabilitation services . . . as a necessary condition of success in social insurance'.

Forty years later, and although the overall health of the population has changed substantially, the measures we employ to assess differences between social groups still demonstrate the inequalities of earlier years. The reasons why this should be so are complex, as are the arguments concerning the strategies of social policy which might influence or reduce them; this Chapter will concern itself with only one limited aspect of the problem in considering whether health *services* have, or may have, value in influencing the health of the urban poor. This issue has a number of different questions within it. Firstly, one might ask whether medical or related services have the potential for altering those measures (such as mortality rates) that are commonly used to describe inequalities of health experience. Secondly, it is appropriate to ask whether — in Blaxter's phrase — health services can serve as 'a defence against the consequences of poverty' (Blaxter, 1983) and, thirdly, but as a separate question, one might ask whether those health services now provided provide an equality of access and participation that is commensurate with the morbidity of the poor.

Poverty and inequality

Continuing variation in the experience of health, and in other areas of social opportunity, has been well-documented recently in a series of reviews undertaken by the Social Science Research Council (see, for example, Rutter & Madge, 1976; Brown & Madge, 1982) and by a Working Group of the Department of Health and Social Security (DHSS) chaired by Sir Douglas Black (the Black Report, DHSS, 1980). Arguments about why inequalities persist take a number of forms but a central issue concerns the changing concept of poverty, the characteristics of those who now constitute the poor and the ways that the structure of society may have changed in order to maintain such observed differentials as class-specific mortality rates.

In considering this argument, it is important to recognise that 'inequality' when applied to measures of health is a very different concept to 'poverty' and that these measures provide little insight into the mechanisms that create observed differences.

In the example of the mortality rates of different social classes, it is necessary to know the extent to which the definition of class has remained constant over time (in Britain, 'social class' is really occupational status), to estimate the degree to which movement into or out of that class may be related to the risk of mortality and — if one is concerned with poverty — to dissociate risks that are attributable to socio-economic status from those that are more directly related to occupation. It is necessary, also, to take account of the *order* of the differences one measures in arriving at a view of the importance of influences such as those listed above. The Black Report's comment that 'men and women in occupational class V had a two-and-a-half times greater chance of dying before reaching retirement age than their professional counterparts in occupational class I' depends on an annual difference of six deaths per 1000 population. Recalling that these data depend on occupation at death rather than during life, it is not difficult to postulate that at least a part of this difference could have its origins in a downward social mobility that is related to health; mortality that is more correctly attributed to occupational hazards rather than socio-economic status will also contribute to this difference in rates (Fox & Adelstein, 1978).

Social mobility

We know surprisingly little about social mobility and health although a clearer picture is beginning to emerge from the longitudinal studies undertaken by the Office of Population, Censuses and Surveys based on the 1971 census (Fox & Goldblatt, 1982; Fox et al, 1982). It is the case, however, that the mix of social classes has changed substantially over the years (social classes IV and V were 38% of the economically active male population in 1951 but only 29% in 1971; the proportions for social class V were 14% and 8%). A survey undertaken by the Oxford Social Mobility Group in 1972 (Goldthorpe, 1980) asked questions about the occupation of the male respondent and about that of the head of his household when he was 14. Only 32% of those whose fathers were semi-skilled or unskilled were in such occupations and only 37% of the fathers of semi-skilled or unskilled workers had been so themselves. Britten (1981), in an analysis of national cohort data, however, has suggested that downward mobility is likely to occur 'to the next class down'.

The most comprehensive empirical analysis of the way that these processes relate to the health of individuals is still that of Illsley (1980) which relates to reproductive performance in Aberdeen in 1951–1954 and in 1969–1975. Table 4.1 provides a synopsis of data for first pregnancies for women in families where the father or husband was in a semi-skilled or unskilled occupation in Aberdeen for the periods 1951–1954 and 1969–1975. In each section of the table, there is evidence that those who leave the class differ in the possession of some favourable attribute from those who enter it or those who remain in it; in 1951–1954 a greater proportion were above average intelligence, were less likely to have a baby of low birthweight and (although the two are connected) had a 40% less chance of perinatal mortality. In 1969–1975, those who left were taller, had about half the rate of low birthweight babies and were as less likely to experience perinatal mortality as their earlier counterparts had been. Those who entered the class, on the other hand, had attributes that were very similar to those who stayed within it.

Illsley concludes, and is supported by more recent work by Stern (1982), that 'we are therefore dealing . . . with a continuous process producing a constant tendency to

Table 4.1 Social mobility and socio-medical characteristics; first pregnancies to Aberdeen women 1951–1954 and 1969–1975

Maternal charactcristics	Semi-skilled or unskilled class of upbringing (father)	Inter-class movement			Semi-skilled or unskilled class at marriage (husband)
		Left	Entered	Stayed	
1951–1954					
Percentage with intelligence above average	31	37	24	21	22
Percentage 160 cm or more in height	23	24	20	21	21
Percentage births less than 2500 g	9	8	12	11	11
Rate of perinatal deaths (per 1000)	41	33	55	55	55
1969–1975					
Percentage 160 cm or more in height	29	32	32	24	28
Percentage births less than 2500 g	7	6	10	9	10
Rate of perinatal mortality	15	12	26	19	24

[Adapted from Illsley (1980): tables 2.2 and 2.3].

widen class differences' (op. cit., p.22). What this means for our understanding of the health of the poor is a need to know much more than we presently do about the way that the correlates of social mobility sustain the differences we measure. This example has concerned mortality but it will be evident that, in the present structure of society, difficulties of this kind will apply with greater force to measures of disability and longer-term illness. It is not difficult to imagine ways that chronic illness — such as asthma — could lead to downward social mobility. There is very little formal evidence in this area; the best example is still that of the downward drift of schizophrenics described by Goldberg & Morrison in 1963. It may also be the case that other behavioural characteristics combine in ways that produce both downward social mobility and unfavourable health outcomes — as, perhaps, in the example of alcoholism.

Perceptions of poverty

The relevance of these considerations to the question of urban poverty is two-fold. In former times it was appropriate to regard the urban poor as comprising a segment of society who had been drawn to cities in the wake of industrial expansion and who were disadvantaged in terms of the absolute resources available to them in this environment. A part of the problem of poverty was the way in which such disadvantage precluded the poor from exploiting opportunities offered by the wider society; in this view, poverty was a feature of the social structure and it was reasonable to equate such concepts as social class with poverty in describing inequalities of health experience.

It would be naive to argue that the effects of social policy in the past half century have made this view wholly redundant but it is increasingly the case that such a framework is inappropriate and unhelpful. It may be more sensible to regard those who are defined as the urban poor as a heterogeneous combination of people who, for different reasons, find themselves living at the margins of society and whose poverty arises as much from this marginality as from any more fixed or inherent cause. In this perspective, urban poverty is a changing (and continuing) by-product of larger-scale changes in society in which the characteristics of the poor reflect the consequences of change and the 'casualties' it creates. This argument has particular significance to the provision of health services for the poor because it suggests that the persistence of inequalities in crude measures of health (for example, those cited in the Black Report) have their origins in the interaction of three broad sets of circumstances:

— first, ill-health which is a consequence of material or social deprivation, *per se*;
— second, ill-health which arises from social circumstances which are also associated with poverty;
— and, third, ill-health which is a characteristic of individuals who, as a consequence, are also poor.

The first category is traditional and self-explanatory; the second will contain people such as the elderly or the mothers of single-parent families whose poverty is a consequence of the other social handicaps that these characteristics imply. The third contains those who are economically handicapped because of ill-health or disability. The categories are not exclusive but an appreciation of the 'mix' of these or similar groupings is necessary for an understanding of the health needs of the poor whether in terms of social policy or for more local service provision.

The second relevance of questions about social mobility is that an understanding of the nature of social change is necessary for the way that issues are perceived for the purposes of policy and thus the strategies that are developed. As an illustration, the SSRC review of 'deprivation' noted above had its origins in speeches by Sir Keith Joseph (then Secretary of State for Health and Social Security) in the early 1970s in which he argued that 'cycles of deprivation' with the transmission of poverty from one generation to the next was a cause of persisting inequalities (Joseph, 1972). This argument had its origins in the American concept of a 'culture of poverty' (Lewis, 1966) and was a stimulus for ideas about 'positive discrimination' which were a feature of the War on Poverty in the 1960s (Valentine, 1968). By emphasising the implied incompetence of family life, it provides a philosophical underpinning for policies which seek to compensate for these deficiencies; programmes such as 'Head Start', for example, had the intent of compensating for inadequacies in the pre-school social and intellectual development of children. The fault in the condition of the poor was thus in the people themselves and not (or not only) in the structural characteristics of society. This is, therefore, an argument not simply for the provision of services but for services of a particular — corrective? — kind, perhaps directed particularly towards children, that would overcome these transmitted deprivations. The contrary view, of course, is that it is the experience of poverty that induces patterns of behaviour that in turn lead, for example, to ill-health. In this perspective, improvements in income would alter life-styles so that individuals would be in a better position to obtain for themselves those services and supports that are appropriate to their circumstances. Illustration of such a strategy is found in those recommendations of the Black Report (DHSS, 1980) which concern increases in child benefit.

It will be evident that support for the concept of a culture of poverty is weakened by evidence of social mobility on any substantial scale. If the 'culture' is to be transmitted, a sufficiently large proportion of the poor must remain so for more than one generation; the processes of demographic change in Britain sketched earlier do not support such a view. Rutter & Madge (1976) review the fairly small number of studies concerned with intergenerational effects in more specifically defined 'problem' families and conclude that they 'do not constitute a group which is qualitatively different from families in the general population. Nevertheless, families with multiple social disadvantages and/or personal problems do constitute a cause for concern . . . in terms of troubles which persist into the next generation' (p. 255). The persistence of these troubles may, of course, be a consequence of poverty and its correlates rather than some more inherent quality of these families. Wedge & Essen (1982) report, for example, that almost three-quarters of those in the National Children's Bureau cohort study who had been in public care were children with additional social adversities. In a study of health attitudes and behaviour across three generations in Aberdeen, Blaxter & Paterson (1982) did not find evidence to support a hypothesis of a culture of poverty but rather described inter-generational differences in views of health and health services which had important implications for service provision. The concept of a culture of poverty is, at best, simplistic and incomplete; in broad summary, a substantial body of research has failed to support it.

THE NATURE OF POVERTY

The condition of being poor may be measured or defined in a variety of ways; one's choice of concept will depend on the motive for doing so and will determine the strategies for alleviation that appear to be appropriate. Sen (1981) argues that there are two requirements that a concept of poverty should satisfy — that it should provide a method of *identifying* people as poor and that it should be possible to *aggregate* the characteristics of a set of poor people in arriving at an overall view of 'poverty'. In this way Rowntree (1901) defined 'primary poverty' as a family income that was 'insufficient to obtain minimum necessities for the maintenance of merely physical efficiency'. In Britain the absolute deprivation of such necessities may not be common today (although reports of hypothermia in the elderly suggest otherwise) but Adam Smith's much older comment is also pertinent:

> By necessaries I understand not only the commodities which are indispensably necessary for the support of life, but whatever the custom of the country renders it indecent for creditable people, even the lowest order, to be without. A linen shirt, for example, is strictly speaking, not a necessary of life. The Greeks and Romans lived, I suppose, very comfortably though they had no linen. But in the present times, through the greater part of Europe, a creditable day-labourer would be ashamed to appear in public without a linen shirt, the want of which would be supposed to denote that disgraceful degree of poverty which, it is presumed, nobody can well fall into without extreme bad conduct. Custom, in the same manner, has rendered leather shoes a necessary of life in England. The poorest creditable person of either sex would be ashamed to appear in public without them (Smith, 1776 — quoted by Sen, 1981).

There is a sense, therefore, in which poverty is given expression by its societal context and is a value judgement within that context. It is then a short step towards the idea of poverty being a circumstance of relative socio-economic deprivation which has two components. One may regard an individual as living in *conditions* of deprivation relative to those of the rest of society but one must also take account of the *feelings* of deprivation that individuals may have. Townsend (1979), reporting his survey of poverty in the United Kingdom, concludes that the two are strongly correlated, especially in old people, and speaks of 'the powerful relationship between objective manifestations of deprivation, and the sheer lack of money resources and wealth, which underlies perceptions of personal deprivation' (p.431).

In distinction to concepts of this kind, but in some sense incorporating ideas about both absolute and relative deprivation, are definitions based on empirical political decisions. These find expression in the day-to-day operation of social security or social welfare systems so that it is common, for example, to speak of a governmental poverty-line determined by contemporary levels of entitlement to income mainten-ance. This is the measure on which most statistical estimates of poverty are based (largely for lack of alternative data) but it is a confused and unsatisfactory approach because it is based on political considerations that are also influenced by other priorities and because it must also depend on the necessary resources being available anyway. There is no reason why either should relate to the actual circumstances of the poor.

Identification and aggregation

If Sen's two criteria for a concept of poverty—identification and the aggregation of characteristics—are to be satisfied, it becomes necessary to add other attributes to measures that derive solely from a lack of economic resources. Economic competitive-ness (or the lack of it) may be the central feature of an individual's poverty but policies for its alleviation also make it necessary to take account of those other kinds of social process that make people poor and of the handicaps associated with them. Traditional (1970s) views of poverty, deriving from a period of relatively full employment, have tended to emphasise the importance of groups who were socially dependent in some other way (such as the elderly) but changes in the industrial structure and the prospect of long-term unemployment for a substantial proportion of the population (Leontieff, 1982) argue the need for a revision of ideas about who constitutes the urban poor. Little is known about the implications of these changes and less about their consequences for health.

Poverty arising from other kinds of social marginality will not, however, become less prevalent; for the rest of this century the numbers of the elderly level off but those aged 75 or more increase. About half will have incomes less than Townsend's 'deprivation standard' and, in any case, the mean resources of people aged 80 are only about 65% of those aged between 65 and 69 (Townsend, 1979, pp. 731, 1061). The elderly poor form a group in society whose presence is largely determined by overt policies. They are there because of employment policies which discourage work beyond a certain age, because of the history of policies regarding pensions, because of political decisions about the level of state pensions and because some of them, so to speak, live longer than their means. A comparable, although very heterogeneous group, comprises those who are in some way disabled and who suffer impairment of income — or who lack economic competitiveness — as a consequence.

In these two illustrations, poverty is a concomitant of the individual's status within society. The other characteristic they share is that their well-being is likely to depend on the (sometimes specialist) services of others. In crude terms one can argue that policies for the alleviation of poverty have focused principally on the maintenance of income at some nationally determined level; given this maintenance, the assumption has generally been that the elderly or disabled poor would then avail themselves of the various services (such as social work or health) provided as part of the social policy of the larger society. While it may be the case that 'positive discrimination' is practised as part of the managerial strategy of some of these agencies (housing is the clearest example), it is difficult to find distinct policies which acknowledge separate or different service needs which arise as a consequence of being both poor *and* socially disadvantaged in some other way. If one extends one's concept of poverty to include both low income and those other incapacities which inhibit the individual's capacity to participate in the ordinary activities of society then it also becomes desirable to consider a poverty of services or social supports which will enable such participation.

There are other examples of ways that social status may have poverty as an outcome. Single parent families are an instance of the way that changes in the norms and values of society may generate social disadvantage if there is not a compensating shift in social policy to accommodate them. (The number of people claiming 'one parent benefit' increased by 150% between 1966 and 1977 and — at 540 000 — by 175% between 1977 and 1983 (Central Statistical Office, 1984).) Social change is here expressed by the trend away from the orthodoxy of the nuclear family that is the accompaniment of different attitudes to divorce and out-of wedlock births. Its effect is that the single parent must fulfil the traditional role of two parents in providing both child care and economic support. The ability to achieve both will depend on occupational skills and the state of the labour market. Evidence on the point is lacking but one might speculate that those who come to be poor for reasons such as divorce will do so with least in the way of other material resources and may also be those least able to provide an appropriate environment for the promotion of health. This could occur in several ways; difficulties in making caretaking arrangements, for example, might in some situations result in a greater likelihood of children being taken into institutional care and thus experiencing the stresses of parental separation.

This illustration contrasts with the example of the elderly and the disabled because it describes a circumstance where the fulfilment of a legitimate social role may have the inability to maintain the economy of the family as its consequence. They differ because, in common with the much larger number of other families who subsist on low incomes, it is difficult to resist the view that the 'handicaps' of single parents would be largely overcome by the provision of sufficient funds to protect the integrity of the family and normal relationships within it. In the context of present policies, this is an unlikely solution but, as is also the case with the elderly poor, it raises another difficulty regarding the provision of services. In a perfect economic world one could postulate that income should provide the means to purchase those services or supports that enable the individual or family to achieve effective social participation. In practice, it is possible to question such an approach on the pragmatic grounds that those who need services may have difficulty in obtaining them (private home help services?) but it is necessary at the same time to be clear about the *intent* of different kinds of service and to acknowledge that some, at least, will be compensatory for lack of income or the opportunity to obtain social support in alternative ways. Although this aspect of service provision is generally recognised, the fragmentation of responsibility between central government for 'income' and local authority and other agencies for 'services' means that it is impossible to achieve a coherent balance between the two.

Services or income?
It will be apparent, for the reasons sketched above, that the debate about policies for the alleviation of poverty (including its associated ill-health) centres on the balance that is to be struck between those which would improve levels of income and those which would focus on more collective forms of action such as service provision and an enhancement of the social environment. 'Health' — or, more precisely, its production — is clearly dependent on a wide range of social and economic attributes which are at present poorly defined in the sense of our understanding of their relative contribution to measured outcomes although this is a topic that has recently interested economists in the United States (for example, Grossman, 1972). Evidence that income is a significant influence on health status is sketchy; Hadley & Osei (1982) have examined the relationship between income and mortality while attempting to exlude the confounding effect of education and conclude that higher income is indeed associated with lower mortality but that 'the strength of the relationship is rather weak'. In another American study, Edwards & Grossman (1982) considered income and race differences in eight measures of the health of children between ages 6 and 11. While finding significant differences in the health of low and high-income children, they suggest that such differences were more likely to be based on parent-reported rather than physician-reported measures and that factors such as parental education may be more important than income in bringing about the differences they observed. One further conclusion of this analysis was the need to regard the health status of children as multidimensional. Findings of this nature, of course, cannot be simply translated into the different social context of the United Kingdom but, without further research, strategies such as the Black Report's recommendations for increases in child benefit stand on insecure foundations.

There has been a scepticism in Britain that investments in health services (and particularly those that might be selectively directed towards the poor) would be of value. This may be because of the powerful contrary view put forward by McKeown (1976) but the fact of the matter is that, in Britain and for recent history, the issue is largely unexplored. Evidence from elsewhere is sparse and difficult to evaluate but Hadley's (1982) study of influences on mortality in the United States concludes that there is indeed such a relationship in which one would expect that between one and two deaths would be averted for each $100 000 increase in medical spending. This is a very much stronger relationship than that between income and mortality. Significantly (and with the exception of white middle-aged males) the number of deaths averted was two to three times greater for blacks than for whites in each age-sex group so that one might argue that such expenditures would have a more useful effect amongst socially disadvantaged populations. Some general support for Hadley's conclusions in the United Kingdom comes from Forbes & McGregor (1984) who have observed a positive relationship between NHS expenditure and mortality rates in Scotland. A more specific association has been reported by Goldman & Grossman (1982) who used infant mortality rates as a health indicator for assessing the American programme of Community Health Centres. These authors found significant reductions in the mortality of both white and black infants but especially so in the latter, a reduction amounting to about 12% of the observed decline. Evidence of a different kind is found in a Report from the State of Michigan (1983) which associates unemployment (with a consequent loss of health insurance) and a substantial reduction in its own service budget with the reversal of a previously downward trend in the rate of infant mortality.

Before turning to the more specific consideration of the health of the poor, it will be useful to come to some conclusions about the nature of poverty. First, is a general confusion about the meaning of the term; quite obviously, the lack of 'necessities' in the sense of both absolute and relative deprivation are central to the concept and it is possible [as Townsend (op. cit.) attempted] to begin to satisfy Sen's (op. cit.) criterion of 'identification'. Thereafter, it becomes necessary to take account of the heterogeneity of those who are poor and to relate their poverty to the other social attributes that are an integral part of their poverty. At this stage any attempt at a 'general model' breaks down and the criterion of aggregation can only be met by defining poverty *within* the categories of these other attributes. This is a conclusion that is central to any discussion of service provision for the poor and it has two components; the first concerns the provision and organisation of services (including health services) which will be compensatory — or enable a more egalitarian social participation on the part of the poor. The second has to do with those that would seek to alter the condition of poverty in a more radical way. The tentative evidence cited above supports the view that a selective investment in health services for the poor could be of value from the utilitarian standpoint of the larger society. The question remaining is that of 'how' or 'in what form' such investments might be deployed.

THE ILL-HEALTH OF THE POOR

The body of literature which catalogues differences in measures of health between those who are poor and the rest of society is substantial. The range is comprehensive and includes most causes of mortality, morbidity measured either by cause or by time lost from work and such wider measures of well-being as are reflected in indicators of intellectual performance or social delinquency. There is little purpose in rehearsing this catalogue or in selecting illustrative examples from it; for the United Kingdom, the topic is reviewed in Rutter & Madge (1976) and in the Black Report (DHSS, 1980). It is, however, pertinent to ask how such differences might come about and thus what strategies might reduce them.

Before specifically addressing this issue, it will be helpful to consider the nature of the measures that are employed. Broadly, these are of three kinds; those that are measures deriving from routine sources, such as mortality rates, those that are measures of shorter-term effects (such as illness or sickness-absence from work) and, thirdly, various measures of social well-being and health-related behaviour.

Mortality and social class
The use of mortality data as an index of the health of the poor raises a number of

difficulties in interpretation mainly because they are based on occupational status at death and so say nothing about the individual's life style or earlier history. Nor do they distinguish between hazards that are a consequence of (presumed) low social status and those related to the occupation itself. In Britain, the contribution of the latter is considerable; Fox & Adelstein (1978) have proposed a method of distinguishing between mortality attributable to broad occupational groups and that which is related to 'way of life' as this is reflected by membership of a particular social class. In this analysis, between 20 and 30% of the variation in mortality from a range of diagnostic groups was attributable to occupation.

The tradition of equating social class and poverty may, in any case, contain an ecological fallacy. In a given time period, one's chance of becoming a member of a particular social class is dependent not only on individual characteristics but on the nature and structure of the local labour market. It will be evident that the opportunities for becoming a member of social class V in the labour market of Surrey are not the same as those of the labour market of Leeds or Liverpool, but these opportunities need bear no relationship to life-style even if it is the assumption of most epidemiologists that they do. The utility of social class, outwith its proper occupational setting, is further weakened when one recalls that the Registrar General's class III encompasses more than 60% of the population and that social class V contributes less than 10% of all deaths. By the criteria adduced earlier, ' the poor' in Britain may now comprise between 15% and 20% of the population (Central Statistical Office op. cit.). From the standpoint of understanding the relationship between poverty and health, there is a serious lack in the British literature of age-specific measures of mortality as it relates to income and this problem will become more important with the need to know more about the inter-relationship between unemployment and health. There is, at the least, a requirement to reappraise the usefulness of the Registrar General's social classes as a measure of social status and, more especially, the values that are imputed to them.

Some specific causes of mortality may reflect observable differences in specific behavioural attributes and thus provide a more plausible chain of causative events; such outcomes may also change over relatively short time intervals and suggest, at least, a process of 'lag' in the adoption of healthier life-styles or the avoidance of hazards to health. Two examples, which may have a common cause, are provided by coronary artery disease and carcinoma of the lung and bronchus. In his analysis of class-related mortality for the years 1949–1953, the Registrar-General for England and Wales (1958) reported standardised mortality ratios (SMR) for coronary artery disease in males aged 20–64 of 144 for the upper social class and of 86 for unskilled workers; the comparable ratios for carcinoma of lung and bronchus were 81 and 118. By 1971–1972 the coronary artery disease gradient had reversed with ratios of 88 and 111, with those for lung cancer having moved further apart at 53 and 143 (OPCS, 1978). Although other changes in the middle-class life-style may have also contributed to the changed pattern for heart disease, changes in habits of cigarette smoking over this period are also striking; in the late 1950s three out of four men and three out of eight women smoked (Cartwright et al, 1959) whereas by 1980 the proportion of professional and managerial workers who were cigarette smokers was nearer one in four for both sexes. By contrast, roughly one in two semi-skilled or unskilled males and two in five women were smokers (OPCS, 1981).

Measures of morbidity

Measures of morbidity derive from two principal sources which also introduce important difficulties in understanding them; statistics deriving from the use of health services are an unreliable measure because the intervening variables of availability of services and attitudes to their use mean that their relationship to actual measures of incidence or prevalence is unknown. The second usual source (self-reported morbidity from such data as the General Household Survey) suffers from similar problems since one can expect both discrepancies between professional and lay ideas about diagnosis or even as to what constitutes illness (Donabedian, 1973, p. 100). In Koos' classic study of 'The Health of Regionsville', for example, low back pain in middle-aged women of low social status was not regarded as illness — it was simply a feature of age and circumstance to be expected and tolerated (Koos, 1954). In a similar way, Blaxter & Paterson (op. cit.), in their study of disadvantaged women in Aberdeen, describe the 'symbolic importance' of the ability to work and of 'the tendency to define health only in functional terms' (p.29).

In general, the morbidity of the poor tends to mirror the pattern of mortality and to suggest that most forms of physical ill-health are indeed commoner (DHSS, 1980). In making this statement, however, it is important to stress that the understanding of morbidity — indeed, of the health status of communities — is seriously inadequate. The principal difficulty in describing the health of the urban poor is simply that data about illness which would permit an epidemiological appraisal of the relevance of social characteristics *within* disadvantaged populations is largely lacking. Comparisons (say) between social classes may suggest that there is a problem to be investigated but they do little to dissect those features of life-style which have causal significance.

This is not entirely true; there are examples in the literature (usually psychiatric) which provide an illustration of the need for a more careful analysis of the kind proposed above. Some understanding of the relationship between social disadvantage and psychiatric disorder in children can be drawn from many studies relating such disorders to the quality of family life and the prevalence of family difficulties in different social classes (reviewed in Rutter & Madge, op. cit.). In a more precise way, Brown and his colleagues have investigated clinical depression in working class women and have proposed an aetiological model which includes general features of the social environment, specific 'vulnerability factors' which are more closely linked to the immediate psychosocial circumstances of the individual and 'provoking agents' — events which are *interpreted* by the individual as a long-term threat to life-style (Brown & Harris, 1978). It is difficult to summarise this study in a brief way; its significance for this discussion is that it provides an example of a methodological approach which allows one at least to begin to contemplate strategies directed at preventive action however complex these may be.

Models of causation which might propose comparable mechanisms for physical disease are hard to find in the contemporary literature although they do exist for older problems such as tuberculosis which are now controlled. An aspect of this difficulty is that scientific habit or tradition tends to insist that one works backwards from specific disease outcomes so that it becomes difficult to achieve a holistic understanding of the effects of poverty except in general comparative terms. Such medical models are useful, of course, but they are also limiting in the sense that what one acknowledges as a disease entity may, in fact, be only the rather narrowly defined outcome of a larger, unrecognised, process. There are few studies which have been designed in ways which would test hypotheses of this kind. Boddy (1976, 1982) has argued from the clinical illustration of a small sample of excessively obese working-class women in middle-age to the effect that fairly small differences in the *prevalence* of circumstances of this kind would be sufficient to explain differences in observed outcomes (in this instance, mortality from cardio-respiratory disease) at later ages. It is, of course, necessary to postulate a variety of such syndromes with different causative pathways but, given the order of magnitude of many observed differences, the prevalence rate of each need not be grossly apart from that of the general population.

Health and well-being

Explanations of the kind sketched above may be of help in understanding measures of health which fit a largely medical taxonomy but health is 'not simply the absence of disease'. A broader concept of health requires one to take account of a further range of measures, when most research tends to concern children and such parameters as educational performance. In a more general way, deprivation or disadvantage in one aspect of life is often associated with 'multiple deprivations' in other areas (Brown & Madge, op. cit., p. 143 et seq.) so that Martin's aphorism that 'not everyone with a health problem has a social problem but most people with social problems also have health problems' is apposite. As Brown & Madge argue (p. 154) the nature of the ill-health that this kind of poverty engenders is complex and difficult to describe; it is perhaps women who bear the greatest brunt of this process, who fight a long battle in maintaining family standards in poor environments and with low incomes, who take the responsibilities for child care, and who may neglect their own health as a consequence of the pressures of day-to-day existence. Blaxter & Paterson's three generation study, for example, recorded 32 chronic conditions in a sample of 47 grandmothers* who averaged a history of two conditions each.

A comparable illustration of this wider expression of health and ill-health as it applies to children is found in the observations of the National Children's Bureau cohort study (Wedge & Prosser, 1973; Wedge & Essen, 1982); although socially disadvantaged 16-year-olds did not show major differences in formal measures of morbidity, but those who were multiply deprived were eight times more likely to have been in public care, 8% were leaving school without being able to do everyday arithmetic and 6% were unable to read adequately.

A causal model?

A 'general model' relating poverty to adverse health status would need to accommodate both the heterogeneity of poverty itself and the conclusion that observed inequalities in health arise more from an increased prevalence of most causes of morbidity rather than an excess of more precisely defined conditions. Clearly such a proposition would not be sensible but it is possible to argue that there may be three broad levels of adverse influence each of which contributes to differences in the experience of health. More speculatively, one might argue further that each succeed-

---

*Who had their first babies in 1950–1953.

ing level contributes — or adds to — the risk inherent in the one above. These levels are:

— risks implicit in the physical or economic environment;
— risks associated with individual characteristics or with specific social stresses;
— risks inherent in patterns of behaviour or life-style induced by — or a consequence of — the experience of poverty.

There is an evident sense in which a broad hypothesis of this kind depends on one's view of the origins of poverty and the argument is to some degree circular. If one is concerned with health service provision, however, these distinctions have the value of suggesting where one might cut into the circle in devising strategies of intervention.

Risks implicit in the environment is a self-explanatory category which, at its simplest, includes the hazards of poor housing, of occupation and, for example, a greater risk of street accidents to children because of the poverty of the wider physical environment. This is the traditional territory of public health but it is possible to give it wider definition and to include hazards to health that may arise from peer group pressures (such as glue-sniffing) or from other forms of drug abuse which may be associated with unemployment amongst adolescents or young adults.

The lack of data which would permit a better appreciation of the way that individual characteristics, including poverty, combine to affect health has already been discussed but this second influence almost certainly provides a basis for understanding differences in observed levels of mental health in which one might include problems associated with alcohol, self-poisoning (or 'para-suicide') and at least some aspects of child abuse and neglect. One area of the problem of urban poverty that has received insufficient attention (but an example is the work of Brown cited above) is that of the significance of social stress for the individual and thus the functioning of that individual within the environment of poverty. Such an interaction could affect health in a number of ways but one might simply be an accentuation of the risks that are implicit in the general environment.

Although it is often claimed, specific hazards to health in the *general* life-style of the poor — other than smoking and, perhaps, alcohol consumption — are not easy to identify. Even so, there is a broad consensus of evidence which suggests that there are sufficient differences in life-style to merit the argument that poverty and the patterns of daily living it induces may pre-dispose to ill-health. In evaluating unfavourable outcomes (of the measurable kind) there are at least two ways in which such general influences could have an effect. The first is by enhancing or potentiating risks to health implicit in individual characteristics, in the simplest example, those who have a 'personal' risk of alcoholism will be at greater hazard in a social environment in which drinking alcohol has an important role and where drunkeness is tolerated. Secondly, a poor appreciation of ways of maintaining health, the neglect of illness or the inability to comply with treatment — all of which may be features of the state of poverty — may conceivably lead to events which become manifest in some statistical formulation or other.

Unemployment and health
Although not directly comparable, present rates of unemployment make the question of whether unemployment has consequences for health one that is relevant to a more

general discussion of poverty. In the time-scale of socio-economic research, present levels of unemployment are too recent for a coherent body of research to have emerged and it may be, of course, that significant health effects also take time to emerge. Conclusions based on rates of unemployment in the 1960s and 1970s (when they were low) need not necessarily apply in contemporary circumstances. One major focus of controversy has been argument over a relationship between unemployment and mortality first proposed by Brenner (1971, 1979). The conclusion that there was such a relationship has been challenged on econometric grounds by Gravelle, Hutchison & Stern (1981) but it is also the case that other studies using comparable methods in different populations have failed to find a consistent association between the two (Spruit, 1982). While supporting this general conclusion, Forbes & McGregor's (1984) study of Scottish rates suggests that there may be some relationship between unemployment and mortality in older age-groups possibly because of a more specific link with ischaemic heart disease.

The difficulty with studies of this kind is that they are concerned with large-scale aggregate measures and provide little insight into the consequences for the individual. In a review of the broad field of research in this area, Warr (1984) concludes 'it is clear that unemployment impairs mental health . . . and that this impairment extends into psychophysical conditions' but 'not everyone is affected negatively . . . '. What is not known is how unemployment may relate to other characteristics and how these other attributes may influence health or ill-health in the context of unemployment.

Areas of deprivation

One other approach to the question of poverty and health which has become fashionable in recent years is that which bases itself on the definition of geographic 'areas of social deprivation' which are themselves derived from the correlation of sets of 'social indicators'. Measures of deprivation commonly have their origin in census data to which other available measures (such as the infant mortality rate) may be added. One classic paper in this field, for example, is that of Holterman (1975) which used centiles of the distribution of variables in the 1971 census to define (on an empirical basis) enumeration districts which were environmentally deprived. From here it is but a short step to such ambiguities as social pathology and the identification of 'Areas for Priority Treatment'.

The deficiencies of these methodologies (both conceptual and technical) are reviewed by Carstairs (1982); the major difficulty, of course, is that although individual measures (such as car ownership or infant mortality) may have meaning in themselves, their statistical manipulation, especially if this involves some implication of ranking, does not necessarily give them any additional meaning. Although it may be the case that activities of this sort may identify some of those areas in which the poor live, the nature of the exercise is such that by no means all of those who live in these areas will be poor or, more importantly, that even a majority of the poor can be corralled in this way. Area-based policies of 'positive discrimination' may have simplistic administrative attraction but the theoretical concept on which they are based (if it can be discerned) is naively close to ideas about a culture of poverty. A more fundamental criticism is that the approach assumes the essential 'rightness' of existing services; by implication, the larger structure of services, their content and the appropriateness of both are largely unchallenged in a strategy which argues for 'more' rather than a reappraisal of what is.

STRATEGIES FOR CHANGE

The alleviation of poverty or an improvement in the health experiences of the poor clearly requires a range of different policies. Some, such as increasing levels of income, are common to poverty in all its forms and others, those that may substitute for income or compensate for its lack, constitute a provision of services that must be directed towards the more precise needs of particular groups. There is then an aspect of policy in which services can have the specific objective of altering or changing the consequences of poverty. The concluding section of this review largely confines itself to this latter topic but, in doing so, does not imply that these activities are any substitute for action in the first two areas. One danger in the attempt to define a more useful approach to service provision is that this kind of strategy can distract attention from other policies which may be of much greater significance. It is easy to be palliative.

Distributing health services

An attempt to influence the health of the poor by the more effective use of health services will depend on three main considerations. These are the structure and organisational assumptions of the services themselves, the ability to deploy or redeploy resources in some useful way and the capacity for implementing strategies that are effective.

Structure

In a recent review of the philosophical assumptions of health service provision, de Jong & Rutten (1983) distinguish four basic principles for the distribution of health care resources; at one extreme they describe a *libertarian* situation in which health care provision is the result of free market negotiation. A *utilitarian* distribution system would concern itself with the maximising of societal benefits over costs; it subsumes many of the ideas favoured by health economists and bases much of its argument on the need to make efficient use of scarce resources. Acceptance of the findings of Hadley (op. cit.) would, in a system of this kind, be a basis for investing selectively in health services for the poor. The provision of health services on the basis of *equal access* is common in most European countries and is that on which the National Health Services (NHS) has been based. This approach has a number of features that are easily recognised by those who are familiar with British health services:

> 'To a large extent, it avoids having to judge the effectiveness of services or the needs of individuals. It does not really matter what is provided, or how much, as long as everyone has equal access. This rule has the obvious advantage of being practical, certainly within policy setting. Policy makers can limit their attention to financial and geographical barriers' (op. cit.).

The fourth principle—described by de Jong & Rutten as *egalitarian* is one which would attempt to equalise the health status of the population to the extent that this is possible. It would thus give priority in the allocation of resources to those most in need even at the expense of the efficiency of resource deployment; the level of service supply should be such as to reflect the prevalence of needs for different services in sub-groups of the population and should also take account of such matters as organisation and location in ways that maximise the access to services and thus their effective use.

Equal access

From the standpoint of services for the poor, the principle of equal access as it is practised in the NHS presents problems of two kinds. The first is that its administrative structure is such as to not only fail to take account of the additional needs of the poor but to create an organisational environment that makes it likely that at least parts of the service will discriminate against the poor. The second is that already noted; it is that policy initiatives concerned with poverty which also accept this principle are thus limited in the scope and extent to which they can be integrated into the overall pattern of services.

Evidence on the first point comes from a number of sources. Le Grand (1978) has examined health care expenditure in relation to social class differences in illness reported to the General Household Survey and concludes that 'there appears to have existed some, possibly substantial, inequality of health expenditure . . . between socio-economic groups'. Cartwright & O'Brien (1976) reach similar conclusions regarding the use and availability of general practitioner services while Brotherston (1976) draws attention to the problem of inequalities in capital provision—for example in the provision of general practitioners' premises. The basic nature of this latter problem is highlighted in the pattern of primary care in inner London described by the London Health Planning Consortium (1981, 'the Acheson Report'). It is probably true, as Tudor Hart (1971) and others have argued, that—on a *per capita* basis—the work-load of an inner-city general practitioner is greater, the problems he is asked to solve are more complex or more time-consuming and (in relation to these difficulties) his supporting resources are less adequate than his counterpart in more prosperous areas. Within the present framework of the NHS, the options that are available for resolving such inequalities are limited. A decision to pursue policies that might favour the poor would most probably be at the expense of some other more general need and, most likely, be made against professional pressures for some other form of service innovation. Decisions of this kind are difficult, in any case, since a high proportion of service revenues is lost to more specific applications in the 'generalist' provisions of the hospital service; administratively, the 'independence' of the general practitioner and the national contracts that regulate his remuneration militates against policies that would appear to favour one doctor at the expense of another. If these are pessimistic conclusions, it is as well to reflect also on the almost complete lack of data which would allow realistic assessments to be made of the equation between the need for health services, the nature and quantity of those services and the resources required to supply them. The major indictment of the NHS as an 'equal access' system has been its success in avoiding judgements about 'the effectiveness of services or the needs of individuals' (de Jong & Rutten, op. cit.). As a consequence, its approach to the problem of inequalities in health has been the largely superficial one of devising specific programmes for particular problems—for example, health education and cigarette smoking, domiciliary programmes of family planning and the pursuit of high immunisation rates. In all of these there is little attempt to adapt the existing structure of services or to alter the conditions of their provision in a significant way. There may be *other* grounds for programmes of this kind, but the usefulness of their effect in modifying the health of the poor should be regarded with scepticism.

Egalitarian approaches

One major philosophical distinction between the egalitarian and equal access principles of health care distribution derives from acceptance of the view that the individual has a right to both health and health care and not simply a right of access to services. In passing, one may note that this distinction includes an interesting comment on the view that health is an 'individual responsibility'; its relevance to this discussion is that the planning of services on this basis should proceed from a holistic appreciation of the different kinds (mixes) of health needs that are found in different populations. Planning is thus a matter of describing the overall pattern of services that is appropriate and of delivering them in ways which are consonant with the characteristics, such as the life-styles and behavioural attributes, of the people for whom they are provided.

This will probably mean that a different emphasis may be given to activities or components within the whole service but it does not necessarily follow that their effectiveness in the narrow sense of the prior evaluation of service elements need be a major constraint. A 'cure' for depression is not a necessary prerequisite for a service that takes the social context of the condition into proper account. In a larger example, one could argue that if antenatal care, defined in medical terms, is regarded as an appropriate form of care for all pregnancies, then an egalitarian strategy should deploy those resources that attempt to ensure the delivery of this care in different ways to different populations. In doing so it would consider such matters as access and the 'costs' of care to the patient and would redirect services to overcome possible handicaps of this kind. But it would go further by attempting to identify and meet needs which were not limited to pregnancy although of consequence to it. It might then appear that other considerations, the health of the family, social isolation, housing, or problems with income, become as significant a part of the health care of pregnancy as its traditional medical context.

One example of recent NHS policy that has had a potential relevance for this approach to service provision has been the Health Centre programme of the 1970s. The impetus for these developments was not, of course, related to the issue of poverty but rather to the separate problem of the more general need to capitalise the provision of primary care services. In Britain, the consequences of these developments have been largely unevaluated, certainly in regard to poverty, but they do not appear to have made a major impact on traditional forms of service delivery (Beales, 1978). One possible reason, which requires formal research, is that Health Centres do not have formal identity within the administrative structure of the NHS and so become simply a structure in which services are situated rather than the focus for the local implementation of service strategies and goals (Robinson & Boddy, 1982). Comparable centres in the United States, established as a more specific response to the health problems of the poor, have, on the other hand, developed more flexible and adaptive programmes of care, have generated a literature concerned with their organisational characteristics and do seem to be effective (Reynolds, 1976; Beckhard, 1972; Zwick, 1972).

It is fairly easy to identify the difficulties that the adoption of a more egalitarian philosophy would create in its practical application. The quality of health information systems, the interrelationship between hospital services and those of the community, the definition of populations which merit additional resources and the ordering and valuing of different kinds of needs all provide the beginnings of a catalogue. If, on the other hand, one wishes to take issues such as inequalities in health seriously, then it is in seeking solutions to these problems that progress can be made. In the meantime, there is much to be said for the standpoint that the egalitarian principle implies and for attempting to manage present services in ways that encourage their operating rules to more closely match the perceptions and attitudes of their patients.

CONCLUSION

This review has had two purposes. The first has been to try to explain some of the confusion that surrounds the debate about the relationship between poverty and health. The conclusion of this part of the discussion is that the relationship is diffuse and indefinite and is one that cannot reasonably be addressed by specific programmes of action that might, for instance, lie within the old tradition of 'public health'. Solutions require a range of different social policies of which a more effective response by the NHS may be one. *If* this is so, then the nature of the problem is such that adaptations to existing services are unlikely to be successful because the present structure of the NHS cannot be responsive to differences in health needs of different population groups. The question of whether health services can adapt to different social contexts is thus central to their relevance to such matters as inequalities in health. It is salutary to recall one of the founding fathers of this debate. Simon (1890) put the matter precisely: 'whether there are ways . . . in which the community can intervene . . . to improvements in the circumstances of life is not a simple question of benevolence. On the contrary, it is a question in which mere good intention would be peculiarly apt to go astray . . .' (p. 447).

REFERENCES

Beales J G 1978 Sick health centres—and How to Make Them Better. Pitman Medical, Tunbridge Wells
Beckhard R 1972 Organisational issues in team delivery of comprehensive health care. Milbank Memorial Fund Quarterly 50: 287–316
Beveridge W H 1942 Social insurance and allied services: Report by Sir William Beveridge. Cmd 6404 HMSO, London
Blaxter M 1983 Health Services as a defence against the consequences of poverty in industrialised societies. Social Science and Medicine 17: 1139–1148
Blaxter M, Paterson E 1982 Mothers and daughters: a three generation study of health attitudes and behaviour. Heinemann Educational Books, London
Boddy F A 1976 Controlling risk factors for coronary artery disease. In: Proceedings of conference on the integration of patient care. Royal College of Physicians, Edinburgh
Boddy F A 1982 Health, health care and the urban poor. WHO Consultation on Poverty, Aberdeen
Brenner M H 1971 Economic changes and heart disease mortality. American Journal of Public Health 61: 606–611
Brenner M H 1979 Mortality and the national economy: a review of the experience of England and Wales, 1936–1976. Lancet ii: 568–573
Britten N 1981 Models of intergenerational class mobility. British Journal of Sociology 32: 224–238

Brotherston J H F 1976 Inequality; is it inevitable? (The Galton Lecture 1975). In: Carter C O and Peel J (eds) Equalities and inequalities in health. Academic Press, London

Brown M, Madge N 1982 Despite the welfare state. Heinemann Educational Books, London

Brown G W, Harris T 1978 Social origins of depression: a study of psychiatric disorder in women. Tavistock Publications, London

Carstairs V 1982 Health and social deprivation. In: Smith A (ed) Recent advances in community medicine 2. Churchill Livingstone, Edinburgh. ch 5

Cartwright A, Martin F M, Thomson J G 1959 Distribution and development of smoking habits. Lancet ii: 725–727

Cartwright A, O'Brien M 1976 Social class variations in health care and in the nature of general practitioner consultations. In: Stacey M (ed) The sociology of the National Health Service. Sociological Review Monograph No 22 University of Keele, Keele

Central statistical office 1984 Social Trends 14. HMSO, London

de Jong G A, Rutten F F H 1983 Justice and health for all. Social Science and Medicine 17: 1085–1095

Department of Health and Social Security 1980 Inequalities in health: the report of a working group. Also published as Townsend P, Davidson N (eds) Inequalities in health: the Black Report. Penguin Books, Harmondsworth

Donabedian A 1973 Aspects of medical care administration. Harvard University Press for the Commonwealth Fund, Cambridge, Massachusetts

Edwards L N, Grossmann M 1982 Income and race differences in children's health in the mid-1960's. Medical Care 20: 915–930

Forbes J F, McGregor A 1984 Unemployment and mortality in post-war Scotland. Journal of Health Economics (in press)

Fox A J, Adelstein A M 1978 Occupational mortality: work or way of life? Journal of Epidemiology and Community Health 32: 73–78

Fox A J, Goldblatt P O 1982 Longitudinal study 1971–75: sociodemographic mortality differentials. Office of Population, Censuses and Surveys, Series LS No 1. HMSO, London

Fox A J, Goldblatt P O, Adelstein A M 1982 Selection and mortality differentials. Journal of Epidemiology and Community Health 36: 69–79

Goldberg E M, Morrison S L 1963 Schizophrenia and social class. British Journal of Psychiatry 109: 785–802

Goldman F, Grossman M 1982 The impact of public health policy: the case of community health centres. National Bureau of Economic Research Working Paper No 1020 Cambridge, Massachusetts

Goldthorpe J H (in collaboration with Llewellyn C, Payne C) 1980 Social mobility and class structure in modern Britain. Clarendon Press, Oxford

Gravelle H, Hutchison G, Stern J 1981 Mortality and unemployment: a critique of Brenner's time series analysis. Lancet ii: 675–679

Grossman M 1972 The demand for health: a theoretical and empirical investigation. Columbia University Press, New York

Hadley J 1982 More medical care, better health? Urban Institute, Washington D C

Hadley J, Osei A 1982 Does income affect mortality? an analysis of the effects of different types of income on age/sex/race specific mortality rates in the United States. Medical Care 20: 901–914

Holterman S 1975 Areas of urban deprivation in Great Britain: analysis of 1971 census data. Social Trends No 6: 33–38, HMSO London

Illsley R 1980 Professional or public health: sociology in health and medicine. Nuffield Provincial Hospitals Trust, London

Joseph K 1972 Speech to the pre-school playgroups association 29th June 1972

Koos E 1954 The health of Regionsville: what the people felt and did about it. Columbia University Press, New York

le Grand J 1978 The distribution of public expenditure: the case of health care. Economica 45: 125–142

Leontieff W W 1982 The distribution of work and income. Scientific American 247: 152–164

Lewis O 1966 La Vida: a Puerto Rican family in the culture of poverty — San Juan and New York. Random House, New York

London Health Planning Consortium 1981 Report of the primary care study group (Chairman: Acheson E D). LHPC, London

McKeown T 1976 The role of medicine: dream, mirage or nemesis? Nuffield Provincial Hospitals Trust, London

Martin F M 1978 Personal communication

Michigan Department of Public Health 1983 Meeting the problem of infant mortality: a plan of action for Michigan. Michigan Department of Public Health, Lancing

Office of Population Censuses and Surveys 1978 Occupational mortality: decennial supplement 1970–72, England and Wales. HMSO, London

Reynolds R A 1976 Improving access to health care among the poor — the neighbourhood health centre experience. Milbank Memorial Fund Quarterly (Health and Society) 54: 47–82

Robinson E T, Boddy F A 1982 Ten years in a health centre: concept and reality. British Medical Journal 284: 1168–69, 1237–38

Rowntree S 1901 Poverty: a study of town life. Macmillan, London

Rutter M, Madge N 1976 Cycles of disadvantage. Heinemann, London

Sen A 1981 Poverty and families: an essay on entitlement and deprivation. Clarendon Press, Oxford

Simon J 1890 English sanitary institutions. Cassell and Company, London

Spruit I P 1982 Unemployment and health in macro-social analysis. Social Science and Medicine 16: 1903–1917

Stern J 1982 Social mobility and the interpretation of social class differentials. Discussion Paper No. 123, Centre for Labour Economics, London School of Economics, London

Titmuss R M 1958 Essays on the welfare state. Unwin, London

Townsend P 1979 Poverty in the United Kingdom: a survey of household resources and the standard of living. Penguin, Harmondsworth

Tudor Hart J 1971 The inverse care law. Lancet i: 405–412

Valentine C A 1968 Culture and poverty: critique and counter-proposals. Chicago University Press, Chicago and London

Warr P 1984 Economic recession and mental health: a review of research. Tijdschrift voor Sociale Gezondheidszong (in press)

Wedge P, Essen J 1982 Children in adversity. Pan Books, London

Wedge P, Prosser N 1973 Born to fail? Pan Books, London

Zwick D I 1972 Some accomplishments and findings of neighbourhood health centres. Milbank Memorial Fund Quarterly 50: 387–420

5. Health promotion in a district

Sheila Adam

INTRODUCTION

Community medicine takes health promotion as one of its central responsibilities. Together with the assessment of health needs, and the planning, implementation and evaluation of health services, the prevention of unnecessary ill-health and the development of a strategy for positive health and well-being form the core of community medicine practice.

The second half of the nineteenth century saw the modern foundation of the medical role in improving social conditions, with consequent dramatic decreases in the mortality from infectious diseases. Similarly, the commitment of Medical Officers of Health to improved maternal and child health in the first part of the twentieth century contributed to the decline in maternal and infant mortality.

Ironically, these successes, whilst establishing one of the traditions of our specialty, may have hampered community physicians in responding to the more taxing demands of the contemporary causes of mortality and morbidity. Their focus of activity before 1974 selectively emphasised the role of local government in promoting or undermining health, and the pragmatic tactic of developing separate health services to meet special and narrowly-defined needs appears to have militated against a comprehensive perception of health care and its full potential for health promotion.

The unification of the health service in 1974 had profound implications for those committed to the promotion of health. On the negative side, it separated community physicians from their strong bases within local government, and from their empires, and made them corporate managers of the health service. This resulted in considerable professional uncertainty, and has been criticised as leading to a reduction in effective public health advocacy (for example, Unit for the Study of Health Policy, 1979). On the other hand, the move to a comprehensive pattern of health care for a defined population offered community physicians the opportunity to co-ordinate previously disparate activities into a more effective health promotion programme. Their role in the management teams of the re-organised health service provided a new power-base within the hospitals; as medical advisers to health and local authorities they maintained their status with the local authority. At the same time, the value of health promotion has been argued by a range of interest groups — for example, the government and Department of Health and Social Security, radical critics of both medicine and the medical profession, and the health consumerism movement. Clearly, each of these groups has a different motivation in advocating more effective health promotion. Yet, with a few notable exceptions, community physicians have failed to capitalise on these sources of support. In the majority of health authorities health promotion remains fragmented, with the inefficient use of existing services, and an allocation of additional resources has not been achieved.

THE CURRENT ADVOCACY OF HEALTH PROMOTION

Prevention has traditionally been divided into three categories — primary, secondary and tertiary. However, this approach tends, as Smith (1983) has pointed out, to present prevention and cure as alternatives or even rivals, a position which is unfortunately still adopted by some senior and influential doctors (for example, Black, 1981; Doll, 1983). Smith argues that this is a misleading dichotomy, and advocates instead the concept of disease control, which has the following levels:

general health promotion
specific prevention
early detection
institution of treatment
rehabilitation and continuing care
terminal care

Clearly, all except the first require a balance of prevention and treatment. The term 'health promotion' used to be employed rather rigidly to describe the category of primary prevention — interceding between a cause of ill-health and the individual, either by eliminating the aetiological agent (for example, air or water pollution) or by specific protection of the individual (for example, immunisation). Such a narrow definition may be counter-productive. For example, a district smoking policy, whilst concentrating on discouraging people from starting to smoke and encouraging others to give up before any lasting harm occurred, would be unlikely to exclude help to smokers whose health was already compromised. In this chapter, health promotion is defined more widely to include those actions taken on behalf of a community to improve their health and well-being, excluding the diagnostic, investigative and therapeutic services provided for those who complain of symptoms.

Community physicians, and before 1974 Medical Officers of Health, have tended to see themselves as lonely advocates of prevention and health promotion. This sense of isolation within the medical profession was exacerbated by the mid-twentieth century wave of therapeutic advances which distracted attention away from health promotion towards the expanding horizons of curative medicine. More recently the balance has shifted, as the limits of therapeutic progress have been appreciated. Many diseases remain resistant to medical or surgical treatment, and the accumulating evidence shows that their aetiology often involves patterns of behaviour which are potentially alterable. Therapeutic successes have been achieved only at the costs of increasing dependency on health professionals, iatrogenic disease and a continued expansion of spending on health. Critiques of modern health care, with its emphasis on acute, curative medicine, have emerged in several Western countries (see, for example, Illich in the USA (Illich, 1974; Illich, 1976), Lalonde in Canada (Lalonde, 1975) and Mahler on behalf of the WHO (Mahler, 1975)). In the UK the most influential writer has undoubtedly been McKeown, in particular, in the Rock Carling Memorial Lecture of 1976 (McKeown, 1979).

In England and Wales, as in other Western countries, the role of health promotion has been endorsed by central government. A range of reports have been published on priorities in health and personal social services (DHSS, 1976a; DHSS, 1977a; DHSS, 1981), prevention and health (DHSS, 1976b; DHSS, 1977b) and follow-up reports about specific areas of prevention (DHSS, 1977c, d, 1978). The Social Services and Employment Sub-Committee of the Expenditure Committee of the House of Commons began a special enquiry into preventive medicine in November 1975, reporting in April 1977 (Expenditure Committee, 1977) and many of their 58 recommendations related specifically to health promotion. The government responded in a White Paper (DHSS/DES/SO/WO, 1977) which aimed to set the 'Sub-Committee's recommendations in the broader context of the Government's total policies and plans on prevention', and did not reject any of the Sub-Committee's proposals about health education. Similarly, the Royal Commission on the National Health Service (Royal Commission on the National Health Service, 1979) included a chapter on 'Good Health' which emphasised the value of health promotion, and recommended its extension and development in areas of proven effectiveness. Many independently-produced reports on specific aspects of health or causes of ill-health have stressed the need for health promotion. These are too numerous to list, but see, for example, the Report of the Committee on Child Health Services (DHSS/DES/WO, 1976), 'Health or Smoking' (Royal College of Physicians, 1977), the third in the Royal College of Physicians' reports on smoking, 'Health Education and Self Help' (Farrell & Robinson, 1980), 'Inequalities in Health' (DHSS, 1980), and five reports published recently by the Royal College of General Practitioners (RCGP, 1981a, b, c, d, 1983).

THE MOTIVES BEHIND THE RENEWED INTEREST IN HEALTH PROMOTION

The recent enthusiasm for health promotion has been demonstrated by widely differing groups — representing both the providers and the consumers of health care. However, although the enthusiasm is shared, each group may argue from a different set of motives and objectives, which often have little in common and may even be in conflict.

Motive 1: economic

The expenditure on health care in Western countries continues to increase (Abel-Smith, 1976). Thus one attractive argument for effective prevention and health promotion is based on the economic savings which might be expected to accrue from the reduced incidence of disease.

The DHSS, however, is clearly ambivalent about the economic consequences of allocating greater resources to health promotion. It has been emphasised in some government documents that prevention is not necessarily cheaper (see, for example, DHSS, 1976b; Expenditure Committee, 1977). On the other hand, a further DHSS document also published in 1976, stated that 'preventive medicine and health education are particularly important when resources are tightly limited, as they can often lead to savings in resources in other areas' (DHSS, 1976a).

This confusion about the economic consequences of programmes of prevention and health education extends beyond the DHSS. The difficulties in assessing the costs and benefits of opportunities in prevention have been summarised (Warner, 1979) as due to:

(i) the lack of precise or definitive empirical evidence on the association between specific preventive activities and health status, attributable not only to the lag between the preventive action and the appearance of any change in health status, but also the difficulties in the valid measurement of either the intervention or any change in health status;

(ii)   the nature of any economic benefits, which are deferred and therefore difficult to attribute to specific action.

The apparent costs and benefits of health promotion programmes are inevitably determined by the assumptions which are made in their assessment. In particular, they will depend on which costs and benefits are included (whether these should include benefits to the individual, to society, or to both, and whether account should be taken of both pecuniary and non-pecuniary benefits) and on the length of time over which they are measured (many preventive activities may result in long-term, rather than short or medium-term benefits). Further complexities in assessing economic costs arise from uncertainty about the extent to which health promotion is or may be provided within the existing framework of health care. For example, one of the recent reports from the Royal College of General Practitioners concludes that the promotion of health and prevention of disease 'require a higher proportion of the general practitioner's attention and time than they appear to receive at the moment' (RGGP, 1981a). The report details various opportunities, but then emphasises (in the only paragraph in bold italic print) that, although prevention is an integral part of primary care, 'it is unlikely to be achieved on a national scale unless additional incentives are offered'. Thus, even if these activities can be absorbed by existing staff, extra costs may still be incurred. Although some types of primary prevention, particularly those which can be applied at a community level, may be judged to have greater benefits than costs (for example, Warner, 1979; Scheffler & Paringer, 1980), many activities remain of doubtful financial benefit. However, apart from the possibility that direct financial benefits may accrue from more effective health promotion, economic arguments may also be used to develop the case that greater individual responsibility for health is the only possible solution to the increasing cost of health care. For example, 'but now the cost of individual responsibility in health has become prohibitive. The choice is, in fact, over the long range, individual responsibility or social failure' (Knowles, 1975), 'much of the responsibility for ensuring his (sic) own good health lies with the individual' (DHSS, 1976b), and indeed the very title of the document — 'Prevention and Health: *everybody's* business' (my emphasis). In discussing this document elsewhere, another DHSS publication emphasises the need 'to bring home to everyone how much they can do to improve their own health and that of their family' (DHSS, 1976a).

The notion of individual responsibility has been criticised, perhaps most extensively by Crawford (1977). He characterises the ideology as one of victim-blaming, in which individuals are seen as guilty, by virtue of at-risk behaviour, of causing their own ill-health. The notion of individual responsibility fulfils the dual functions of justifying the control of public expenditure on health-related services, and of diverting attention from society's role in the production of morbidity and mortality. Thus the advantages of the deliberate promotion of individual responsibility might, at least partially, explain the recent government enthusiasm for health promotion. The economic benefits will not necessarily be direct, but may occur indirectly through an alteration in the expectations of health care consumers. This critique has been applied specifically to health education, which is seen as over-emphasising individual change (Brown & Margo, 1978).

Such reasoning is exemplified in some recent, influential medical reports — for example, the phenomenon of 'self-destruction' (Medical Services Study Group, 1978). In a series of 250 deaths among medical in-patients aged under 50 years, they found that 'in no fewer than 98 cases the patients contributed in large measure to their death'. These self-destructive acts included self-poisoning (8 cases, of whom 7 had a history of psychological problems), excessive alcohol consumption (6 cases), smoking (38 cases), over-weight (12 cases), delay in seeking medical treatment (9 cases) and inadequate compliance with medical advice (37 cases). Two case histories are detailed to demonstrate that not only did these patients die through their own shortcomings, but that in the process they consumed inordinate quantities of NHS resources. However, since one patient had 'irretrievable brain damage', and the other was in an intensive care unit, it seems unlikely that they were in a position to demand that expensive investigations and a teaching hospital bed be provided for them. The apparent ingratitude of the patients is also highlighted: one who died of self-poisoning 'had had every conceivable treatment for schizophrenic depression', and others were considered to demonstrate 'fecklessness or a psychopathic attitude to life and to doctors in particular'.

Another report of a confidential enquiry, that of maternal deaths in England and Wales during 1973–1975 (DHSS, 1979) includes similar assumptions. In apportioning the responsibility for the total of 230 avoidable factors which were judged to be present in 140 (60%) cases of maternal death, the responsibility was considered to lie with the women themselves in 48 (21%) instances. During the antenatal period one-third of the avoidable factors were 'the responsibility of the patient or her relatives'. Ten deaths resulted from illegal abortion, and in all cases the avoidable factor was ascribed to the patient — an interesting professional decision when the geographical (Maresh, 1979), and social (DHSS, 1980) inequalities in obtaining an abortion are now well-established.

Thus the economic motive may be an important argument in favour of increased resources for health promotion, although, at the present time, there may be relatively weak evidence that a direct financial benefit would result. The justification may be less concerned with substituting prevention for cure, than with engendering new attitudes about individual responsibility for health, and culpability for illness.

Motive 2: medical disillusionment with therapeutic progress

Medical education since the Second World War has emphasised the doctor's role in diagnosis and cure, rather than the prevention of disease and the promotion of health. Inasmuch as this was considered to be useful, it was usually judged to be the responsibility of others — those outside the spheres of direct patient care, for example, the legislators, health education officers, teachers and the medical and nursing staff employed in the community health service.

Perhaps the first signal of change from within the medical establishment was the publication by the Royal College of Physicians in 1962 of 'Smoking and Health', and the subsequent establishment by the Royal College of Physicians of Action on Smoking and Health (ASH) in 1971. A succession of reports from expert advisory committees have reinforced this shift. For example, the Report of the Committee on

Child Health Services (DHSS/DES/WO, 1976) recommended that the primary health care team should play a greater role in promoting better health amongst children; one means of accelerating this would be the relocation of the clinicians working in the community health service from clinic to primary care premises. A report from the Royal College of Psychiatrists in 1979 (RCPsych, 1979) has defined the extent of problem drinking, and identified the different types of prevention available, many of which involve the medical profession. The Royal College of General Practitioners (RCGP, 1981a, 1983) advocates a similar increase in the practice of prevention by their members, with the recruitment of additional primary care health workers, whose work would be entirely preventive.

'Doctors have been saying for years that the causes of many of the killing diseases of middle life are not mysteries, but are contributed to by over-eating, excess alcohol and tobacco' (Medical Services Study Group, 1978). Now, instead of making rather obvious and unoriginal assertions, doctors, faced with the limited therapeutic measures available, are acknowledging the importance of their own involvement in attempting to reduce preventable mortality and morbidity.

Motive 3: limiting the power of the medical profession
Perhaps the most vocal proponent of this motive is Illich (Illich, 1974, 1976). His opening sentence in Medical Nemesis, 'The medical profession has become a major threat to health', sets the tone of his argument, which develops an analysis of the sickening qualities of a professional and physician-based health service (Illich, 1974). As well as the inevitable tendency of medical intervention to cause iatrogenic disease, and to deflect interest from the social causes of much ill-health, he identifies the way in which individuals are deprived of the ability to maintain their own health or to shape their environment. To reverse these trends, Illich stresses the need for individuals to be 'self-governing' rather than 'administered', and to assert their rights to cope autonomously with pain, sickness and death. This considerable over-simplification of Illich's critique may appear to imply some similarities between him and the advocates of individual responsibility for the maintenance of health.

Superficially it seems that similar arguments are used. However, the contexts within which the changes are proposed are obviously radically different. The simple promotion of the concept of individual responsibility is as a pragmatic adjunct to the existing health service within the present framework of society. Illich advocates a reclamation not only of health but also of all other areas of life, and a fundamental re-ordering of the levels of power within society. This emphasis on the dangers to health of medicalisation, or medical imperialism, exemplified by Illich, has been expanded by other writers, most notably Marxist writers such as Navarro (for example, Navarro, 1976) and Waitzkin (for example, Waitzkin, 1979).

Motive 4: the growth of health consumerism
The previous three motives are attributed mainly to professionals — politicians and civil servants, doctors and the academic observers of medicine. At the same time there has been a large popular, albeit middle-class, movement towards a greater awareness about health and participation in health promotion, with parallels seen in other spheres of life. The health service has been criticised, both in terms of the quality of

specific services and the management of patient-professional interaction, and in terms of the sole claims to expertise which tend to be made by the health professions.

The women's movement has played a prominent role in articulating these criticisms, and, not surprisingly, many have focused on obstetric care. The management of antenatal consultations, with their emphasis on the doctor's rather than the patient's convenience, and the conduct of the delivery, have been systematically attacked. There has also been a questioning of the basis on which obstetric care is provided, namely, that pregnancy and childbirth are primarily medical events, that the women are therefore defined as patients and the doctors and midwives are experts, who will automatically be in the best position to make decisions (see, for example, Oakley, 1980). Obviously, the merits and otherwise of both the pattern of care and these criticisms can be debated, but it is difficult to refute many of the specific points. However, what is perhaps more interesting is that such a substantial literature is emerging.

The authors include social scientists and workers in pressure groups, but much of the evidence is produced by individual women detailing their own experiences. Certain popular publications have traditionally maintained an interest in health— especially women's magazines, although many newspapers also have health correspondents or medical columnists. The newer magazines have maintained this interest, although they tend to adopt a rather more campaigning style and to be less dependent on experts (see, for example, Spare Rib or Mother Jones). Books on health intended for the lay public have rapidly increased in number, with similar indications of a change in emphasis. The newer books tend to be more explicit, provide more detailed explanations (including interpretations of relevant medical jargon), to consider health within a broader context and to encourage a rather more critical attitude towards health care (see, for example, McKeith, 1977; Stimson & Stimson, 1978; Boston's Women's Health Book Collective, 1978; Vickery et al, 1979; Guillebaud, 1980; Open University, 1980). Many are written by non-experts, from the consumer's point of view. These changes, and the apparent commercial success of publishing books about health and health care, indicate a considerable interest among the lay public and a growing sophistication in their understanding of and participation in health care and health promotion.

Despite this, the professional understanding of health beliefs, attitudes and behaviour remain incomplete, and sometimes fragmentary. Very little work has been done on lay versions of health and health behaviour in Western societies. Health professionals tend to assume that they are responsible for providing the totality of health care, whereas in the majority of episodes of illness official health practitioners are not even consulted (Hannay, 1979), and health care is provided by relatives and friends, usually female. Similarly, studies of antenatal care have shown that working class women have extensive lay networks of information and advice (McKinlay, 1972).

A recent study of the health attitudes of second generation working class women in Aberdeen demonstrated the existence of complex theories about health and illness (Blaxter & Paterson, 1980). Of particular interest was the very negative definition of health which many of the grandmothers (women in their 40s and 50s) used. Health was seen as the ability to 'carry on' (a phrase which recurred), and being healthy was not so much a positive state, or even the absence of symptoms, as the determination not to admit to having a health problem. The implications of this definition are considerable, as it suggests that these women be unlikely to seek advice for the very early symptoms of disease and would probably be reluctant to attend for screening. Health apparently figured relatively low in their hierarchy of problems — illness in itself was an inconvenience rather than anything more serious. Other areas of their life (such as their family, housing or money) seemed to present more immediate difficulties, and conventionally defined health-threatening behaviour might, within this framework, be seen as health-promoting (by helping them to cope or carry on, which they considered to be healthy). Eating a nutritionally poor, but undemanding, diet, collapsing in a chair for 10 minutes rather than going for a jog, even a cigarette may all be re-defined as coping or healthy behaviour.

Unfortunately, very few studies have looked in similar detail at the layer of beliefs, attitudes and behaviour which predate and may counteract health promotion strategies. Meanwhile many health professionals still tend to assume that, if they give information with sufficient authority, they will achieve appropriate change.

Conflicting motives?

There is little dissent from the view that health promotion designed to inform individuals about their body and how to look after it, and about health services and how to use them, is a good thing. More serious disagreements emerge over proposals to educate people about the wider environment in which health choices are made, the potential influence of this environment on health, and ways in which the environment can be changed to enhance rather than to threaten health. This has been categorised as Type III health education by Peter Draper and his colleagues (1980), and implies the need for political change at both the macro and micro level. The providers of health care tend to see health promotion, at least to some extent, as a means of making health care more effective and efficient. The consumers, and those who wish to limit the powers of the medical profession and to alter some of the underlying structures of health care, may see health promotion as one means of achieving far-reaching and much more radical change.

Those who accept Type III health education tend to dismiss much current health promotion as at best somewhat naive, and at worst dangerously misleading. Those who see a more limited role for health promotion are suspicious of what they see as attempts to politicise health, what appears to them to be the simple transmission of information. Health promotion is thus invested with a range of different and conflicting aspirations, all of which could not be realised, even if unlimited resources were available.

THE SCOPE FOR HEALTH PROMOTION

'All will agree that the health of the nation may be improved in many ways, not only by the activities of our profession as we strive to prevent and treat disease, but also by the social and economic changes that result in better nutrition, smaller families, less overcrowding, and better education' (Doll, 1983). Richard Doll reviewed the present prospects for prevention in his 1982 Harveian ovation. He summarised the opportunities for action as:

socio-economic improvements

modification of personal habits (smoking, alcohol and addictive drugs, diet and
   physical exertion)
protection against trauma
control of infection
control of pollution
population screening (antenatal and postnatal)
prophylactic medication
mental illness   (Doll, 1983)

This list serves to emphasise the inter-relationship between specific health services
and their social context. The health education units of district authorities provide
information about the health hazards of smoking; the impact of this is always
susceptible to the more expensive, sophisticated and manipulative exercises carried
out by the tobacco companies, under the guise of voluntary agreements. Population
screening may have considerable resource and ethical implications; for example,
although screening for hypertension is relatively cheap and easy, the management and
follow-up is much more complicated and expensive. Abortion may be the only
'treatment' available for some diagnoses made by antenatal screening, and the
abortion of foetuses because of their future disease or disability may not be readily
acceptable to either the individual or to society. Although the health service can
alleviate the effects of many illnesses and accidents, their origins may lie, at least in
part, in the life style which society allocates to different individuals. Inequalities in
health due to geography, gender, ethnicity, marital status and social class are
well-documented, and demonstrate the impact of an individual's characteristics on
their place in society and their health.
   Despite a widespread agreement that much disease is potentially preventable, there
is surprisingly little evidence of the effectiveness of different health promotion
strategies. However, this is perhaps not so surprising given the complexities of this
type of evaluation.
   Figure 5.1 shows a very simple framework for health promotion. An effective
health promotion strategy would achieve a positive change among health beliefs,
attitudes and behaviour, with a consequent improvement in health status, although
this improvement might not be apparent for years or even decades. The problems in
evaluating health promotion are both practical and theoretical. For example, collecting and analysing data about health beliefs and behaviour is time-consuming and
expensive. The data are usually self-reported, and may cover long periods of time,
thus leading to inaccuracies and incompleteness, and a possible lack of validity. There
are also problems in the assessment of health status, and proxy measures such as
morbidity or disability may be used instead. Alternatively, the time scale between a
change in health behaviour and an improvement in health status may be so long, that

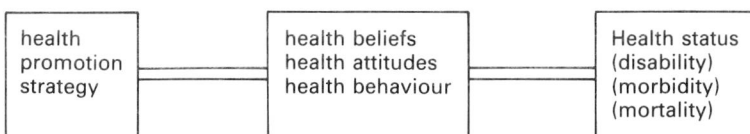

Fig. 5.1   The framework of health promotion.

this relationship is assumed on the basis of previous studies, and health behaviour itself is the outcome measure. Thus, although a growing number of research projects have addressed the evaluation of specific health promotion strategies, many doubts and uncertainties remain. Although a wide range of diseases are *potentially* preventable, the most effective ways of preventing them are far from clear.

THE PRESENT STATE OF HEALTH PROMOTION

The UK manifests a range of different approaches to health promotion. On the whole, the emphasis tends to be individualistic, with the thrust being through the work of the health education unit. This creates two main problems — a neglect of the impact of societal factors on health, and a disregard of the potential role of all NHS staff as health educators — and an inevitably reduced effectiveness. Some authorities, although active in a wider range of areas, have yet to unite these into a district programme for health promotion. For example, screening for cervical cancer is offered in isolated clinics, and the opportunities within primary care and hospital practice are not fully exploited. Other district health authorities have evolved comprehensive policies — for example, for smoking or for food and health — although not all have achieved full implementation and evaluation.

Some regional health authorities, notably Wessex, have attempted to take the lead. Wessex Regional Health Authority has established a Regional Positive Health Team, with a specialist in community medicine as secretary. The team includes 'representatives of various interested disciplines within the region' (Catford & Nutbeam, 1983), and works as a ginger group to stimulate health promotion activity throughout the region. Various problems have been identified including a lack of defined responsibility and co-ordination, a lack of information and professionalism, a lack of resources and, perhaps most importantly, a lack of real commitment (Catford & Nutbeam, 1983). Richard Doll (1983) argued for more central direction and leadership from the DHSS, in requiring district health authorities to submit 'detailed programmes for preventive services, with specified minimum budgets'. Although equally convinced of the importance of health promotion, Ashton (1982) has criticised an overtly centralised approach on the grounds that it tends to operate in isolation from the operational level of health care, and the specific interests of each community. Health promotion activities should be carried out as locally as possible, unless the action will be more effective if taken elsewhere.

The tension between a position which is essentially responding to a community's wishes and one which seeks to be pro-active is most keenly felt at district level. It is exacerbated by the difficulties inherent in defining appropriate goals for health promotion, and in ensuring that progress is evaluated, but that the process of evaluation is not out of proportion to the health promotion activity itself. For example, the implementation of a district health promotion policy should effect a change in knowledge, attitudes and behaviour throughout a whole community, with consequent improvements in health. Endless meetings can pass in ultimately fruitless discussions about the appropriate methods of evaluation, and to what extent changes in knowledge, attitudes, reported behaviour and health status can be ascertained. There are many opportunities for clinicians, accustomed to end-points which are much more susceptible to accurate and valid measurement, to make cheap capital over the allegedly impoverished state of professional practice within health promotion.

Within the sphere of positive health, the development of health goals and objectives has been pioneered in the USA, with the publication of 'Healthy People' (US Department of Health Education and Welfare, 1979). A recent workshop and conference on the prevention of coronary heart disease developed the approach beyond indices of mortality, and included goals relating to individual knowledge and behaviour — for example, about smoking, diet and excercise (Health Education Council, forthcoming).

ACTION WITHIN DISTRICT HEALTH AUTHORITIES

The opportunities for health promotion within district health authorities exist despite the present constraints upon the health service. However, plans must be developed, implemented and evaluated in a professionally-competent manner, which will demonstrate the justification for investing energy and resources in health promotion. The environment will vary from district to district. In some there will be enthusiasm and encouragement from region, and possibly examples of good practice from other nearby districts. Others will be operating much more in isolation. Similarly, there will be differences within the district — for example, in the levels of interest among members and senior officers, in the strength of key departments, including the health education unit, and in the degree of local awareness about health and health care. Districts also vary in the extent to which they prefer to work formally, and within teams and working parties. It is impossible, therefore, to prescribe an ideal approach, although obviously this should draw on all the available talent, and should be appropriate for each individual health authority.

The advantages of a district health promotion policy

A comprehensive district policy ensures that maximum advantages is taken of the scope for health promotion within all the existing range of activities, and that action at an individual level is located within the conceptual framework of the totality of factors which affect health.

District health authorities are allegedly accountable to the population living within their boundaries, and their responsibilities include the promotion of health. The planning of services, and the information and research on which the plans are based, should reflect the local needs and priorities for health promotion. At the level of individual patient care, both inside and outside hospital, each interaction offers the opportunity to include an element of health promotion. Some of these interactions, especially those with health visitors, are already used to practise prevention, but in many others the chance is missed. There is also evidence of neglected opportunities within the management of health service premises — for example, a failure to implement no-smoking areas or to ensure that patients and staff are offered healthy food. District health authorities relate to both local and central government, and are thus capable of influencing the political decisions which will affect health, as well as any measures which might be taken within their own organisation.

Despite the advantages of a district policy in increasing the effective and efficient use of resources, a number of objections are likely to be raised, including the following.

(i)   Philosophical issues: an effective district policy may be considered to be authoritarian, and likely to deprive individual patients or members of the community of choice. This is a familiar argument to anyone who has worked in this field, and appears to indicate an objection to health promotion strategies which are at risk of proving effective; if the activity remained fragmented and inefficient there would probably be much less protest. This argument is produced by a wide range of people, and may require extensive discussion. It stems from the mistaken belief that health promotion policies seek to restrict rather than extend choice, and the misapprehension that individuals living in a society are able to exercise a free choice whenever they so wish.

(ii)   Priority issues: community physicians are all too familiar with the experience of attempting to justify additional expenditure on health promotion at a time when health service resources are in effect being cut. Any hint of additional costs, including hidden costs, will fuel arguments to erode the policy, thus emphasising the need for those district health authorities which have implemented health promotion policies to estimate and make public the costs and savings. Nevertheless, the problem of diverting resources from services which provide immediate and obvious benefits, to those where the benefit will inevitably be delayed and might not happen, remains and is real.

(iii) Scientific and medical issues: although most clinicians are not famed for evaluating their clinical practice, many expect this of health promotion. Extensive proof is required, not only of the links between a risk factor and a disease, but also that the proposed health promotion strategy is capable of reducing the incidence or prevalence of the disease. In addition, anxieties will be raised that, not only might the planned reduction in disease not be achieved, but the intervention itself may be responsible for further health problems. When these arguments have been dealt with, the spectre of evaluation may well be raised, with unrealistic expectations about the quantity and quality of such work which an average district health authority can undertake.

Although the arguments about district health promotion policies are usually conducted at a level of academic abstraction, they may well cover other anxieties. Many staff will feel threatened by the prospect of change, both for themselves and for the staff they manage. They may fear that the policy will compromise their status, increase their workload, reduce their autonomy, put greater demands on their budget or test their own ability to change their own work pattern. These objections may never be raised explicitly, but might explain the dogged and quite irrational stances which may be taken.

Developing a district health promotion policy

Whether the policy is intended to cover the totality of health promotion within the district, or only one part of it, there are several distinct stages which have to be undertaken in its formulation.

Define the problem

This should be done using a combination of local and national information. District mortality and hospital morbidity statistics should be available, together with the results of any special studies undertaken or reports prepared. Some information on activities can also be obtained — for example, immunisation rates, the numbers of cervical smears taken, the number of women receiving family planning services and attendance for antenatal, perinatal and postnatal care. Such information gives a woefully partial view of a health district and its problems. Frequently it is impossible to disaggregate district-wide data to small areas, and much useful information is therefore lost (Scott-Samuel, 1982). There is unlikely to be local information on non-hospital morbidity, or on disability or health status, and no routine linking of preventive activities to outcome.

A more rounded view can be gained by extrapolating from studies carried out in other districts or nationally, but care must be taken in the interpretation of such findings. For example, the best source of prevalence information on disability is still Amelia Harris's study, which was carried out in the late sixties (Harris et al, 1971), and these data are increasingly historical. Extrapolation of national data to districts with very distinct characteristics (such as inner city deprivation or rural dispersal) may be misleading. However, such exercises do at least give an idea of the order of magnitude of particular health problems, and strengthen the argument to develop health promotion activities.

It may be necessary to collect additional information locally, in order to plan appropriate interventions. This may seem a daunting task, but there are a number of sources of potential assistance in the collection of data — for example, university or college students undertaking attachments, research nurses, medical students and trainees in the various disciplines within the health service. It may also be possible to use local groups to collect information. For example, school children may work on health-related projects, or a local women's group might examine the views of service users or their knowledge and attitudes about a particular health issue.

Such assistance can be invaluable, but must be properly supervised and supported. Additional help may be necessary for the analysis, interpretation and presentation of the data. The definition of the problem should also include an explanation of why it should receive priority in the allocation or redistribution of resources.

Selecting health promotion priorities is initially a complex issue. On purely pragmatic grounds there is a preference for interventions which are likely to produce certain and short-term gain. However, in the longer term other strategies may prove to be more effective, although the benefits may not be obvious for 40 or 50 years. There are also value judgements, often implicit, about the relative values of avoiding different events — for example, measles in a 2-year-old, cervical cancer in a 40-year-old and stroke in a 60-year-old. There is also the tendency, common within organisations, to favour a health promotion programme which is underway, in preference to a new proposal; thus, a practical proposal to divert resources may need to be included in the definition of the problem.

Analyse the problem and potential interventions
Once a specific problem has been defined, then further epidemiological and clinical evidence on its prevention and treatment must be collected. The problem might be a particular disease (for example, coronary heart disease) or a type of behaviour (for example, lack of exercise) which predisposes to ill-health.

If health promotion is to gain professional credibility, then this stage is crucial. It should include a summary of the relationship between causal factors and disease process, and review the range of interventive strategies which have been implemented and evaluated. For example, if coronary heart disease were selected as the priority, the evidence about smoking, poor nutrition, hypertension, lack of exercise and any other aetiological factors should be presented, with indications of the benefits of reducing these risk factors, and the methods by which this has been achieved. Again, this may seem an overwhelming task, and again it is important to mobilise any available expertise, which may be among local clinicians.

Set health goals and objectives
As the report of Working Group D (community health services) of the Steering Group on Health Services Information (DHSS, 1983) highlighted, health service activities are all too rarely goal-orientated. Once the problem has been defined and analysed, clear, explicit and measurable health goals must be set — for example, to reduce the mortality from coronary heart disease by 25% over the next 10 years. On the available evidence such a goal looks to be realistic, and failure to achieve it should lead to a re-appraisal of the intervention programme. Intermediate goals should also be set — for example, to reduce smoking among 20–64-year-olds to 30% in three years, to ensure that all men aged 35–64 years have had their blood pressure checked at least once within the next five years, or to press the government within two years to require food manufacturers to label their food so that people can choose to eat healthily. Goals and objectives are only useful if they can be measured. 'To encourage people to eat less sugar' is not a helpful objective, as the district health authority would have little idea about whether it had been achieved. Methods of measurement must be considered at the time of establishing the goals — many types of information which ideally would be used to assess health promotion programmes may not be practicable to collect, and surrogate measures, and thus surrogate goals, may be needed instead.

Outline a policy and strategy
The policy and strategy should be outlined bearing in mind the wide range of individuals, groups, and agencies which may have either a positive or a negative influence on health. Health promotion must not be seen as the function only of the health education unit. All NHS staff are potentially health educators, and should be involved in health promotion, if only for the benefit of themselves and their families. At the same time, the district health authority should identify those areas on which it can have little impact without additional external change. For example, however well informed people are about nutrition and health, they will still find it difficult to choose to eat healthily if processed food is not clearly labelled, and if a healthy range of foods is not relatively easily available to them — and access depends on income as well as transport.

The policy and strategy should consider a 5–10 year timetable for implementation, and define areas of activity. It may be wise to pick off some relatively easy areas to begin with — for example, a smoking policy might begin with NHS premises as no-smoking areas, or a hypertension policy with a pilot study in a few interested primary care practices. Estimates of costs and savings should be given, together with proposals for finding any additional resources.

Selling the policy

Depending on the district, the emergent policy may be the work of a group of professional staff, all of whom are committed to it, or it may have been produced almost single-handed by one enthusiast. Support will be needed from the local medical staff, the district management team, other managers who may be particularly affected and, finally, members of the district health authority. This support is more likely, if consultation has been relatively wide, if community groups have been involved and if it can be seen to be relevant to the needs of the health district. However, extensive lobbying may be necessary, emphasising the extent of the problem, the value of a co-ordinated approach to health promotion and the likely benefits.

Implementation and evaluation

The successful implementation of a district health promotion policy requires the commitment of all the staff groups likely to be involved. It will almost certainly be necessary to constitute a team or working group, which should encompass key members of staff, as well as additional staff with specialist skills — for example, an information office might be included. It is also essential to ensure that some members are skilled in group work, as other members may have relatively little experience of multi-disciplinary work and there may well be a reluctance to participate or even an explicit conflict of interest. The working group must be clearly located within the organisation, and have a close link with the district management team. The participation of the local community must be ensured, either through the district health authority, community health council or a specific local group or groups. The community physician, as a senior manager and with their range of clinical, epidemiological and social science skills, is likely to play a central role.

CONCLUSION

There are clear roles for central bodies, such as the DHSS and the Health Education Council in stimulating and facilitating health promotion. By means of the planning timetable and the district review programme, regional health authorities can ensure that all districts prepare realistic and costed plans for health promotion, and allocate an agreed budget to implement and evaluate these plans. One or more of these bodies may provide additional resources for health promotion, which should be geared to local initiative and innovation rather than national campaigns or programmes. However, the opportunities are potentially greatest within the district health authority with its accountability to a defined population, range of existing activities and chances for implementing effective health promotion strategies.

REFERENCES

Abel-Smith B 1976 Value for money in health services. Heinemann Educational Books Ltd, London
Aston J R 1982 Towards prevention — an outline plan for the development of health promotion teams. Community Medicine 4: 231
Black D 1981 Inequalities in health. Birmingham, University of Birmingham (Christie Gordon Lecture, 1981)
Blaxter M and Paterson E 1982 Mothers and daughters: a three generational study of health attitudes and behaviour. Heinemann Educational Books Ltd, London

Boston Women's Health Book Collective 1978 Our bodies ourselves: a health book by and for women: British edition by Angela Phillips and Jill Rakusen. Penguin Books and Allen Lane

Brown E R, Margo G E 1978 Health Education: can the reformers be reformed? International Journal of Health Services 8: 3

Catford J C and Nutbeam D 1983 Promoting health, preventing disease: What should the NHS be doing now? Health Education Journal 42: 7

Crawford R 1977 You are dangerous to your health: the ideology and politics of victim blaming. International Journal of Health Services 7: 663

Department of Health and Social Security 1976a Priorities for health and personal social services in England: a consultative document. HMSO, London

Department of Health and Social Security 1976b Prevention and health: everybody's business. HMSO, London

Department of Health and Social Security 1977a Priorities in the health and social services: the way forward. HMSO, London

Department of Health and Social Security 1977b Prevention and health: everybody's business — report of a symposium on 'Involvement in Prevention', 22 July 1976, Imperial College London. GLR Offset Ltd

Department of Health and Social Security 1977c Prevention and health: reducing the risk: safer pregnancy and childbirth. HMSO, London

Department of Health and Social Security 1977d Prevention and health: occupational health services: the way ahead. HMSO, London

Department of Health and Social Security 1978 Prevention and health: eating for health. HMSO, London

Department of Health and Social Security 1979 Report on confidential enquiries into maternal deaths in England and Wales 1973–1975. HMSO, London

Department of Health and Social Security 1980 Inequalities in health: report of a research group. London

Department of Health and Social Security 1981 Care in action. HMSO, London

Department of Health and Social Security 1983 Steering group on health services information: a report from Working Group D, community health services

Department of Health and Social Security, Department of Education and Science, Welsh Office 1976 Fit for the future: report of the committee on child health services: Cmnd 6684. HMSO, London

Department of Health and Social Security, Department of Education and Science, Scottish Office, Welsh Office 1977 Prevention and health: Cmnd 7047. HMSO, London

Doll R 1983 Prospects for prevention. British Medical Journal 286: 445

Draper P, Griffiths J, Dennis J, Popay J 1980 Three types of health education. British Medical Journal ii: 493

Expenditure Committee 1977 First report from the expenditure committee, session 1976/77: Preventive Medicine Volumes I–III. HMSO, London

Farrell C, Robinson D 1980 Health education and self help: based on working papers of the Royal Commission on the National Health Service (Number RC8). Kings Fund Centre, London

Guillebaud J 1980 The pill. Oxford University Press

Hannay D R 1979 The symptom iceberg: a study in community health. Routledge and Kegan Paul, London

Harris A I, Cox E, Smith C R W 1971 Handicapped and impaired in Great Britain. Office of Population Censuses and Surveys: Social Survey Division. HMSO, London

Health Education Council 1984 The prevention of coronary heart disease: plans for action. Report of a conference held at the University of Kent 28–30 September 1983

Illich I 1974 Medical nemesis: the expropriation of health. Calder and Boyars, London

Illich I 1976 Limits to medicine. Marion Boyars, London

Knowles J 1975 Conference on future directions in health care: the dimensions of medicine. Sponsored by Blue Cross Association, the Rockefeller Foundation and Health Policy Program, University of California. New York

Lalonde M 1975 A new perspective on the health of Canadians: a working document. Information Canada, Ottawa

McKeith N (ed) 1978 The new women's health handbook. Virago

McKeown T 1979 The role of medicine: dream, mirage or nemesis? Basil Blackwell, Oxford

McKinlay J B 1972 Some approaches and problems in the study of the use of services — an overview. Journal of Health and Social Behaviour 13: 115

Mahler H 1975 Health — a demystification of medical technology. Lancet ii: 829

Maresh M 1979 Regional variations in the provision of NHS gynaecological and abortion services. Fertility and contraception 3: 41

Medical Services Study Group of the Royal College of Physicians of London 1978 Deaths under 50. British Medical Journal ii: 1061

Navarro V 1976 Medicine under capitalism. Croom Helm

Oakley A 1980 Women confined: towards a sociology of childbirth. Martin Robertson, Oxford

Open University 1980 The good health guide. Harper and Row, London

Royal College of General Practitioners 1981a Health and prevention in primary care: report from General Practice 18. Royal College of General Practitioners, London

Royal College of General Practitioners 1981b Prevention of arterial disease in general practice: report from General Practice 19. Royal College of General Practitioners, London

Royal College of General Practitioners 1981c Prevention of psychiatric disorders in general practice: report from General Practice 20. Royal College of General Practitioners, London

Royal College of General Practitioners 1981d Family planning an exercise in preventive medicine: report from General Practice 21. Royal College of General Practitioners, London

Royal College of General Practitioners 1983 Primary prevention: occasional paper 22. Royal College of General Practitioners, London

Royal College of Physicians 1977 Smoking *or* health: third report from the Royal College of Physicians of London. Pitman Medical, London

Royal College of Psychiatrists 1979 Alcohol and alcoholism: report of a special committee. Tavistock, London

Royal Commission on the National Health Service 1979: report of the Royal Commission on the National Health Service: Cmnd 7615. HMSO, London

Scheffler R M, Paringer L 1980 A review of the economic evidence on prevention. Medical Care 18: 473

Scott-Samuel A 1982 Community medicine and the politics of health. In: Smith A (ed) Recent Advances in Community Medicine Volume 2. Churchill Livingstone, London

Smith A 1983 Epidemiology and prevention. Paper presented to the Anglo-French section of the Society for Social Medicine 5–7 April 1983

Stimson G, Stimson B 1978 Health rights handbook: a guide to medical care. Prism Press, London

Unit for the Study of Health Policy 1979 Rethinking community medicine: a report from a study group. Unit for the Study of Health Policy, London

US Department of Health Education and Welfare 1979 Healthy people: Background Papers. Bethesda, Maryland, US DHEW

Vickery D M, Fries J F, Gray J A M, Smail S A 1979 Take care of yourself: a practical do-it-yourself guide to medical care. George Allen and Unwin, London

Waitzkin H 1979 Medicine, superstructure and micropolitics. Social Science and Medicine 13A: 601

Warner K E 1979 The economic implications of preventive health care. Social Science and Medicine 13C: 227

6. Geographical epidemiology

Michael Alderson

This chapter provides a brief section on the history of mapping of disease. There is then a lengthier section on methods, which deals with the validity of the data and various ways of handling geographical epidemiology, there are then two hypothesis testing examples.

Three topics are then presented: the first describes some of the descriptive studies on multiple sclerosis; the second is on descriptive and hypothesis testing studies on the aetiological relationship of hardness in drinking water and cardiovascular disease; the final section indicates how geographical studies may be relevant to issues of medical care.

THE HISTORY OF THE MAPPING OF DISEASE

This brief section indicates the development of tabulation in the official reports stemming from vital registration in England and Wales and the pioneer work of various individuals.

Official publications

Since the first annual statistics report of the Registrar General for 1837, data have been presented by local areas; these were subsequently supplemented by decennial analyses, the first of which covered the period 1851–1860. This included tables of deaths by sex and age for 23 selected causes, which included cancer—and were presented for 623 separate districts in the country. In this Farr (1864) pointed out that it had 'been compiled to show in detail from the consecutive records of 10 years the causes of deaths and the comparative salubrity of every part of the country'. Further analyses were presented at 10-yearly intervals; more limited material was presented annually. Table 6.1 sets out the extent of the tabulations published in the period 1851–1973.

The Decennial Supplement Part III for 1931 was not published until 1952. This presented data by sex and age for 205 causes of death, but this only provided for twelve subdivisions of the country (four regions classified into County Boroughs, other urban areas and rural areas). Data by specific local authority districts was only available for 16 causes of death.

The Decennial Supplement for 1951 presented 12 causes for males and 14 causes for females for each Administrative County and County Borough in England and Wales by sex and six age-groups. Again it was suggested that such analyses drew attention to areas with particularly unfavourable mortality experience, so that local factors could be looked for and remedial measures taken. It was also considered that the material might reveal geographical patterns of disease incidence that may provide clues about the causation of these diseases.

Table 6.1   Area mortality in the decennial supplements of the Registrar General, England and Wales 1851–1973

Years	Causes	Areas*	Sex/Age (+)	SMR
1851–1860	23	623 Districts	Sex × Age (16)	
1861–1870	25	623 Districts	Sex × Age (16)	
1871–1880	26	44 Counties	Age (15)	
		630 Districts		
1881–1890	24	44 Counties	Sex × Age (15)	
		631 Districts	Age (15)	
1891–1900	24	45 Counties	Sex × Age (15)	
		631 Districts	Age (15)	
1901–1910	24	55 Counties	Sex × Age (17)	
		634 Districts	Sex × Age (13)	
1911–1920	189	CB/ UD/ RD × 4 Regions	Sex × Age (18)	Yes
	30	29LBs; 82CBs; UD, RD × County	Sex × Age (8)	
1921–1930	205	CB/ UD/ RD × Regions	Sex	
	105	London/ CB/ UD/ RD	Sex × Age (18)	
		London/ CB/ UD/ RD	F × MS × Age (9)	
	16	61 Counties (CB/ UD/ RD)	Sex × Age (4)	
1950–1953	12	29LBs; 83CBs; 62ACs	× Age (6)	Yes
	14	29LBs; 83CBs; 62ACs	× Age (6)	Yes
1959–1963	12	29LBs; 83CBs; 62ACs	× Age (6)	Yes
	16	29LBs; 83CBs; 62ACs	× Age (6)	Yes
1969–1973	100	34LBs; 81CBs; 59ACs	Sex × Age (11)	Yes
	100	255MBs; 525UDs; 469RDs	Sex × Age (11)	Yes

*AC = Administrative County, CB = County Borough, LB = London Borough, MB = Municipal Borough, RD =Rural District, UD = Urban District.

The data in the 1961 Area Mortality Supplement were presented for exactly the same classification of the material as for 1951. No text was provided.

The supplement for 1971 had the same objectives, but broke new ground by providing more detailed tables on microfiche. The microfiche gave the opportunity to present a much more extensive set of tabulations; the extent of the cross-tabulations is however not just an issue of the number of tables or the table size that can be published. The robustness of the population estimates and the desire to reflect local variations in disease patterns has to be balanced against random fluctuations due to few or very few events.

With postcoding of event data, and improvement of soft-ware for computing, it is now possible for OPCS to map event data at any areal level from region down to local level such as ward. The quality of the computer drawn maps is also improving, with digitised boundaries being drawn — for example for counties. Figure 6.1 shows an example of plotting congenital malformation statistics.

A major special analysis was performed in the General Register Office in the 1930s. Stocks (1936, 1937, 1939) provided three linked reports on the distribution of cancer of various organs in England and Wales. He pointed out that the Registrar General's reports had contained statistics of cancer deaths in different counties for over 80 years, but only recently had serious attention been paid to the distribution. A major activity was carried out using deaths for 1921–1930 and the populations from the censuses of 1921 and 1931. There were over $\frac{1}{2}$ million deaths from cancer in England and Wales in this period; for a range of sites for males and females, age and locality standardised rates were produced. Age standardisation was based on 10 age-groups for those 25 and over, or six age-groups for those aged 25–64. Separately the data were standardised for

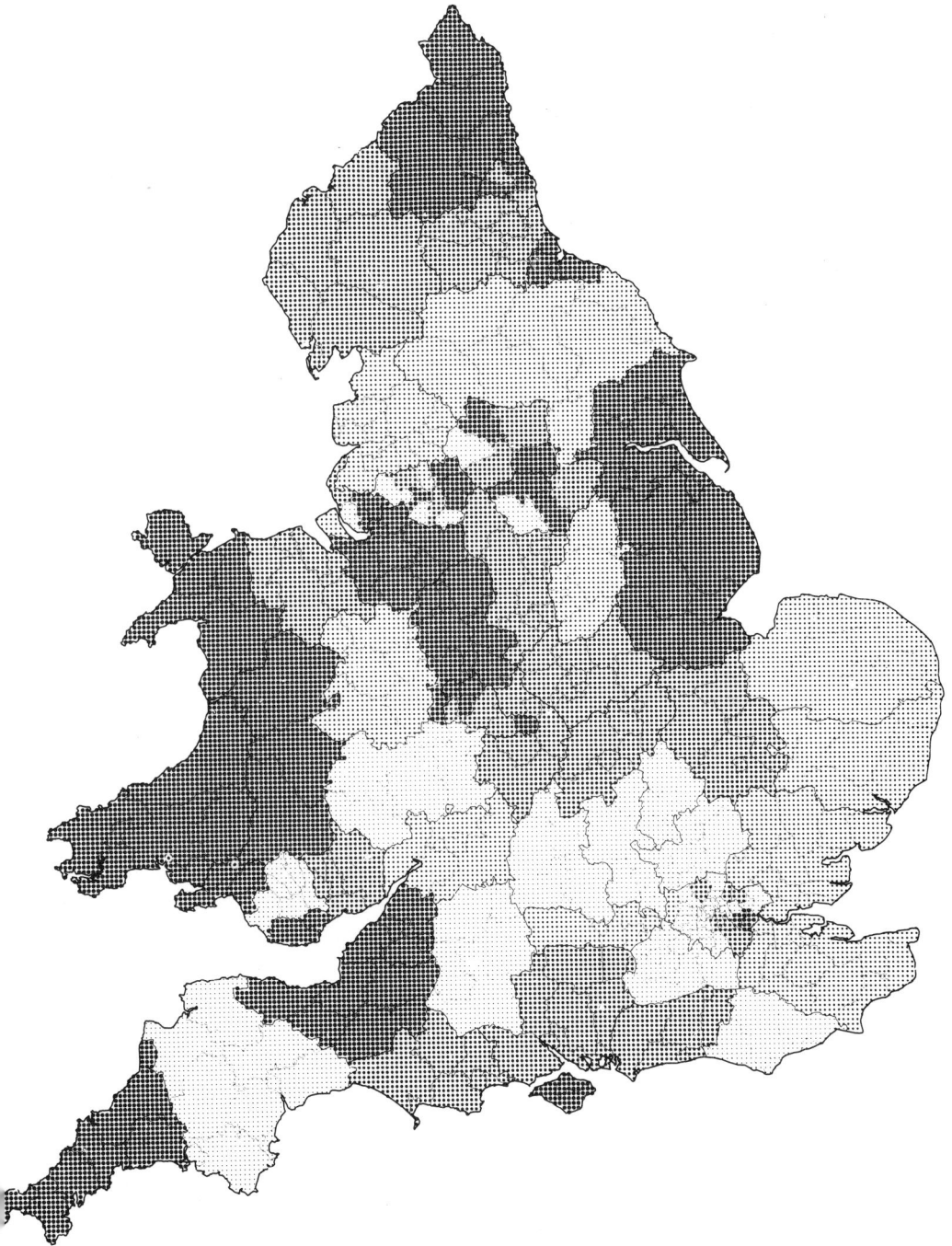

Fig. 6.1 Congenital malformations, central nervous system 1976–1980 England and Wales counties and metropolitan districts. Notifications per 10 000 total births: ▦ 32.7+; ▦ 27.3–32.6; ▦ 24.3–27.2; ▦ 0–24.2.

the proportion of residents in each county living in: county boroughs, other urban districts, or rural districts. The data are presented predominantly depicting the mortality ratios in the counties; there is a commentary on each of the sites. For example, cancer of the stomach is presented for males and females (maps 2, 3 and 4). A significant excess was noted in Wales and adjacent English counties. Attention was drawn to the possible errors from certification of stomach cancer due to imprecise diagnosis, reluctance to use the word 'cancer' on death certificates in North Wales (medical certificates prior to 1927 always being given to the relatives), and variation in facilities for diagnosis. It is suggested that the differences found could not be explained by death certification or distribution in the social classes, but that dietary habits may be involved. The third report discussed this further, drawing attention to the cancer excess in North Wales which might solely account for the enormous stomach cancer excess (Stocks, 1939). It was suggested that this may be due to the ingestion of irritant foods or substances in certain foods that tend to be preventive — reference is made to lack of fresh milk and vegetables in the diet of those in North Wales, and the predeliction for use of the frying pan. Stocks suggested that it was the medical statisticians' function not only to check statistical claims in fitting together information from different specialists studying the cause of cancer, but also to search for the 'bridges between one island and another'.

Studies by individuals

Barker (1981) suggested that doctors in Norfolk, England had long been aware that bladder stones were remarkably common in their county, with records going back to about 1600. Morris (1975) has referred to Sir George Barker's 'consummate proof' that Devonshire colic was due to lead poisoning. This colic, which often terminated in palsy and epilepsy, was recognised by Baker in the eighteenth century as resembling lead poisoning. Such symptoms were rare in other English cider-producing counties and investigation showed a unique construction of the apple presses in Devonshire, which used lead. However, Howe (1970) pointed out that the main early examples of disease mapping were related to infectious disease. Seaman (1798) showed the distribution of yellow fever in New York at the end of the eighteenth century, whilst there was a major expansion of mapping of the distribution of cholera in the early nineteenth century — in London (1832), Leeds (1833), Exeter (1849), and the whole of the British Isles (1852). The great outbursts of cholera in the first half of the nineteenth century seem to have been the factor which stimulated work of this kind, and the mapping of diseases began in England during those years, as also did the mapping of the distribution of population. Perhaps the most famous work is that of John Snow (1855), who mapped the deaths from cholera in the Soho locality of London in September 1854. This made a major contribution to his hypothesis of the mode of infection.

Haviland (1875) produced maps of the distribution of various diseases in Great Britain for 1851–1860: heart disease, cancer in females, tuberculosis in females. An enquiry, fostered by the Medical Congress in 1884 and supported by the British Medical Association was published by Owen in 1889. A questionnaire had been sent to every medical practitioner in the UK asking: 'Are the following diseases common in your district?' The diseases involved were cancer, cholera, rheumatism, rickets and urinary calculus. More than 3000 completed returns were analysed (the report gives no details of the sample size or exact responses but there were 25 998 doctors on the Medical Register in 1885). The responses were sorted into localities and transferred on to maps which showed towns and villages with positive, doubtful and negative responses to the questions (where there was a disagreement in the responses of individual practitioners the result was coded according to the two-thirds majority). It was suggested that cancer was in general spread from end to end of the island, with a tolerably uniform distribution, apart from some suggestion of more negative responses in the south of Scotland than in the north. There was no evidence of the cancer following the sea coast, mountains, rivers, plains, or other geographical features of the country. Owen concluded: 'On the whole one cannot claim to have made much out of the distribution of cancer'. This work was extended towards the end of the nineteenth century when Booth (1889) produced a series of 'poverty maps' as part of his survey of social conditions in London.

Hoffman (1915), in a major statistical study of cancer throughout the world, devoted a chapter to its geographical incidence. He indicated the evidence suggesting there was geographical variation in incidence, and suggested that the conditions or methods of living which typify modern civilisation might be responsible for higher levels of cancer. He discussed various specific aetiological factors that might be influential, including genes, diet and occupation.

Veitch Clark (1928) provided a general survey of the incidence of cancer and drew attention to an appreciable variation in mortality for specific sites of cancer in different countries. In 1923 the health committee of the League of Nations began to review the available mortality statistics for certain sites in different countries, using data from long-established vital statistics systems. Examining data for breast and cervical cancer, they found that sources of error existed which seriously affected the proper comparison between countries. They also concluded that it was impossible to assess the influence of race on mortality from cancer.

Pickles (1939) demonstrated the use of (a) a chart of five infectious diseases recorded daily for eight villages, (b) a map showing the position of the individual villages. This was used to investigate such aspects as the incubation period of various infections. Other classic and more recent examples of studying the geographical distribution of disease are given in the three topics chosen for special comment later in this chapter.

METHOD

Aim

Analysis of routine mortality and morbidity statistics are based on the three classic axes of: persons, places, or time. The exploration of geographical variation is thus central to much epidemiological work; the analysis of the routine statistics being followed by appropriate analytical studies. Such work has four rather different aims.

1. Descriptive: where is there variation in the incidence, prevalence, survival, or mortality from disease?
2. Hypothesis generation: what might be the factors related to the observed distribution of disease? (For example, why is lung cancer more common in urban rather than rural locations?)

3. Hypothesis testing: do specific aetiological factors influence the risk of a particular disease? (For example, does alcohol intake influence the risk of cirrhosis of the liver?)
4. The evaluation of medical care: is a particular campaign controlling the disease? (Is variation in uptake of cervical cytology in different locations influencing the incidence or mortality from the disease?)

Validity of data

This subsection discusses five aspects of validity: the distortion from migration, place of death versus place of residence, differential survival, certification of death, and population estimates.

Distortion from migration

Farr (1864) suggested 'the bulk of the immigrants to towns from the country are probably in good health but a certain number of sick resort to the town hospitals: upon the other hand, of the emigrants, some are consumptive, seeking health in the country and abroad, or returning home to die; but the emigrants are less numerous in the aggregate than the immigrants, and so have less effect on the mortality.'

Welton (1872) suggested that (1) migrants were generally stronger than those who remained behind, (2) some migrants, having lost their health in the towns, returned home to die, and (3) longstanding town dwellers might move to the countryside on becoming ill. Though there was lower mortality in rural areas, this did not apply to the young adult. Stevenson (1913) suggested this was due to a tendency for recent migrants to return to rural areas when ill, particularly females who did not move so far from their initial place of residence before becoming ill. The difficulty that these biases could cause in interpreting area mortality was emphasised by Stevenson (1919).

The Decennial Supplement Part 3 for 1921 (Registrar General, 1933) discussed the urban–rural and north–south variation in mortality from specific cancers. There had previously been the suggestion that the urban excess of deaths from malignancy was a reflection of ease of access to diagnostics. However, the excess of female breast cancer and male bruccal cancer in urban areas, the increase in intestinal and brain cancer in the south, the increase in skin, stomach and liver cancer in the north, and the negligible variation in female genital organ malignancy suggested an appreciable contribution from environmental factors with different distributions.

A specific study on the health of migrants (Hill, 1925) showed that the healthy migrate whilst the weaker element tend to remain at home. Increase in earnings in the towns might then secure a better environment for those who went there, whilst those remaining in the country are subjected to poor housing and deficient diet. However, Hill found clear evidence that some migrants to the towns returned to their place of origin to die.

Starting with a 1% sample of the population of England and Wales enumerated in the census of 1971, a cohort file of events was assembled, including births to sample parents, cancer registrations, emigrations, and deaths. Migration histories between 1966 and 1971 were ascertained from census questions on address one and five years before the 1971 Census. As a group, migrants so identified had raised mortality in the few years after census. However, this is shown to depend on distance migrated and time since migration; mortality levels decreased with distance moved and this differential narrowed with time. High mortality among short distance movers was thought to be associated with ill-health because those moving included people migrating to obtain support either from relatives or institutions. Low mortality in private households and mortality differentials according to household composition were explained by this differential in prevalence of illness in those making up different types of household (Fox & Goldblatt, 1982). People who lived in the North and West of the country, in either 1966 or 1971, and who migrated between regions during that period had raised mortality from circulatory diseases, but not from other causes of death. This excess occurred several years after migration. However, migrants between regions were generally healthy, and this type of movement did not make a major contribution to regional gradients in mortality except among young adults.

Place of death or place of residence

Early in the twentieth century, it was recognised that tabulating deaths by place of occurrence was introducing possible errors. The Registrar General (1909) pointed out that nearly one fifth of deaths in England and Wales occurred in public institutions and frequently the subjects had been admitted from outside the administrative authority in which the institution was located. With the advent of the 1911 Census electrical sorting of punch cards was introduced; with collaboration of medical officers of health a system commenced of 'transferring' deaths back to the original place of residence from the institution in which the subject died (Registrar General, 1912).

The definition of usual residence was modified in 1953; inmates of hospitals for the chronic sick, mentally ill, and mentally deficient who died in such hospitals were regarded as having died at their place of residence. (From 1910 until 1952, such deaths had been transferred back to the address from which the subject had been admitted, even if this was many years before death.) This change substantially increased the death rate in some small areas with large institutional populations; for example, the locality of Epsom and Ewell had nearly a two-fold increase in mortality (Registrar General, 1958). The general impact of this change in processing was described by Hewitt (1957). In 1958, a new approach was introduced; for deaths in chronic sick, psychiatric and mental subnormality hospitals the event was only transferred back if it had occurred within six months of admission.

The problem that can occur with deaths in institutions was shown in mapping malignancy by local authority districts in 1968–1978. The rural district of Stone had very high figures for 19 out of 23 sites of malignancy (Gardner et al, 1983). Stone is on the outskirts of Stoke-on-Trent; for three years deaths in a newly established terminal-care home had been included in the rural district figures rather than being transferred back to the neighbouring large towns in which the patients had lived. If these deaths had been transferred back, the mortality rate in Stone rural district would have been unexceptional.

Regional variation in survival

In a limited probe of the variation in cancer survival across the regions in England and Wales, the Standardised Registration Ratio in 1978, age-adjusted 5 year survival in 1975–1980, and SMR in 1979 have been compared for (a) lung cancer in males, and (b) breast cancer in females. These showed no clear evidence that the variation in SMR was a reflection of variation in survival in the regions.

Validity of cause of death

Many studies on the validity of death certificates have shown that error rates are associated with factors such as characteristics of the deceased or the certifier. Perhaps the clearest is the increase in the proportions of errors with increase in age of the deceased (e.g. Alderson, 1964; Heasman & Lipworth, 1966). There are also suggestions that the social class of the deceased may be relevant. As far as the certifier is concerned, it has been suggested that the age, place of training, or possession of post-graduate qualifications may be relevant. There is no hard evidence that fashions of terminology can be passed round by colleagues.

There is a very limited data on variation in certification by locality. In 1926 analysis of pneumonia deaths showed that the proportion certified as pneumonia undefined was lowest in London (13%), slightly higher in county boroughs (16%), higher in urban districts (20%), and highest in rural districts (22%). This is one of the few examples indicating variation in certification practice across the country. In 1935 examination of an appreciable sample of non-coroner death certificates looked at the quality of certification. The proportion with a single cause entry was lowest in London, and highest in parts of Wales, whilst there was very little difference in the small proportion (1 or 2%) with either a double or an inverted entry in Part I of the certificate.

A number of authors have made the general point that the characteristics of certifiers may vary in different localities (age, place of training, access to diagnostic facilities, use of terminology, etc.) and this might influence the validity of area mortality statistics (Robb Smith, 1967; Markus et al, 1967). Diehl & Gau (1982) circulated case histories to a number of doctors in England, but found the ascribed cause of death did not vary by region, place of medical training, or type of practice.

A number of international studies have been carried out which do show greater between county variation in certification and coding practice. Of histories circulated to British, Norwegian, and US doctors, the Norwegian ascribed only 13.8% to arteriosclerotic heart disease, whilst the US doctors 'certified' 24% to this cause (Reid & Rose, 1964). Major variation between six countries in coding of 1000 sample certificates was identified by WHO (1967). Puffer & Griffith (1967) found that access to detailed case histories for over 40 000 deaths in 10 countries produced relatively small changes in death rates, partly due to compensating errors.

The coroner, in non-inquest deaths he investigates, usually transcribes the cause of death directly from the pathologists' report. In comparison to certifying medical practitioners, each coroner's pathologist may be responsible for a large number of cause of death certificates. If the pathologists incorporate set expressions for different diseases (particularly for deaths from cardiac and respiratory disease), there is greater chance of local variation in coding of the certificates.

Population estimates

It must be remembered that population estimates are not entirely valid and the lower the level of area disaggregation used the greater the bias may become. The errors in the census may be biased for different age-groups, household sizes, or ethnic sub-groups in the population. In addition, those locations with high levels of internal migration may pose difficulties for establishing annual population estimates.

The likely error levels are small compared with the random fluctuation that may occur in event rates even for moderately common health problems. However, Davies (1980) showed how a previously reported significant excess of stomach cancer in females in the Worksop area could be attributed to: (a) use of inappropriate population estimates, and (b) failure to adjust the local population data for the known confounding with social class and mining occupations. Re-analysis of the data showed adjustment for the three aspects removed the significant excess.

Presentation
Once the geographical distribution of the disease has been identified, the material may be presented in a variety of ways. One facet to consider is the geographical level at which the comparisons are made — between one country and another, or within a country, between one region and another, or within regions between particular localities. There are various problems in using international comparisons such as whether the validity of mortality statistics differs in the different countries, which can influence the statistics used; regions within a country may have statistics based on large numbers, but the use of data at this level may obscure contrasting mortality in small areas. In some studies the distribution may even be plotted at ward or another local level. Another aspect to be considered is whether conventional (choropleth) maps are used, with boundaries and shapes that the reader is used to, which have the disadvantage that sparsely populated areas may create a major visual impact due to their relative size on the map. An alternative is a 'demographic based map', on which the area plotted for each locality is proportional to the resident population. This distorts the boundaries and may confuse the reader, limiting his immediate reaction to the environmental differences that may be associated with spatial distribution of the disease. This will particularly occur when contiguity of neighbouring areas is lost.

In the 1970s technology was advancing from the laborious hand-drawn maps to the use of computer graphics. However, though this initially introduced an increase in speed, efficiency, and reliability of processing (and avoided the lengthy and repetitious calculations and plotting of the data), the early material used computer line printer output, with a mixture of symbols to indicate the statistical index of mortality. However, this has now been overcome with the introduction of more sophisticated plotting equipment; an example has already been given of a map drawn by computer.

An alternative to actually plotting the data on maps is to provide lists of localities with high and low incidence or mortality. These may be easier to produce, but have the major disadvantage of providing less stimulus to thought than a map. The contribution of this simpler form of presentation will depend upon the quality of the accompanying text.

Collation studies
Data can be collated either graphically or statistically to examine the interrelationship between various environmental factors and the distribution of disease. Localities (regions or counties) can be plotted by their incidence of, or mortality from, a particular cancer and the associated *per capita* intake of particular dietary nutrients. For example, various aspects of diet and breast cancer have been examined; the linear relationship, with an increase in mortality for higher levels of fat intake, has been one of the pointers to the aetiology of this disease. Instead of examining the data graphically, it is possible to calculate the statistical association between a wide range of

variates and the frequency of disease; the geographical level selected will depend on the availability of the environmental material; many studies have been carried out on a national level. These may explore a wide range of dietary and comparable information in relation to the distribution of different sites of malignancy in both males and females. An alternative to this general exploratory study is the more specific probing of a particular hypothesis, such as the examination of the relationship between varying measures of alcohol intake and the risk of cancers such as those of the oesophagus, liver, pancreas, or large bowel. There are obvious pitfalls in such studies; the quality of both the mortality and the environmental data have to be carefully considered. Again, when using data from many different countries, the differences may reflect the quality of the data rather than the direct relationship between a particular variate and the disease. In such studies the number of comparisons made can be very large; in one study on diet and cancer over 4000 correlation coefficients were calculated (Knox, 1977). There is then the problem of distinguishing the genuine positive from the positives that result purely from the large number of comparisons made.

A more powerful probe is the examination of the trends of the disease in relation to trends of the environmental factor in several countries over as long a period as the data allow. McMichael (1978, 1979) used this technique in studying alcohol intake and various sites of malignancy.

One problem with such studies at local level is obtaining the 'environmental' data for areas coterminous with those for which mortality statistics are available.

Migrant studies

In aetiological studies a recurring topic of interest is the separation of environmental from genetic factors. One preliminary approach has been the international comparison of mortality rates; however, these are subject to bias owing to differences in diagnostic habit and certification. Around the time of a national census it may be possible to use a count of the population by place of birth as a denominator in mortality rates for immigrants. This has enabled a number of studies to be carried out on the death rates of those born abroad. When the mortality rates in the country of birth are very different, but the rates of long-stay immigrants are similar to those of the 'native' population, it has been suggested that environmental factors are of greater importance than genetic ones (Haenszel, 1961; Krueger & Moriyama, 1967; Stenhouse & McCall, 1970).

Studies have been carried out for groups of migrants into America during the past 30 years, looking in particular at cancer mortality in the Japanese and Chinese, but also in migrants from European and other countries. Other studies have been done on migrants into Israel, Australia, England and Wales. If there is a long history of migration and appropriate population statistics exist, it may be possible to look not only at the mortality of those born abroad who migrate and then die in another country, but also at the mortality of the second generation (i.e. those born to parents who had migrated from other countries).

A recent publication of migrant mortality for England and Wales (Marmot et al, 1984) uses the material (1) to check the validity of international mortality differences, (2) indicate variation in mortality as a guide to possible aetiological factors, and (3) as a gauge of health care problems in sub-groups of the population.

Statistical analysis

The first consideration with descriptive material is whether numbers, crude rates, age-specific rates, or indices such as an SMR should be used. When handling incidence, prevalence, or mortality an age-adjusted index is most commonly used. However, the final decision will depend upon the particular topic and the purpose of the presentation. Medical care studies may more frequently involve attack rates or case fatality rates.

In mapping an SMR, a choice will have to be made of the number of classes to be presented; these may be equal interval on a scale, present the top/bottom 10 and 20% categories, or those localities differing from the average value with significance of 1 and 5%.

For maximum visual effect the choice or shades need to be chosen with care — aiming at clear 'separation' of the sub-groups and avoiding an approach that highlights the middle range values.

The number of events recorded per year and the stability of the rates over time will determine the level of disaggregation of the areal data and the span of years covered. With very many events per year it may be possible for very local variations in frequency to be probed (searching for micro-clusters of disease). The fewer the number of events the larger the area and the greater the time span that must be studied. The power of the area comparisons may be enhanced by searching for differential trends over time. The next subsection deals with space-time clustering.

Pocock et al (1982) cautioned that simple geographic associations need to be interpreted cautiously, and methods of simple regression could be used to allow for the effects of factors influencing mortality. However, no matter what statistical methods are employed, the interpretation of geographical mortality studies remains difficult. Inevitably, there will be variables one would like to include in the study, which cannot be measured at local level (for example, diet and tobacco consumption are available at a regional level). Whatever statistical technique is utilised, it must be remembered that these are carrying out analyses at area level, rather than handling data based on statistics for individuals. This is obviously a weaker epidemiological tool.

Selvin et al (1982) suggested, as an alternative to regression analysis of geographic data, that the material might be aggregated for equal person-years at risk in each group and then the event rate be examined for these new groupings. As an example, they investigated leukaemia mortality in children in relation to average earnings in each sub-group of the population — searching for a gradiation in mortality in relation to income level. Until more experience is gained with this approach, care is required as a gradient may appear significant but be due to concentration of events at one end of the distribution of the classifying variate.

Space-time clustering

At the beginning of the century a limited amount of work was done on the distribution of cancer between different houses in a given locality; Pearson (1913), using appropriate statistical techniques, sought to discover whether there were cancer houses in which a higher than expected proportion of residents died from malignant disease. A major extension of such work occurred in the 1960s when improved statistical techniques facilitated examination of the distribution of cancers by locality and also by time (Knox, 1964). An early application looked at clustering in leukaemia and found some positive evidence of this. Subsequent studies did not confirm these findings. Similarly, for Hodgkin's disease, a degree of clustering has been reported but not substantiated by repeat studies in other localities or of larger numbers of events.

The statistical technique for clustering may be an inefficient examination of topic, if the contact between one case and another did not occur in the place of residence. The approach was refined by looking not only at the residence of children with leukaemia, but at the place and date of birth of the children (Pike & Smith, 1968), but even with this refinement there was no evidence of clustering (Till et al, 1967). However, the contact between one case and another need not necessarily relate to the place of residence of the mother during her pregnancy, or the child during its early life. A rather different technique was therefore introduced which examined the network of contacts between cases; this was studied in Oxford for subjects with Hodgkin's disease (Smith et al, 1977).

One important point is whether these statistical techniques give positive results for patients with known infectious disease. Barton et al (1965) studying infectious diseases in this country, Pike et al (1967) and Williams et al (1978) studying Burkitt's Lymphoma in East Africa, and Goldacre (1977) studying meningococcal disease found evidence of space-time clustering. There have been negative findings for Mononucleosis (Nye & Spicer, 1972), *Haemophilus* meningitis (Goldacre, 1977), Multiple Sclerosis (Mantel et al, 1977), and Neural Tube Defects (Siematycki & McDonald, 1972). Mann et al (1978) observed a striking cluster of juvenile diabetes, but lack of space-time clustering in Oxfordshire.

Discussion on method

Some of the problems of studying variations in small area mortality were discussed by Davies & Chilvers (1980). They identified difficulty caused by: (1) small numbers of events, (2) migration, (3) the advantages and disadvantages of mortality versus morbidity events, (4) matching localities to availability of statistics on 'aetiological' factors, (5) boundary changes, (6) lack of ready availability of historical data for events or population estimates for small areas.

Obviously in considering geographical distribution of disease, great care needs to be paid to the validity of the material. Periodically reference is made to the 'classic study' in Devon of distribution of cancer in relation to the water supply (Allen-Price, 1960). However, Shaper (1981) pointed out that the data were based on very small numbers of events, and did not take any account of the age and sex distribution of the population. There was therefore great need for caution in interpreting the material, and Shaper emphasised the need to have regard to the basic principles of epidemiology.

Robertson (1982) discussed how environmental pollution may be localised — often smaller groups being exposed than are covered by reliable mortality or morbidity statistics. Special surveys may therefore be required to assess an hazard — only after some 'clinical' observation has raised suspicion.

Potential bias in the material may stem from other biases in the local regional or national systems for handling the data. Hayes et al (1982) showed that in the Netherlands and Belgium there was an excess mortality from stomach cancer along the common border of these two countries in 1972–1975. They suggested it is unlikely that this was an artefact, as biases would not so readily affect the adjacent parts of the two countries with different vital statistics systems. However, no obvious environmental factor was known for the excess they observed.

The topic of fluoridation of water supplies and cancer mortality provides an ideal case study of the false conclusions that can be drawn from incorrect handling of local statistics. Cook-Mozaffari & Doll (1983) show how the erroneous suggestion that Birmingham had had an increase in cancer mortality following fluoridation of water was due to:

(1)   incorrect aggregation of event data prior to boundary changes,
(2)   minor arithmetic errors,
(3)   incorrect population estimates after boundary changes,
(4)   restriction of the trend data to a short span of years, involving an aberrant year's data, and
(5)   use of a single comparison city rather than the six appropriate ones.

A comprehensive atlas of cancer mortality in England and Wales has been published by Gardner et al (1983). Its 69 maps are based on statistics on the cause of death for 1968–1978. For the 21 sites with over 10 000 deaths in the 11-year period, these have been plotted down to pre-1974 local authority district level (1366 in the country), whilst for the 44 less common causes of death the data are presented at county level. The other four maps give the distribution of mortality from all causes, and for mesothelioma.

Such maps are clearly good at depicting what we already know, but they are much more interesting for the questions they raise. The cautious have worried in the past that presentation of data at low level, where the statistics are based on small numbers, may be so subject to chance fluctuation in the figures that the pattern revealed is misleading. Some of the maps that support previous evidence are reassuring from this point of view; but do the unexpected findings point to genuine environmental variation, or are they statistical quirks thrown up by the technique? In general, the patterns do not suggest distortion by the small numbers, difficulty in determining the population at risk, bias from migration, or variation in the accuracy of the cause of death statistics (Lancet, 1983).

It appears that a lot of the work carried out on 'geographical pathology' has been done either by epidemiologists or by geographers—but one discipline working in isolation from the other. The epidemiologist reading the recent series of essays edited by McGlashan & Blunden (1983) will be struck (1) by the extensive range of work being pursued by geographers, (2) the fact that much of this is published quite separately from the main stream epidemiological work, and (3) the apparent lack of collaboration between biostatisticians, epidemiologists and geographers in this work. Improvement in the collaboration of these disciplines should facilitate a wider range of sound studies.

MULTIPLE SCLEROSIS

This is a disease where striking geographical variation has been observed and migrant studies have indicated the importance of exposure to some environmental agent after the age of 15. The following brief notes indicate how the geographical studies have contributed towards identification of the aetiology of multiple sclerosis (MS).

Geographical variation

Spillane (1972) pointed out that there had been impressions of an uneven geographical distribution of multiple sclerosis expressed at the beginning of the present century, and epidemiological surveys have established that there are high risk, medium risk, and low risk areas across the world. He provides a list of the countries coming into these categories (but does not appear to discuss the validity of the material). It is interesting that a consultant neurologist is thus satisfied with the epidemiological data on variation in diagnosis. There are surprising local variations in Southern Europe; there is a high prevalence of MS in Sicily, but a very low prevalence in Malta (Dean et al, 1979; Vassallo et al, 1979).

In addition to noting the variation in prevalence of the disease throughout the world, there have been many papers on the impact of migration. Dean (1967) showed that MS was common in South Africa amongst immigrants from Europe, but occurred less frequently in Afrikaans-speaking whites. It had not been recognised in the Bantu. In Israel the disease is five times more prevalent amongst immigrants from Europe than those from the more southerly Afro–Asian countries. However, native Israelis of either European or Afro–Asian origin have the same prevalence rates. It was suggested that these findings support the hypothesis that environmental factors play a role, and that the migrants must bring their high risk with them (Leibowitz et al, 1969).

The advent of a wave of migrants can affect the prevalence of the disease in the indigenous population. This was observed on the Faroe Islands where MS was not recognised until the advent of British Forces during the Second World War. Since this time, there has been an appreciable 'epidemic' of the condition, which is not thought to reflect change in clinical detection of the condition (Kuntzke & Hyllested, 1978).

Examination of the development of multiple sclerosis in migrants to the United Kingdom was investigated through the hospital discharge statistics for England and Wales. It was suggested that residents in Greater London from Europe, Ireland, the USSR, the Old Commonwealth, North and South America, Egypt, Turkey, and Iran had a high or moderately high hospital admission rate. However, migrants from India, Pakistan, and other Asian countries, and the New Commonwealth including West Indies, had a low incidence of hospital admission for MS (Dean et al, 1976). Kutzke (1976) queried the validity of the data, including such factors as latent interval and the difference between having a disease and being admitted to hospital.

Genetic susceptibility

A number of studies have shown that patients with MS in Europe, Japan, and the United States are more likely to possess histocompatibility antigens of HLA types A3, B7, and DW2 than the general public. In many studies on these HLA haplotypes, there has been linkage of two or all three types of these determinants of risk (Poskanzer et al, 1980a). There appears to be confounding between HLA type and latitude, which indicates the genetic predisposition to MS operates independently of any environmental agent (British Medical Journal, 1977).

Association with an environmental factor

In an attempt to identify the geographical factor, Agranoff & Goldberg (1974) compared the age adjusted mortality from multiple sclerosis in 48 states in the US for the period 1949–1967, against data on milk consumption, 'wealth', medical services available, and climate. They were using the ratio of observed to expected deaths adjusted for age, sex, and race.

They concluded that milk production or consumption was the environmental factor associated with variation in mortality. This was after they had looked at other data on environmental factors. For 20 OECD countries they looked at the relationship of multiple sclerosis (they just say maps of density and don't indicate the specific statistic) against per caput daily consumption of 12 dietary variates, and also an index of medical care (population per hospital bed) latitude, and calorie consumption. Again, they felt this supported the relationship with milk consumption. Dean (1974) commented that the general geographical distribution fits more closely with the level of hygiene — in particular he suggested that their hypothesis would not hold up when considering white South African born who had very high milk consumption but low prevalence of multiple sclerosis. He also referred to the important point about immigration, where those coming from high risk countries below the age of 15 have a relatively low risk subsequently than those who emigrate after the age of 15 (he was referring to those going to South Africa, subsequently having a diet rich in animal fat and dairy produce, and there being a fourfold difference in risk of sclerosis depending on age at migration).

In discussing the geographical distribution of MS in England and Wales, Greenham & Peacock (1975) queried whether lead ore deposits might be relevant. This was not generally accepted, though Dean (1983) has pointed out that the peculiar 'epidemic' of MS in scientists studying swayback in sheep occurred in the vicinity of long established lead mines in Derbyshire.

Nathanson & Palsson (1978) examined the areal distribution of canine distemper in Iceland during the present century, and observed that MS has occurred in regions where distemper has been absent for 70 years, and the MS prevalence overall is high in their country despite the absence of distemper. Epidemics of canine distemper at three periods in the present century have not been associated with alteration in the prevalence of MS.

The work of Poskanzer and his colleagues (1980b) shows how the crude leads from geographical epidemiology need to be studied by laboratory and field studies collecting further information on the factors associated with variation in risk. These workers investigated mortality statistics for a 100-year period, and the incidence and prevalence for most recent years. The influence of demographic changes, migration and case ascertainment were examined. A clinical study checked whether the disease was similar to that in other countries. Case-control studies were mounted to check on (1) lifetime events, (2) histocompatibility differences, (3) variation in viral antibody titres, and (4) the interrelationship of HLA and viral titres. A sociological study on migration was also carried out.

CONCLUSIONS

The Lancet (1976) discussed the laboratory data on the aetiology of MS; this was compatible with a transmissable factor (which might be a virus) either being the cause, or perhaps a passenger virus. In review of the work on this topic, Dean (1983) concluded that there was genetic disposition to the disease, and an environmental factor causing the condition. Though MS probably results from a virus infection of the central nervous system, further studies are required involving collaboration between scientists from different disciplines.

HARDNESS OF WATER AND CARDIOVASCULAR DISEASE

Koyabashi (1957) reported that the mortality from cardiovascular disease was unusually high in Japan in prefectures where the river water was particularly soft. This observation stimulated workers in other countries to look at material; Schroeder (1960) demonstrated an association between mortality from hypertensive and arteriosclerotic heart disease and the degree of softness of municipal water in the United States. Further support for this came from Morris et al (1961). Using death rates and average hardness of water for county boroughs in England, they showed a striking negative correlation between water hardness and cardiovascular mortality. Excluding those localities where there was very soft water (and where the industrial revolution had begun) still resulted in highly significant correlations for the remaining 51 county boroughs. There was no indication that local social indices were the primary determinants of the association and it appeared that temporary hardness was more important than measures of permanent hardness, whilst the highest negative correlation was found with calcium levels. Work in Sweden showed a highly significant negative correlation between calcium in drinking water and death rates from degenerative heart diseases in males (Biorck et al, 1965).

The authors that examined many causes of death found some other correlations, but there was consistency with each of the four countries showing some relationship with cardiovascular disease. However, there were dissimilarities in detail: in Japan the association was greatest for cerebrovascular disease; in the US it was most marked for hypertensive and coronary disease; in Britain for cerebrovascular and degenerative heart disease, rather than coronary disease. In Britain Sweden, and the US the correlations were greater with calcium concentration, but in Japan where the calcium content of the water was low the correlation was strongest for the ratio of sulphates and bicarbonates in the water (British Medical Journal, 1966). In addition, there was an absence of an association in a study carried out in Ireland (Mulcahy, 1964). Further work in England and Wales (Crawford et al, 1968) extended the positive findings previously reported and concluded that there was no acceptable explanation for the associations between water hardness and mortality. An interesting extension of this was the examination of the death rates in 11 county boroughs, where the hardness of the water supply was substantially changed at some time in the preceding thirty years (Crawford et al, 1971). In general, cardiovascular death rates showed a favourable effect in the towns where water had become harder, and an unfavourable effect where the water supply had become softer. These changes were not reflected in the death rates from other conditions.

Six years mortality data for male deaths aged 35–64 in municipalities in Canada showed a negative association between water hardness and risk of death in general, rather than cardiovascular causes in particular. The degree of association depended on the geographical unit studied in the analysis (Neri et al, 1972).

Some local studies found no association between water hardness and components of mortality (for example, in the Los Angeles location—Allwright et al, 1974). In contrast a study suggested that the atypical findings in Kansas was due to confounding with other important variates such as cadmium levels (Bierenbaum et al, 1975). Comparisons of two Australian cities, Brisbane and Melbourne, showed higher mortality in Brisbane for components of ischaemic heart disease and this was the city with the higher water hardness (Meyers, 1975). Further work in South Wales showed that in 48 local authorities, there was a closer association between calcium levels and total mortality, rather than ischaemic heart disease, which was thought to be inconsistent with the general hypothesis (Elwood et al, 1974).

In a review Heyden (1976) discussed the suggestion that there was something in drinking water or associated with drinking water that affects the rate of heart attacks and strokes. He pointed to some inconsistences in the data and queried whether the positive results might not be a reflection of association with unidentified factors rather than a causative relationship.

A major project was reported by Pocock et al (1980), studying regional variation in cardiovascular mortality in 253 towns in Great Britain in 1969–1973. The negative relationship between water hardness and cardiovascular disease was quantified, though climate and socio-economic conditions also were recognised as important influences. On average, very soft water towns have about 10% higher cardiovascular mortality than medium hard, or hard water towns, after adjustment for socio-economic and climatic factors.

The second phase of this British regional heart study involved examination of risk factors for cardiovascular disease in a random selection of men aged 40–49 drawn from group general practices in each of 24 towns with population varying from 50 to 100 000. Results from this work are now beginning to appear (see Cook et al, 1982). Shaper et al (1983) have put the issue in perspective by commenting on the relatively small size of the water effect compared with that of smoking, which may double the risk of a cardiovascular event compared with the 10% increment from the water factor.

Though some of the results raise queries rather than provide answers, the practical implications of this work have been discussed by Shaper et al (1983), who provide a statement on the policy implications. They suggest that domestic water softener manufacturers should provide a hard water supply for drinking and cooking, there is no justification for recommending water hardening as a policy, and there is no rational basis for introducing specific water treatment to reduce the risk of cardiovascular disease.

APPLICATION TO MEDICAL CARE STUDIES

This brief section begins with a warning about possible biases in data from different sources. Infant mortality has been selected as a topic where geographical studies have been of value; a brief note on some of these is provided. The section ends with some aspects of method, which use surrogates of 'address' for indicators of need.

A cautionary tale
Alderson (1976) drew attention to the contrast between (a) hospital discharge statistics, which showed considerably higher rates for urban than rural populations,

and (b) general practice statistics which indicated higher consultation rates and higher referral rates to hospitals in rural practices. There may have been differences in the way practices and hospital patients were classified to urban or rural localities; the survey practices may not reflect the overall pattern of care in the country due to biases in selection of collaborating doctors; there might be differences in use of ancillary staff in urban and rural areas, or direct approach of patients to Accident and Emergency Departments (which was not documented in the study). However, the explanation of the differences in the general practice and hospital statistics data did not seem compatible with suggestions that the hospital statistics reflected higher prevalence of disease in urban areas.

Morrell et al (1970) in a study in Lambeth, had shown evidence that the distance between a patients' home and their general practice's surgery was inversely related to frequency of surgery and home visits. Further study (Parkin, 1979) showed that this applied to all categories of patient except males aged 15–64. The effect was particularly marked for women, the elderly, and those in Social Classes III, IV and V.

Taken together, these two examples indicate how published data may give an imprecise index of the distribution of morbidity or need for care. The discrepancy between the national statistics from hospital discharge and general practice suggest that neither provide an absolute measure of urban/rural variation in 'need', whilst the local study demonstrated the barrier that distance from a health care facility could have upon 'met demand'.

Studies on infant mortality

Infant mortality and its components has long been used as an index of the health problems of a community. Stevenson (1912) presented infant mortality rates (sub-divided into four components of the first year of life) in a histogram for the 55 counties of England and Wales showing over a two-fold variation (with low values in the South and high values in the North and Wales).

In a review of the vital statistics for London from 1901–1951, Martin (1955) particularly emphasised the changes in the relation between infant mortality and three social indices (% males in Social Classes IV and V, and two measures of overcrowding). In 1911–1913 there had been a high positive correlation, which became non-significant by 1950–1952. This appeared to be predominantly due to the increasing proportion of infant deaths in the neonatal period, the difference in the association of neonatal and post neonatal deaths to these social indices, the difference in the statistics for large and small boroughs, and impact of reduced overcrowding. Many studies have been carried out on the determinants of perinatal mortality, where an essential component in comparisons of input, process, and output data between localities (e.g. see Ashford et al, 1973; Ashford, 1981; Knox et al, 1980).

Perinatal mortality rates were examined for the parishes in Gloucestershire for the period 1968–1979; the material for contiguous parishes were aggregated if the rate remained significantly high or low. This resulted in 106 parishes being identified with a rate of 4.7/1000 births and 54 with a rate of 29.6/1000 births. Data were assembled on the factors known to be associated with risk of a perinatal death, and this material compared for the parishes with high and low rates (Shaw, 1982). Some differences were observed; for example, high mortality localities had a significant excess of low birth weight babies or children with severe congenital malformations. However, there was an excess of families with the head of the household in unskilled work in the mortality localities. It was concluded that the known factors did not account for this variation in perinatal mortality and one or more potent local factors might be responsible. This posed a major problem for investigation; examination of small area statistics results in appreciable chance variation in the statistics, and yet the additional factors altering risk of perinatal mortality may only operate in defined small localities.

Aspects of method

Scott-Samuel (1977) emphasised the difficulties of appropriate presentation of socio-economic data to guide resource allocation and service planning. He described the use of Social Area Analysis, with a variety of methods for classifying small areas from census and other sources of data. Carstairs (1981a) used census variates to classify the 37 Glasgow and 23 Edinburgh wards on degree of 'deprivation'; this was then related to: mortality for all and selected causes; perinatal deaths; infant deaths; discharges and bed days in general hospitals for all and selected causes; admissions to mental hospitals; low birth weight. There were fairly strong associations with mortality, hospital discharges and bed days, and low birth weight; perinatal and infant deaths were not related and this could not be explained by small numbers of events. There was no evidence of variable availability of hospital beds influencing use of such facilities. The general aspects of small areas analysis of health and associated data have been discussed by Carstairs (1981b). She emphasised: the advantage of more homogenous populations; the ability of allocating some events to areas, the ability to study aetiology and health care issues; the difficulty of allocating some events to areas, unless postcodes are used; the lack of population estimates, which can be overcome in studying infant mortality, with births as the denominator; the need for age-adjustment, and the distorting effect of long-stay institutions; the variation from use of events based on small numbers, which can be partly overcome by aggregation over several years; the difficulty of aligning some of the environmental data to the selected small areas.

Morgan (1983) reviewed the various measures of social inequality, pointing out that the choice will depend on (1) the number and size of sub-groups required, (2) particular aspects of inequality requiring emphasis, (3) the age/sex composition of the population, (4) any specific constraints on data collection. Webber & Craig (1978) have described a method of socio-economic classification of local authority areas, from which developed A Classification of Residential Neighbourhoods (ACORN). The latter classification was used to examine the health experience of primary school children and was adequate to identify small areas which were extremely disadvantaged in terms of illness of the children (Morgan & Chinn, 1983). In comparison with area codes, Morgan & Chinn (1983) used information from 5500 children aged 5–11 on: height; weight; history of asthma, bronchitis, any respiratory illness or hospitalisation in the previous 12 months; consultation with the general practitioner in the two weeks prior to interview. ACORN was found to differentiate as well as social class and to identify small 'areas' with particularly high rates of morbidity. One advantage of the ACORN classification is that it only requires postcodes as a key to the locality classification from the last census.

Charlton et al (1983) selected causes of death which were (a) largely available and (b) numerically large enough to permit analysis for 98 area health authorities.

Age-adjusted SMRs were calculated, which were refined by controlling for social factors from available data. Computer maps were then produced to provide a visual demonstration of the geographical pattern of variation for each disease group; both sextile and equal-interval shading were used. The authors drew attention to the appreciable variation between localities and the need to consider variation in health service provision in addition to possible errors and biases in the material.

REFERENCES

Agranoff B W, Goldberg D 1974 Diet and the geographical distribution of multiple sclerosis. Lancet ii: 1061–1066
Alderson M R 1964 The accuracy of the certification of death and the classification of the underlying cause of death. MD thesis, London
Alderson M R 1977 An introduction to epidemiology. Macmillan, London
Allen-Price E D 1960 Uneven distribution of cancer in West Devon, with particular reference to the divers water-supplies, Lancet i: 1235–1238
Allwright S P A, Coulson A, Detels R, Porter C E 1974 Mortality and water-hardness. Lancet ii: 860–864
Ashford J R, Read K L Q, Riley V C 1973 An analysis of variations in perinatal mortality amongst local authorities in England and Wales. International Journal of Epidemiology 2: 31–46
Ashford J R 1981 Trends in maternity care in England and Wales 1963–1977. In: McLachlan G (ed) Matters of Moment, Oxford University Press, Oxford, p 71–106
Barker D J P 1981 Geographical variations in disease in Britain. British Medical Journal 283: 398–400
Barton D E, David F N, Merrington M 1965 A criterion for testing contagion in time and space. Annals of Human Genetics 29: 97–102
Bierenbaum M L, Fleischman A I, Dunn I, Arnold J 1975 Possible toxic water factor in coronary heart disease. Lancet i: 1008–1010
Björck G, Boström H, Widström A 1965 On the relationship between water hardness and death rates in cardiovascular diseases. Acta Medica Scandinavica 178: 239–252
Boot C 1889 London life and labour. Williams Norgate, London
British Medical Journal 1966 Cardiovascular disease and water supply. British Medical Journal i: 438
British Medical Journal 1977 Multiple Sclerosis. British Medical Journal i: 530–531
Carstairs V 1981 Multiple deprivation and health state. Community Medicine 3: 4–13
Carstairs V 1981 Small area analysis and health service research. Community Medicine 3: 131–139
Charlton J R H, Hartley R M, Silver R, Holland, W W 1983 Geographical variations in mortality from conditions amenable to medical intervention in England and Wales. Lancet i: 691–696
Cooke D G, Cummins R O, Bartley M J, Shaper A G 1982 Health of unemployed middle-aged men in Great Britain. Lancet i: 1290–1294
Cook-Mozaffari P, Doll R 1983 Fluoridation of water supplies and cancer mortality II Mortality trends after fluoridation. Journal of Epidemiology and Community Health 35: 233–238
Crawford M D, Gardner M J, Morris J N 1968 Mortality and hardness of local water supplies. Lancet i: 827–832
Crawford M D, Gardner M J, Morris J N 1971 Changes in water hardness and local death rates. Lancet ii: 327–329
Davis J M 1980 Stomach cancer mortality in Worksop and other Nottinghamshire mining towns. British Journal of Cancer 41: 438–445
Davies J M, Chilvers C 1980 The study of mortality variations in small administrative areas of England and Wales, with special reference to cancer. Journal of Epidemiology and Community Health 34: 87–92
Dean G 1967 Annual incidence, prevalence and mortality of multiple sclerosis in white South African-born and in white immigrants to South Africa. British Medical Journal ii: 724–730
Dean G 1974 Diet and geographical distribution of multiple sclerosis. Lancet ii: 1445
Dean G, McLoughlin H, Brady R, Adelstein A M, Tallett-Williams J 1975 Multiple sclerosis among immigrants in Greater London. British Medical Journal i: 861–864
Dean G, Grimaldi G, Kelly R, Karhausen L 1979 Multiple sclerosis in Southern Europe I prevalence in Sicily in 1975. Journal of Epidemiology and Community Health 33: 107–110
Dean G 1983 The epidemiology of multiple sclerosis. Talk given to International Federation of Multiple Sclerosis Societies, 12–16/9/83.
Diehl A K, Gau D 1982 Death certification by British doctors: a demographic analysis. Journal of Epidemiology and Community Health 36: 146–149
Elwood P C, Abernethy M, Morton M 1974 Mortality in adults and trace elements in water. Lancet ii: 1470–1472

Farr W 1864 Supplement to the 25th Annual Report of the Registrar General p 440, HMSO, London

Fox A J, Goldblatt P 1982 Socio-demographic differences in mortality. Population Trends 27: 8–13

Gardner M J, Winter P D, Taylor C, Acheson E D 1983 Atlas of cancer mortality in England and Wales, 1968–1978. Wiley, Chichester (in press to be published in 1983).

Goldacre M J 1977 Space-time and family characteristics of meningococcal disease and haemophilus meningitis. International Journal of Epidemiology 6: 101–105

Greenham L W, Peacock D B 1975 Geographical distribution of multiple sclerosis. Lancet i: 106

Haenszel W 1961 Cancer mortality among the foreign-born in the US. Journal of the National Cancer Institute 26: 37–132

Haviland A 1875 The geographical distribution of heart disease and dropsy, cancer in females, and phthisis in females in England and Wales. London, Swan Sonnenschein

Hayes R B, Swaen G M H, Ramioul L, Toyns A J 1982 Stomach cancer mortality: geographic comparisons in the Netherlands and in Belgium. European Journal of Cancer 18: 623–627

Heasman M A and Lipworth L 1966 Accuracy of certification of cause of death. General Register Office, Studies on Medical and Population Subjects No 20. HMSO, London

Hewitt D 1957 Vagaries of local mortality rates under the 1953–1954 rules for transfer of deaths. British Journal of Preventive Social Medicine 11: 45–49

Heydens S 1976 The hard facts behind the hard water theory and ischaemic heart disease. Journal of Chronic Diseases 29: 149–157

Hill A B 1925 Internal migration and its effect upon the death-rates: with special reference to the county of Essex. Medical Research Council Special Report Series, No 95, HMSO, London

Hoffman F L 1915 The mortality from cancer throughout the world. Prudential Press, Newark NJ

Howe G M 1970 Some recent developments in disease mapping. Journal of the Royal Society of Health i: 16–20

Knox G 1964 Epidemiology of childhood leukaemia in Northumberland and Durham. British Journal of Preventive Social Medicine 18: 17–24

Knox E G 1977 Foods and diseases. British Journal of Preventive Social Medicine 31: 71–80

Knox E G, Marshall T, Kane S, Green A, Mallett R 1980 Social and health care determinants of area variations in perinatal mortality. Community Medicine 2: 282–290

Kobayashi J 1957 On geographical relationship between the chemical nature of river water and death rate from apoplexy. Berichte des Ohara i.f. laudwirtschaftlichte biologie, Okayama Universität 2: 12

Krueger D E, Moriyama I M 1967 Mortality in the foreign born. American Journal of Public Health 57: 496–503

Kurtzke J F 1976 Multiple sclerosis among immigrants. British Medical Journal i: 1527–1528

Kurtzke J F, Hyllested K 1978 Multiple sclerosis in the Faroe Islands. Annals of Neurology v: 6–21

Lancet 1976 A milestone in multiple sclerosis. Lancet i: 459–460

Lancet 1983 Cancer mapping. Lancet ii: 832–833

Leibowitz U, Kahana E, Alter M 1969 Multiple sclerosis in immigrant and native populations of Israel. Lancet ii: 1323–1325

Mantel N, Brown C, Byar D P 1977 Tests for homogeneity of effect in an epidemiologic investigation. American Journal of Epidemiology 106: 125–129

McMichael A J 1978 Increases in laryngeal cancer in Britain and Australia in relation to alcohol and tobacco consumption trends. Lancet i: 1244–1247

McMichael A J 1979 Laryngeal cancer and alcohol consumption in Australia. Medical Journal of Australia. i: 131–134

McGlashan N D, Blunden J R 1983 Geographical aspects of health. Academic Press, London

Mann J I, Thorogood M, Smith P G 1978 Space clustering of juvenile-diabetes. Lancet i: 1369–1370

Markush R E, Schaff W E, Siegel D G The influence of the death certifier on the results of epidemiological studies. Journal of the National Medical Association 592: 105–113

Marmot M, Adelstein A, Bulusu 1984 Immigrant mortality in England and Wales, 1970–78. Studies on Medical and Population Subjects No 47, OPCS, HMSO, London

Martin W J 1955 Vital statistics of the county of London in the years 1901–1951. British Journal of Preventive Medicine 9: 126–134

Meyers D 1975 Mortality and water hardness. Lancet i: 398–399

Morgan M, Chinn S 1983 ACORN group, social class and child health. Journal of Epidemiology and Community Health 37: 196–203

Morgan M 1983 Measuring social inequality: occupational classifications their alternatives. Community Medicine 5: 116–124

Morrell D C, Gage H G, Robinson N A 1970 Patterns of demand in general practice. Journal of the Royal College of General Practitioners 19: 331–342

Morris J N, Crawford M D, Heady J A 1961 Hardness of local water i: 860–862

Morris J N 1975 Uses of Epidemiology, p 46, Edinburgh, Churchill Livingstone

Mulcahy R 1964 The influence of water hardness and rainfall on the incidence of cardiovascular and cerebrovascular mortality in Ireland. Journal of the Irish Medical Association 55: 17–18

Nathanson N, Palsson P A, Gudmundsson G 1978 Multiple sclerosis and canine distemper in Ireland. Lancet ii: 1127–1129

Neri L C, Mandel J S, Hewitt D 1972 Relation between mortality and water hardness in Canada. Lancet i: 931–934

Neutel C I, Walter S D, Mousseau G 1977 Clustering during childhood of multiple sclerosis patients. Journal of Chronic Diseases 30: 217–224

Nye F J, Spicer C C 1972 Space-time clustering in infectious mononucleosis. British Journal of Preventive Social Medicine 26: 257–258

Owen I 1889 Geographical distribution of rickets, acute and subacute rheumatism, chorea, cancer, and urinary calculus. British Medical Journal i: 113–116

Parkin D 1979 Distance as an influence on demand in general practice. Journal of Epidemiology and Community Health 33: 96–99

Pearson K 1911–1912 On the appearance of multiple cases of disease in the same house. Biometrika 1911–1912 8: 404–412; 430–435 1913; 9: 28–33

Pickles W N 1939 Epidemiology in country practice. Wright, Bristol

Pike M C, Smith P G 1968 Disease clustering: a generalisation of Knox's approach to the detection of space-time interactions. Biometrics 24: 541–556

Pocock S J, Shaper A G, Cook D G, Packham R F, Lacey R F, Powell P, Russel P F 1980 British Regional Heart Study: geographic variations in cardiovascular mortality, and the role of water quality. British Medical Journal 280: 1243–1249

Pocock S J, Cook D G, Beresford S A A 1981 Regression of area mortality rates on explanatory variables: what weighting is appropriate? Applied Statistics 30: 286–295

Poskanzer D C, Terasaki P I, Prenney L B, Sheridan J L, Park M S 1980 Multiple sclerosis in the Orkney and Shetland Islands III Histocompatibility determinants. Journal of Epidemiology and Community Health 34: 253–257

Puffer R R, Griffith G W, Curiel D and Stocks P 1965 International collaborative research on mortality. p 113–130 in Trends. In the Study of Morbidity and Mortality, Public Health Papers No 27 WHO, Geneva

Registrar General 1909 Annual report of the Registrar General of Births, Deaths and Marriages in England and Wales for 1908, p vi–vii. HMSO, London

Registrar General 1912 Annual report of the Registrar General of Births, Deaths and Marriages in England and Wales for 1910, p vi–vii. HMSO, London

Registrar General 1933 Decennial supplement for England and Wales, 1921, Part III, p cxix. HMSO, London

Registrar General 1958 Statistical review of England and Wales 1956, Part III Commentary p 65. HMSO, London

Reid D D and Rose G A 1964 Assessing the comparability of mortality statistics. British Medical Journal 2: 1437–1439

Robertson J S 1982 Aspects of environmental monitoring, p 111–125. In Recent Advances in Community Medicine, ed Smith A. Churchill Livingstone, Edinburgh

Robb-Smith A H T 1967 The enigma of coronary heart disease. Lloyd-Luke, London

Schroeder H A 1960 Relation between mortality from cardiovascular disease and treated water supplies. Journal of American Medical Association 172: 1902–1908

Scott-Samuel A 1977 Social area analysis in community medicine. British Journal of Preventive Social Medicine 31: 199–204

Seaman V 1798 An enquiry into the cause of the prevalence of yellow fever in New York. Medical Repository 1: 315–322

Selvin S, Merrill D, Sacks S T 1982 An alternative to ecologic regression analysis of mortality rates. American Journal of Epidemiology 115: 617–623

Shaper A G 1981 A classic in cancer epidemiology. Lancet i: 1318

Shaper A G, Pockock S J, Packham R F, Lacey R F, Powell P 1983 Softness of drinking water and cardiovascular disease — practical implications of recent research. Health Trends 15: 22–24

Shaw C D 1982 A study of perinatal mortality in Gloucestershire parishes. Part II report of MFCM Faculty of Community Medicine

Siemiatycki J, McDonald A D 1972 Neural tube defects in Quebec. British Journal of Preventive Social Medicine 26: 10–14

Smith P G, Pike M C, Kinlen L J, Jones A, Harris R 1977 Contacts between young patients with Hodgkin's disease. Lancet 2: 59–62

Snow J 1855 On the mode of communication of cholera. 2nd Edn Churchill, London

Spillane J D 1972 The geography of neurology. British Medical Journal ii: 506–512

Stenhouse N S, McCall M G 1970 Differential mortality from cardiovascular disease in migrants from

England and Wales, Scotland and Italy, and native-born Australians. Journal of Chronic Diseases 23: 423–31

Stevenson T H C 1912 Review of the vital statistics of the year, p xxxv. In Annual Report of the Registrar General of Births, Deaths and Marriages in England and Wales for 1910, HMSO, London

Stevenson T H C 1913 Mortality in town and country, p xlix–lii, In Annual Report of the Registrar General of Births, Deaths and Marriages in England and Wales for 1911, HMSO, London

Stocks P 1936 Distribution in England and Wales of cancer of various organs. British Empire Cancer Campaign 13th Annual Report: 240–280

Stocks P 1937 Distribution in England and Wales of cancer of various organs. British Empire Cancer Campaign, 14th Annual Report: 198–223

Stocks P 1939 Distribution in England and Wales of cancer of various organs. British Empire Cancer Campaign, 16th Annual Report: 308–343

Till M M, Hardisty R M, Pike M C, Doll R 1967 Childhood leukaemia in Greater London: a search for clustering. British Medical Journal iii: 755–758

Vassallo L, Elian M, Dean G 1979 Multiple sclerosis in Southern Europe II prevalence in Malta in 1978. Journal of Epidemiology and Community Health 33: 111–113

Veitch Clark R 1928 General survey of the incidence of cancer. Manchester Committee on Cancer, Manchester

Webber R J, Craig J 1978 Socio-economic classification of local authority areas. Studies on Medical and Population Subjects No 35, HMSO, London

Welton T A 1872 The effects of migration in distributing local rates of mortality as exemplified in the statistics of London and the surrounding country for the years 1851–1860. Journal of the Institute of Actuaries 16: 153–186

Williams E H, Smith P G, Day N E, Geser A, Ellice J, Tukei P 1978 Space-time clustering of Burkitt's lymphoma in the West Nile district of Uganda. British Journal of Cancer 37: 109–119

World Health Organisation 1967 The accuracy and comparability of death statistics. WHO Chronicle 21: 11–17

7. Diet and related factors in the aetiology of cerebrovascular disease

D. R. R. Williams

Despite the fact that mortality from the cerebrovascular diseases (International Classification of Diseases, 9th Revision, 430–438) has fallen in many countries over the last two or three decades, this group still represents one of the major public health problems of industrialised countries and an increasing health burden in developing countries. Trends in mortality rates in the USA and England and Wales have been published and commented upon in some detail (e.g. Acheson & Williams, 1979). Trends in hospital admission rates in England and Wales from 1968 to 1979 are shown in Figures 7.1 and 7.2. Admission rates in all the age groups considered have risen steadily since the routine collection of these hospital data began in 1968. Rates for all causes have also been rising during this time, and the proportion which admissions for the cerebrovascular diseases make up of all admissions has remained at around 2% (Table 7.1). More importantly, however, the proportion of hospital bed days which are used by patients with cerebrovascular disease has increased from around 8% in 1968 to 11% in 1979.

Table 7.1 Hospital admissions (in England and Wales) with cerebrovascular disease as principal cause for admission as a percentage of all admissions and of average daily occupied beds (ADOB)

Year	1968	1969	1970	1971	1972	1973
Percentage of all admissions	1.8	1.8	1.8	2.3	1.9	2.0
Percentage of all ADOB	8.1	8.1	8.3	8.4	9.0	10.2
Year	1974	1975	1976	1977	1978	1979
Percentage of all admissions	2.0	2.2	2.1	2.4	2.4	2.0
Percentage of all ADOB	9.7	9.6	9.5	10.3	11.4	11.0

About 60% of patients suffering their first attack of stroke may be cared for at home (Oxfordshire Community Stroke Project, 1983) so that the use of hospital resources is but part of the burden of cerebrovascular disease. Whether at home or in hospital, these patients usually impose heavy demands on medical, nursing, remedial and social services and on voluntary organisations and relatives so that consideration of the causes and possible prevention of this group of diseases is of considerable importance.

117

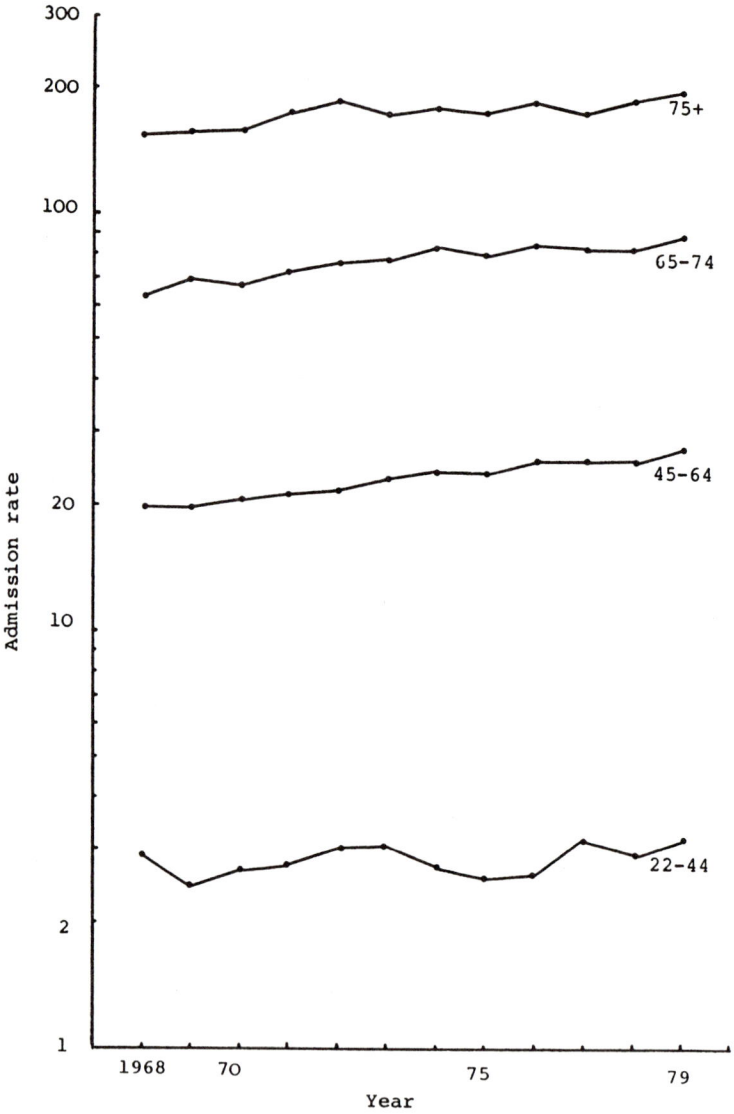

Fig. 7.1   Hospital admission rates (/ 10 000/year) for the cerebrovascular diseases (ICD 430–438) in England and Wales — Males.

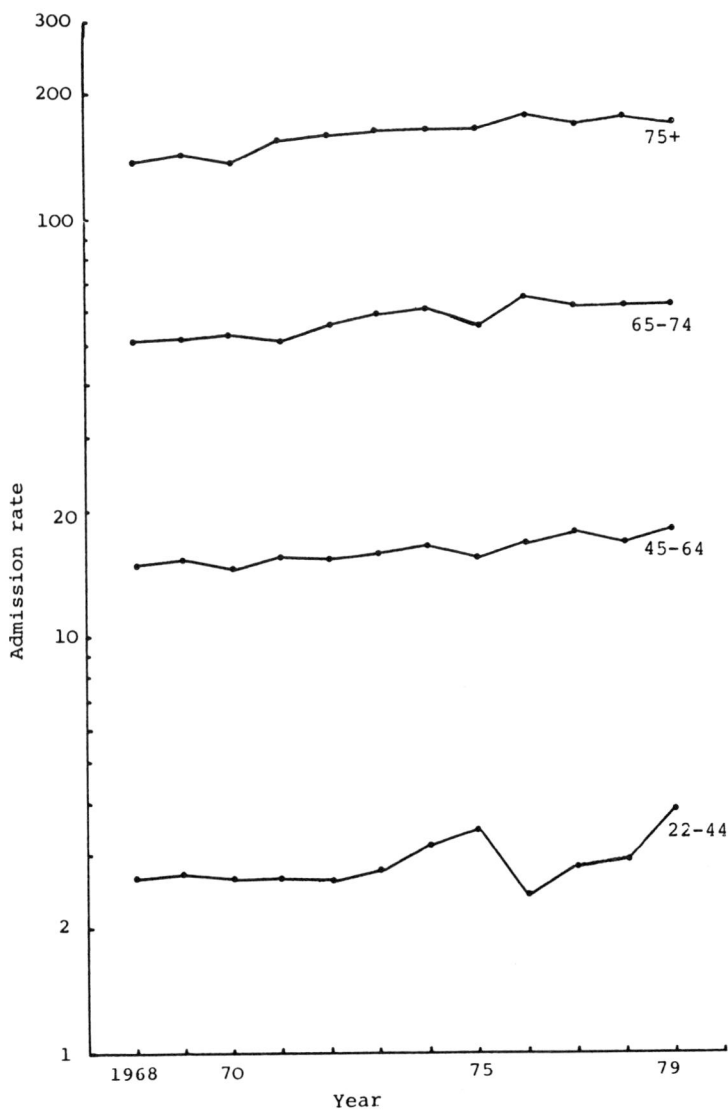

Fig. 7.2   Hospital admission rates (/10 000/year) for the cerebrovascular diseases (ICD 430–438) in England and Wales — Females.

SALT AND HYPERTENSION

Central to the issue of diet and cerebrovascular disease is the question of whether sodium intake is an important cause of essential hypertension — the most important identified risk factor for this group of diseases. The debate is long standing, extending, some would maintain, from at least the third century BC. The often quoted passage from the Yellow Emperor's Classic in Internal Medicine* is sometimes used as support of this antiquity. The debate is still in progress and, like most, has generated its evangelists and sceptics who sometimes appear to draw opposite conclusions from the same sets of data.

Rather than produce yet another appraisal of the evidence (there are many comprehensive reviews both evangelical and sceptical), this chapter will examine four of the reasons why the debate has continued for as long as it has. There are several lessons to be drawn concerning, particularly, the framing of hypotheses and the conduct of field studies. These lessons apply not only to the salt and hypertension debate but to any epidemiology investigation of an association between a dietary exposure and a disease which is difficult to define. As in all epidemiological investigations, the problems of confounding and interaction are present as is the possibility that different combinations of causal factors are operating in different populations and at different times in the same populations.

(1) Aetiology or therapy?

In the salt and hypertension literature there has frequently been a failure to distinguish clearly between evidence on aetiology and evidence on the therapeutic efficacy of low salt diets (see, for example, Dustan, 1983). Although the current interest in the role of sodium in the *aetiology* of hypertension arose largely from observations concerning the efficacy of a virtually sodium free diet (the Kempner rice-fruit diet) in the *treatment* of the disease, it is important, until there are compelling reasons to believe the contrary, to extrapolate neither from therapeutic trials to aetiological questions nor from epidemiological studies to questions of therapy. This same disassociation should be applied to all epidemiological debates. The most compelling reason for this is the asymmetry with which evidence is, in practice, applied from one field of investigation to the other. It is tempting (though not necessarily justified) to conclude from a positive therapeutic finding (i.e. in this instance that sodium restriction reduces blood pressure) that sodium is also involved in the causation of the disease. Conversely a negative therapeutic finding is usually dismissed from the aetiological debate because, it is claimed (perhaps correctly), that though sodium may have been an initiator in the pathological process, once the disease process has begun, removing one of the causes is not necessarily an effective treatment. Such reasoning can obscure rather than illuminate the debate on aetiology.

(2) Failure to define the correct hypothesis

As has been pointed out by others (see for example Watt & Foy, 1982; Lever et al, 1981), studies of the relationship between sodium intake and blood pressure have frequently failed to distinguish at the outset between several crucially different hypotheses. Do all subjects when exposed to a high sodium intake develop hyperten-

* 'If too much salt is used in food the pulse hardens.'

sion or is this a feature only of a susceptible sub-group? Is it a high sodium intake *per se* which is influential or is the sodium/potassium ratio a more important determinant?

The possibility of a salt-susceptible sub-group within the population has been ignored by most of the studies examining associations between sodium intake and blood pressure or sodium intake and the presence or absence of hypertension. Whereas *between* population comparisons have demonstrated a convincing association between sodium intake and systolic and diastolic blood pressures (Gleiberman, 1973), *within* population studies have, in general, failed to do so. The combination of observations on a small number of susceptible individuals with those on a large number of non-susceptibles may have been one of the reasons for this.

Inherited susceptibility to the effects of sodium on blood pressure are well described in the rat (Bianchi et al, 1974; Dahl et al, 1974). Similar differences may be present in humans and when the observations on sodium ion exchanges across the cell membrane have been clarified (Lancet, 1982), these may provide an explanation of one of the mechanisms which cause susceptible individuals to suffer in an environment where sodium intakes are high whereas those who are not susceptible escape without developing hypertension. Few studies have taken this possible inherited susceptibility to sodium intake into account. An early attempt to do this (Pietinen et al, 1979) used the presence of a family history of hypertension to distinguish susceptible individuals from non-susceptible. The results showed a statistically significant positive relationship between blood pressure and 24 h sodium excretion, the Na/K ratio and overnight sodium excretion in subjects with a positive family history but no relationship in those without. Unfortunately, the study was small, the presence of hypertension in the subjects' relatives was corroborated neither by objective measurements nor by the examination of medical records and, in any case, a 'positive' or 'negative' family history is an exceptionally crude index of susceptibility. Nevertheless, this sort of approach deserves to be further explored.

(3) Problems with measurement

The methods of assessment of sodium intake in field studies varied greatly in the 27 population studies reviewed by Gleiberman (1973). Mean population sodium intakes were estimated from urinary collections in 11 studies; in 10, intakes were determined by quantitative observations of food intake, and, in the remaining six, estimations had to be made from non-quantitative dietary information.

Measurements of sodium intake in free living human subjects can only satisfactorily be performed by measuring urinary sodium excretion. In the steady state, dietary intake and urinary output are virtually equal with minimal loss in the faeces. Assessment of sodium intake from dietary records, on the other hand, is liable to gross error since, even when assessment of food intake is accurate, the calculation of the sodium content of foods is liable to considerable inaccuracies as a result of deviations from the available tabulated values of electrolyte content. These differences are produced by variations in the growing conditions of plants, recipe variations, differing cooking methods and, of course, the addition of variable quantities of table salt by the subject.

The methodological problems of estimating sodium intake *within* populations are of a different nature and in general more difficult to overcome than those encountered in measuring differences *between* populations. Liu et al (1979) in a paper of crucial importance in this field, pointed out that seven to fourteen 24-hour urine samples are required to accurately characterise an individual's sodium intake—a number far larger than that which is usually employed in epidemiological studies (one or two samples only). This problem is a consequence of the large day to day intra-individual variation in sodium intake compared with the observed inter-individual differences in industrialised populations It is a difficulty which has also, in an analogous fashion, affected the within population study of the relationship between fat intakes and ischaemic heart disease (Liu et al, 1978).

The further problem of ensuring complete 24-hour urine collections in such studies has never satisfactorily been overcome though now a harmless urinary marker (4-aminobenzoic acid), which can be used to distinguish complete collections from incomplete collections and which is suitable for use in population studies, has been developed (Bingham, 1983).

Two epidemiological studies which have been widely quoted as refuting the salt hypothesis (Malhotra, 1970; Whyte, 1958) are unfortunately based on inadequate or unevaluable population assessments of sodium intake in the samples studied. The first of these compared railway employees living in North and South India (Delhi and Madras), measuring their blood pressures, serum cholestrol and faecal urobilinogen. Mean blood pressures, by age, were higher in the South than in the North, though not when ponderal index (weight/height^2) was taken into account—Southerners are more frequently obese than Northerners. The prevalence of hypertension in the South was more than double that in the North and Northern Indians were stated to consume 12–15 g of NaCl/day compared to 8 g/day for the Southerners. Unfortunately, the dietary data used in the study for the North do not refer to the same group of subjects as the blood pressure data but to 28 pairs of healthy railway employees who were involved in another study. These were inhabitants of Udaipur, a North Indian city some distance from Delhi.

Whyte (1958) compared a group of subjects living in the Central Highlands of New Guinea with a group from the coastal region of the same country. The coastal group, unlike the highland group, had experienced contact with Europeans over a long period. Mean blood pressures in the younger natives of both groups did not differ significantly from those considered normal for European populations but blood pressures did not rise with subsequent age in either group. The means for coastal natives were not greater than those for highland natives, in fact, mean diastolic pressures were slightly (but significantly) higher in the latter. The assessment of dietary intake in the highland group was performed by Vekatachalam (quoted by Whyte as a personal communication) but the details of this survey have not appeared in the literature and no assessment of the validity of the data can therefore be made. The diet of the coastal natives was assessed by an Australian Government Survey [Hipsley E. H. & Clements F. W. (1947) 'Report of the New Guinea Nutrition Survey Expedition', Department of External Territories, Canberra] but this makes no *quantitative* reference to sodium intake. Daily sodium excretion was measured on a small sample of highlanders (20 subjects — mean 30 mEq/24 h) and the coastal natives were 'assumed to have a greater (salt) intake' than the highlanders.

In addition to the considerable difficulties of measuring electrolyte intake, difficulties also exist in the measurement of blood pressure in population studies (see, for example, Armitage et al, 1966). These relate particularly to observer error and machine error but also to day to day intra-individual variation in blood pressure values. Few studies can be said to have satisfactorily dealt with these important problems. Reports which deal with 'hypertension', rather than 'blood pressure' also encounter the serious problem of disease definition which is still not (and perhaps never will be) satisfactorily resolved.

(4) Reliance on studies with insufficient statistical power
Watt & Foy (1982) have reviewed the published reports which explore the relationship between blood pressure and electrolyte excretion or seek a difference in electrolyte excretion between hypertensives and nonhypertensives (the standard case control design). Of the five studies cited by them in the former group only two (Cooper et al, 1980 and one of the studies described by Joossens et al, 1970) showed a statistically significant positive relationship between blood pressure and sodium excretion. However, of the five which failed to show such a relationship none were statistically powerful enough to have had a greater than 90% chance of detecting a linear relationship with a slope of 0.1 mm Hg per mmol of Na. In fact the statistical power $(1-\beta)$ of all five of these studies was below 30%.

Of the case control studies considered by Watt & Foy seven showed no difference, one showed higher sodium excretion in normotensive subjects and two showed higher excretion in hypertensives. However, of the seven studies which showed no difference none could be considered sufficiently powerful to exclude a case control difference of 20 mmol and in only one (Miall, 1959) was there a greater than 90% chance of detecting of 40 mmol difference if present.

This lack of statistical power in studies which report 'negative' findings is analogous to that found in the analysis of randomised control trials published by Freiman et al (1978) where a large number of trials suggesting 'no difference' between given treatments were insufficiently powerful to constitute an acceptable test of the hypothesis under consideration. The importance of the type II (or beta) error in the epidemiological literature on salt and hypertension cannot be over-emphasised and none of the hypotheses which have been put forward in this field can yet be regarded as exhaustively tested. It should be noted, however, that *most of the few studies that have possessed sufficient statistical power have supported the proposition that blood pressure levels and sodium excretion are positively associated.*

INTERACTIONS WITH SODIUM

(1) Potassium
A protective role for potassium in human hypertension has been strongly argued by authors such as Meneely & Batterbee (1976). There is almost invariably a reciprocal relationship between sodium intake and potassium intake in human populations. The Yanomamo Indians of Brazil, for example, when first described, showed no rise in blood pressure with age (and no hypertension) and excreted large quantities of potassium (200 mEq/24 h) with a very small sodium output (1 mEq/24 h) (Oliver et al, 1975). Population samples drawn from industrialised countries like Finland show low potassium excretion and high sodium output (Tuomilehto et al, 1981).

Animal experiments have been described which support a protective effect of potassium in the face of a high sodium intake. Meneely, Ball & Youmans (1957), for example, reduced the hypertensinogenic effect of sodium feeding in rats by simultaneously feeding large quantities of potassium.

The possibility that a high potassium intake may counteract any hypertensinogenic effect of a high sodium intake in humans is obviously of considerable public health importance but it is unlikely that this question can be answered satisfactorily by the results of descriptive epidemiological studies alone. In general, population studies that have estimated electolyte excretion or dietary intake or both have concentrated on the sodium–hypertension hypothesis and not a potassium-hypertension hypothesis or one postulating sodium–potassium interaction. A few, such as Simmons (1983), have addressed the question of relationships with sodium, potassium and the sodium/potassium ratio. Simmons found an association between raised blood pressure and the sodium/potassium ratio in Creoles of Central America but no convincing relationship with either sodium or potassium alone. Such studies taken alone are unlikely to determine the relative importance of sodium and potassium intake in the development of the disease and an adequate examination of these more sophisticated interactive models has not yet been carried out outside the laboratory. To do so in free living human populations would require a very large study indeed.

In the laboratory, Lever et al (1981) testing more precisely framed hypotheses than are characteristic of most of the epidemiological literature, obtained data suggesting that potassium lack rather than sodium excess is important in the early stages of the development of hypertension. This conclusion was based on a failure to find a correlation between exchangeable sodium and blood pressure in younger hypertensives (though a relationship was found in older patients) contrasted with negative correlations of blood pressure with exchangeable potassium ($r = -0.15$, $p < 0.01$), plasma potassium concentration and total body potassium in the same group of patients.

There is no convincing evidence to suggest that increasing the potassium intake of populations while their sodium intakes remain high will be effective in the prevention of hypertension. However, an increase in potassium intake at the same time as a decrease in sodium may well be more effective than the latter alone. These simultaneous changes are inevitable if suggested increases in fruit, vegetable and cereal products (Health Education Council, 1983) accompany suggested decreases in the consumption of foods with high sodium contents.

(2) Fat

A direct influence of dietary fat on blood pressure has not yet been established in humans. There is a suggestion that an increase in the P : S ratio can decrease blood pressure experimentally (Iacono et al, 1975), though the effect noted might have been the result of decreasing total fat intake. There is no convincing mechanism for an influence of specific dietary fatty acids on blood pressure, though these same authors have suggested that an effect on prostaglandin synthesis might provide a mechanism for such a relationship. Rabbits fed fat-enriched diets show an increase in arterial blood pressure, especially when the fat is of animal origin (Burstyn & Firth, 1975). Individual rabbits differ in the magnitude of this response which seems to be independent of weight gain.

The population data on fat and hypertension and stroke are confusing. Death rates from hypertensive diseases in Japanese prefectures are positively correlated with total fat intakes (Sasaki, 1962) as are death rates from the cerebrovascular diseases in Standard Regions of Britain (Acheson & Williams, 1979). Shaper's work on the Samburu, however (Shaper et al, 1969), showed lower blood cholesterol and phospholipid levels in soldiers with their higher blood pressures than in native warriors, who consume between 2 and 15 pints of milk per person per day. It seems unlikely that fat consumption plays a significant part in determining international differences in the occurrence of hypertension in view of the fact that the Japanese, for example, have strikingly high prevalences but have low fat intakes. The possibility that, in some populations with high fat and high salt intakes, fat contributes to the pathogenesis of hypertension perhaps by interaction with sodium, cannot, however, be ruled out.

(3) Stress
The idea that stress, or, more correctly, the physiological reaction to stress, causes hypertension has been cited by many authors. Objective measurement of this across linguistic and cultural barriers is difficult and has not been satisfactorily undertaken in conjunction with studies of blood pressure. There are some indications, however, that noise, which may be regarded as a particular form of stress, is hypertensinogenic in humans since, when subjected to loud noise in the laboratory, human subjects show a rise in blood pressure and hypertension is more frequently encountered in population samples chronically exposed to the noise of low flying aircraft (Knipschild, 1977).

In animals, a rise in blood pressure has been produced by stressful situations such as the food-shock conflict (Friedman & Iwai, 1977). Strains of salt sensitive rats are rendered moderately hypertensive by exposure to such a conflict even in the absence of a high salt diet. Resistant rats, however, show no rise in blood pressure in this situation. When salt sensitive rats are simultaneously exposed to a moderately high salt diet (2% NaCl) and a stressful situation the level of blood pressure shown is greater than that seen either with stress or a high salt intake alone. One possible conclusion from such animal experiments is that stress can act synergistically with such factors as dietary sodium but that, in the absence of sensitivity to these factors, its effect may be slight. Skrabal et al (1981) have suggested that a reduction in sodium intake (from 200 to 50 mmol/day) reduces the hypertensive effects of intravenous infusions of noradrenaline in normotensive human volunteers. Such an effect may be part of the basis of an interaction between the physiological effects of stress and the effect of dietary sodium in both humans and animals.

(4) Sucrose
The role of dietary sucrose and its possible interaction with sodium has been the subject of several recent experimental studies. Ahrens et al (1980), studying the laboratory rat, have shown that the substitution of sucrose for starch in the diet can elevate mean blood pressure when the effect of a 10% sucrose/30% starch diet (fed for 6 weeks) is contrasted with no sucrose in a 40% starch diet. The same authors studied the effect of sucrose on sodium excretion in this same experimental animal and found, in general, that the higher the sucrose intake (up to 20% of total energy) the lower the rate of urinary sodium excretion (constant sodium content of diets and constant body

weight) thus at least part of the effect of sucrose on blood pressure may be the result of sodium retention.

Srinivasan et al (1980) have also considered the interaction between sucrose and sodium but using the spider monkey as an experimental model. After 100 days of feeding, monkeys on a high sodium diet (3% NaCl, 9.9 mg/Kcal) showed systolic blood pressures 21 mmHg higher than controls while monkeys fed the same quantity of NaCl but with 38% of energy from sucrose (compared with 0% in the comparison groups) showed a mean blood pressure consistently higher (by about 2–3 mmHg) than the means of the high salt only group. Thus, in an analogous fashion to a possible stress-sodium interaction, sucrose intake may have an effect on any hypertensive action of sodium.

An increase in sucrose intake almost inevitably accompanies the social changes that human populations undergo when they are 'industrialised'. Any effect of sucrose intake on blood pressure or any synergistic action it may have with dietary sodium have not been taken into account in published epidemiological studies, nor is it likely that future observational studies on human populations will be able by themselves to unravel this interrelationship.

CONCLUSION

Though it is extremely likely that dietary sodium intake is one of the most important aetiological factors in essential hypertension in many populations, as far as the biological mechanisms are concerned and, particularly, as far as possible interactions with other factors are concerned, it is probably true to say that 'to every question there is a simple answer but that answer is usually wrong'.

DIRECT EFFECTS OF DIET ON THE CEREBROVASCULAR DISEASES

In contrast to the extensive epidemiological research on diet and hypertension, very few population studies have been carried out in direct effects of dietary factors on the occurrence of cerebrovascular disease. One of the reasons for this is undoubtedly the large clinical, pathophysiological and, aetiological heterogeneity encompassed by the term (Table 7.2). It is unlikely that such a heterogeneous group of diseases will, when studied together, reveal any clear pattern of occurrence. One of the difficulties with cerebrovascular disease epidemiology is that, in the absence of sophisticated modern

Table 7.2 International Classification of Diseases (I.C.D.) rubrics for the cerebrovascular disease (I.C.D. 9th edition)

Disease	I.C.D.
Subarachnoid haemorrhage	430
Cerebral haemorrhage	431
Occlusion of pre-cerebral arteries	432
Cerebral thrombosis	433
Cerebral embolism	434
Transient cerebral ischaemia	435
Acute but ill-defined cerebrovascular disease	436
Generalised ischaemic cerebrovascular disease	437
Other and ill-defined cerebrovascular disease	438

diagnostic techniques, subdivision into discrete diagnostic entities is of extremely dubious accuracy. This applies particularly to the analysis of mortality data which is commonly the subject of epidemiological discussion and which is one of the subjects of this section.

Mortality rates from this group of diseases taken as a whole show virtually no relationship with mortality rates from ischaemic heart disease (ICD 410–414) when rates in 31 countries are compared (Tunstall Pedoe, 1983). Within England and Wales mortality rates from all cerebrovascular disease taken together and from two of the major sub-divisions — cerebral haemorrhage (ICD 431) and cerebral thrombosis (ICD 433) — show clear North West to South East declining gradients. These are qualitatively similar to that seen for ischaemic heart disease but a similar geographic gradient is, of course, seen for most chronic diseases. It has been demonstrated (Acheson & Sanderson, 1978) that, although death rates from cerebral haemorrhage and cerebral thrombosis also show a marked social class gradient, and the social class make up of populations in the North and West of England and Wales differ from those in the South and East, the observed geographic gradients in mortality are not the results of social class admixture but persist even when social class is taken into account (Table 7.3).

Table 7.3   Standardised mortality ratios (means S.E.) for males aged 15–64 by grouped social classes (based on occupation) and by grouped hospital boards (1970–1972)

Regional hospital board grouping	Cerebral haemorrhage (I.C.D. 431) Social class grouping			Cerebral thrombosis (I.C.D. 433) Social class grouping		
	I and II	III	IV and V	I and II	III	IV and V
Newcastle and Wales	120 ± 9	135 ± 6	157 ± 9	132 ± 12	191 ± 10	209 ± 13
Birmingham, Manchester, Liverpool, Leeds and Sheffield	99 ± 4	112 ± 3	127 ± 4	100 ± 6	123 ± 4	152 ± 6
East Anglia, Oxford, South Western and Wessex	89 ± 6	97 ± 5	99 ± 6	68 ± 6	72 ± 5	87 ± 7
Metropolitan	76 ± 4	80 ± 3	92 ± 5	47 ± 4	57 ± 7	62 ± 5

Though the Registrar General's social class groupings have stood the test of time, they are comparatively crude indicators of exposure to factors which may be concerned in the aetiology of cerebrovascular disease and which may explain the observed geographic gradients. Exposure to these risk factors presumably differs depending on place of residence, even within social classes. These factors may include the prevalence and treatment of hypertension, cigarette smoking, fasting blood glucose and body mass (factors known to be associated with cerebral thrombosis (Kannel et al, 1974)) but may also include dietary factors, not only those involved in the aetiology of hypertension, but others which may be more immediate precipitating factors for these diseases.

Some preliminary data on associations with fruit and vegetable consumption have been reported (Acheson & Williams, 1983). When cerebrovascular disease death rates between 45 and 65 are considered, statistically significant negative correlations with consumption figures (based on National Food Survey estimates) are seen for geographic areas (significant correlations with female rates only) and population density groupings (correlations with male rates only). These are illustrated in Table 7.4. Although such correlations form the weakest epidemiological evidence for a causal relationship, biological mechanisms for a relationship between vitamin C intake (one of the many possible active constituents of fresh fruit and vegetables) and both cerebral haemorrhage and thrombosis have been suggested. Intake of this vitamin is related to collagen biosynthesis and therefore, perhaps, to the fragility of cerebral and other small blood vessels. Platelet adhesiveness has also been suggested to fall with reduced vitamin C intake (Born & Wight, 1968), so that a relationship with cerebral haemorrhage is possible. The suggested effect of vitamin C intakes of fibrinolytic activity (Bordia et al 1978), may be the basis of a pathophysiological relationship with both thrombotic and embolic cerebral events. Equally speculative at present is the inference that may be drawn from experimental work such as that of Verlangieri & Stevens (1979), that low vitamin C intake may increase the likelihood of atherogenesis in humans as well as the rat (which was their experimental model).

Table 7.4   Correlation coefficients (r) and statistical probability (p) between mortality for all cerebrovascular diseases (at ages 45–64) and fresh fruit and fresh vegetable consumption (as estimated by the National Food Survey (all data for 1970)

	Scotland, Wales and Standard Regions of England (n = 11)				Population aggregations*			
	Males		Females		Males		Females	
	r	p	r	p	r	p	r	p
Fresh fruit	−0.68	0.04	−0.74	0.02	−0.85	0.03	−0.66	0.15
Fresh vegetables	−0.55	0.12	−0.80	0.01	−0.92	0.01	−0.69	0.12

* Rural, urban, metropolitan etc.

PREVENTION

Intervention studies which have sought to reduce cerebrovascular disease incidence and mortality in defined populations are potentially useful sources of evidence on dietary causes. In 1972 the North Karelia project set out to identify known hypertensives, to improve the control of hypertension in them and to reduce the other known cardiovascular disease risk factors of cigarette smoking and serum cholesterol in this Finnish province. Although the results from this study suggest a substantial decrease in cerebrovascular disease mortality and incidence (though this was not significantly different from the control population), it is not possible to ascribe this to the changes produced in local dietary habits as opposed to changes in other risk factors or a combination of several effects. Since 1979 an additional study is in progress in the same population aimed at reducing sodium intake and also increasing potassium intake partly by encouraging the use of a NaCl/KCl table salt substitute. Although the results in established hypertensives have been published, and suggest that, while reduction in fat intake may have lowered blood pressure, sodium restriction probably did not, results in the prevention of hypertension and cerebrovascular disease are awaited.

A study by Farquhar et al (1979), however, has reported modest success in that a reduction in blood pressure did occur when sodium intake was reduced in a North American intervention study and it has been claimed (Joossens & Geboers (1983) that the acceleration of declines in cerebrovascular disease death rates in Belgium after 1968 was the result of a reduction in NaCl intake from about 15 g/day in 1966 to about 9 g/day in 1981.

The period of life during which such interventions are carried out may be crucial. There have been few attempts to explore the effects of intervention in early infant life but Hofman et al (1983) have recently reported the effect of placing a cohort of newborn children on a low sodium diet from birth compared with a similar cohort raised on a 'normal-sodium' diet. At the end of 25 weeks of life, the systolic blood pressure in the low sodium group was 2.0 mmHg lower than that of the normal-sodium group ($p < 0.05$) and there was a statistically significant difference in the rate of increase of blood pressure from birth. Given the 'tracking' phenomenon of blood pressure in human groups, the results of this study deserve to be considered seriously.

Despite falling mortality rates, the impact of the cerebrovascular diseases on society is increasing. Despite its complexity and several unresolved and important questions, the aetiological link between diet and these diseases especially through hypertension is likely to be important. Preventive nutrition, as well as the strategies of the early detection and effective treatment of hypertension should be seriously considered as a means of reducing this impact.

ACKNOWLEDGEMENTS

The Health Promotion Committee of the Faculty of Community Medicine has recently commissioned a report on dietary salt and health. The discussions which I have had with the three colleagues with whom I worked on this have been an important stimulus for the writing of this chapter. As always, Mrs Doreen Ashpole's patience in compiling the manuscript is much appreciated and Dr Liz MacDonald's help in preparing the data used for Tables 7.1 and 7.2 is also gratefully acknowledged.

REFERENCES

Acheson R M, Sanderson C 1978 Strokes: social class and geography. Population Trends HMSO 13–17
Acheson R M, Williams D R R 1979 The epidemiology of stroke: some unanswered questions. Proceedings of Symposium on neuro-epidemiology held at Medical Society of London. Pitman 88–104
Acheson R M, Williams D R R 1983 Does consumption of fruit and vegetables protect against stroke? Lancet i: 1191–1193
Ahrens R A, Denrith P, Lee M K, Majtcouski J W 1980 Moderate sucrose ingestion and blood pressure in the rat. Journal of Nutrition 110: 725–731
Armitage P, Fox W, Rose G A, Tinker C M 1966 The validity of measurements of casual blood pressure II Survey experience. Clinical Science 30: 337–344
Bianchi G, Fox U, Di Francesco G F, Giovanetti A M, Pagetti D 1974 Blood pressure changes produced by kidney cross-transplantation between spontaneously hypertensive rats (SHR) and normotensive rats (NR). Clinical Science and Molecular Medicine 47: 435–448
Bingham S, Cummings J H 1983 The use of 4-aminobenzoic acid as a marker to validate the completeness of 24 h urine collections in man. Clinical Science 629–635
Bordia A, Paliwal D K, Jain K, Lothari L K 1978 Acute effect of ascorbic acid on fibrinolytic activity. Atherosclerosis 30: 351–354
Born G V R, Wight H P 1968 Diminished platelet aggregation in experimental scurvy. Journal of Physiology 197: 27P–28P

Burstyn P G, Firth W R 1975 Effects of three fat-enriched diets in the arterial pressure of rabbits. Cardiovascular Research 9: 807–810

Cooper R, Soltero I, Liu K, Berkson D, Levinson S, Stamler J 1980 The association between urinary sodium excretion and blood pressure in children. Circulation 62: 97–104

Dahl L K, Heine M, Thompson K 1974 Genetic influence of the kidneys on blood pressure. Evidence from chronic renal homografts in rats with opposite predispositions to hypertension. Circulation Report 40: 94–101

Dustan H P 1983 Nutrition and hypertension. Annals of Internal Medicine 98: 660–662

Farquhar J W, Wood P D, Haskell W L, Williams P, Fortmann S P 1978 Relationship of urinary sodium/potassium ratio to systolic blood pressure: The Stamford Three Communities Study. Abstract 18th Conference of Cardiovascular Disease Epidemiology, Dallas. CVD Epidemiology Newsletter No. 25 American Heart Association

Freiman J A, Chalmers T C, Smith H, Kuebler R R 1978 The importance of beta, the type II error and sample size in the design and interpretation of the randomised control trial. Survey of 71 'negative' trials. New England Journal of Medicine 299: 690–694

Friedman R, Iwai J 1977 Dietary sodium, psychic stress and genetic predisposition to experimental hypertension. Proceedings of the Society of Experimental Biology and Medicine 155: 449–452

Gleiberman L 1973 Blood pressure and dietary salt in human populations. Ecology of Food and Nutrition 2: 143–156

Health Education Council 1983 Proposals for nutritional guidelines for health education in Britain: a consultative document prepared for the National Advisory Committee on Health and Nutrition Education

Hofman A, Hazebrock A, Valkenburg H A 1983 A randomized trial of sodium intake and blood pressure in newborn infants. Journal of the American Medical Association 250: 370–373

Iacono J M, Marshall M W, Dougherty R M, Wheeler M A, Mackin J F, Canary J J 1975 Reduction in blood pressure associated with high polyunsaturated fat diets that reduce blood cholesterol in man. Preventive Medicine 4: 426–443

Joossens J V, Geboers J 1983 Salt and hypertension. Preventive Medicine 12: 53–59

Joossens J V, Williams J, Claessens J, Class J, Lissens W 1970 Sodium and hypertension. In: Nutrition and cardiovascular disease. Proceedings of 7th International Meeting of Centro Studi Lipidi Alimentaria Biologia e Clinica Delta Nutrisione. Rimini. Fondazione Sasso 91–110

Kannel W B, Gordon T, Dawber T R 1974 Role of lipids in the development of brain infarction: the Framingham study. Stroke 5: 679–685

Knipschild P 1977 Medical effects of aircraft noise: Community Cardiovascular Survey. International Archives of Occupational and Environmental Health 40: 185–190

Lancet Editorial 1982 Cells, ions and blood pressure. Lancet ii: 965–967

Lever A F, Beretta-Piccoli C, Brown J J, Davies D L, Fraser R, Robinson J I S 1981 Sodium and potassium in essential hypertension. British Medical Journal 283: 463–468

Liu K, Cooper R, McKeever P, Byington R, Soltero I, Stamler R, Gosch F, Stevens E, Stamler J 1979 Assessment of the association between habitual salt intake and high blood pressure: methodological problems. American Journal of Epidemiology 110: 219–226

Liu K, Stamler J, Dyer A 1978 Statistical methods to assess and minimize the role of intra-individual variability in obscuring the relationships between dietary lipids and serum cholesterol. Journal of Chronic Diseases 31: 399–418

Malhotra S L 1970 Dietary factors causing hypertension in India. American Journal of Clinical Nutrition 23: 1353–1363

Meneely G R, Ball C O T, Youmans J B 1957 Chronic sodium chloride toxicity: the protective effect of added potassium chloride. Annals of Internal Medicine 47: 263–273

Meneely G R, Battarbee H D 1976 High sodium, low potassium environment and hypertension. American Journal of Cardiology 38: 768–785

Miall W E 1959 Follow-up study of arterial pressure in a population of a Welsh mining valley. British Medical Journal ii: 1205–1210

Oliver W J, Cohen E L, Neel J V 1975 Blood pressure, sodium intake and sodium related hormones in the Yanomamo Indians, a 'no salt' culture. Circulation 52: 146–151

Oxfordshire Community Stroke Project 1983 Incidence of stroke in Oxfordshire: first year's experience of a community stroke register. British Medical Journal 287: 713–717

Pietinen P I, Wong O, Altschul A M 1979 Electrolyte output, blood pressure, and family history of hypertension. American Journal of Clinical Nutrition 32: 997–1005

Sasaki N 1962 High blood pressure and the salt intake of the Japanese. Japanese Heart Journal 3: 313–324

Shaper A G, Leonard P J, Jones K W, Jones M 1969 Environmental effects on the body build, blood pressure and blood chemistry of nomadic warriors serving in the army in Kenya. East African Medical Journal 46: 282–289

Simmons D 1983 Blood pressure, ethnic group and salt intake in Belize. Journal of Epidemiology and Community Health 37: 38–42

Skrabal F, Aubock J, Hortnagl H 1981 Low sodium/high potassium diet for prevention of hypertension: probable mechanisms of action. Lancet ii: 1293

Srinivasan S R, Berenson G S, Radhakrishnamurthy B, Dalferes E R, Underwood D, Foster T A 1980 Effects of dietary sodium and sucrose on the induction of hypertension in spider monkeys. American Journal of Clinical Nutrition 33: 561–569

Tunstall Pedoe H 1983 Stroke. In: Epidemiology of Diseases Ed. Miller D L and Farmer R D T. Blackwell 136–145

Tuomilehto J, Puska P, Tanskanen A, Karppanen H, Pietinen P, Nissinen A, Enlund H, Rustsalainen P 1981 A community-based intervention study on the feasibility and effects of the reduction of salt intake in North Karelia, Finland. Acta Cardiologica 36: 83–104

Verlangieri A J, Stevens J W 1979 L-Ascorbic acid: effects on aortic glycosaminoglycan 35S incorporation in rabbit induced atherogenesis. Blood Vessels 16: 177–185

Watt G C M, Foy C J W 1982 Dietary sodium and arterial pressure: problems of studies within a single population. Journal of Epidemiology and Community Health 36: 197–201

Whyte H M 1958 Body fat and blood pressure of natives in New Guinea: reflection on essential hypertension. Australian Annals of Medicine 7: 36–46

8. Giving up smoking for life

John C. Catford   Martin C. Woolaway

INTRODUCTION

One of the few success stories in health promotion this decade in this country has been the dramatic decline in cigarette smoking. This fall is unprecedented in an international setting and is attributable to health education and health promotion in their widest sense (Royal College of Physicians, 1983). In 1972 there were approximately 19.5 million adult smokers in Great Britain but 10 years later this had fallen to 15 million (OPCS, 1983). The reasons are twofold — fewer people are starting to smoke and more people are giving up.

There are now about 10 million British people who at one time smoked but have now given up. Three million of these have given up smoking in the last 10 years. Not only will this change of behaviour have a major impact on the health of those individuals and their families, but also the nation will gain. The avoidance of an appreciable proportion of premature deaths and handicaps (for example from cancer, respiratory disease and heart and peripheral vascular disease) will have considerable financial benefits for the NHS and Industry (Wells, 1982; Elkan, 1982).

Since the publication of the first Royal College of Physicians report on smoking in 1962, doctors have been concerned with the smoking problem. However this interest has rarely been matched by a real commitment from within health authorities. Whilst some have formulated policies, often little action has been taken in practice. This led ASH (Action on Smoking and Health) to produce a model smoking plan for health authorities in 1981 (Olsen et al, 1981). At this time approximately £243 per head of total population was spent on health services per year of which no more than 12 pence per head was spent on all types of health promotion by NHS Health Education Units. In contrast the tobacco industry spent of the order of £2 per annum per man, woman and child on promoting the consumption of tobacco.

With recent advances in knowledge about giving up smoking, there is an urgent need for health authorities to reconsider their role in promoting smoking cessation. Community physicians can play an important part in these discussions both as senior officers of health authorities and as doctors charged with the protection and improvement of the public health.

This chapter first examines which groups of smokers have given up the habit and for what reasons. Why people smoke and why ex-smokers relapse are then considered. The final sections discuss how more smokers can be motivated to try to give up, how they can be helped in their attempt to give up, and how ex-smokers can be prevented from relapsing. Concluding remarks argue that there is now sufficient knowledge to mount, as one of the highest priorities, large scale smoking cessation programmes of various kinds in a co-ordinated and integrated way.

WHO IS GIVING UP SMOKING?

The majority of adults in Britain are now non-smokers. Information from the most recent General Household Survey (OPCS, 1983) shows that in 1982, 38% of men and 33% of women over the age of 16 were cigarette smokers. Table 8.1 gives the proportion of current smokers, ex-smokers and never-smokers for both sexes between the periods 1972 and 1982. There has been a steady decline amongst men who smoke cigarettes averaging 1.4% per annum. Amongst women who smoked less than men the decline was 0.8% per annum. However between 1980 and 1982 both sexes experienced a dramatic 2% drop in smoking prevalence. Sales of cigarettes have also declined over this period after a peak in 1973/1974. By 1982 sales had fallen to 102 000 million, a decline of 26%. Between 1978 and 1982 sales fell by almost 20%.

Table 8.1   Percentage of current, ex- and never-smokers of cigarettes by sex amongst adults (16 years and over) in Great Britain 1972–1982

	Men			Women		
Year	Current smokers	Ex-smokers	Never smokers	Current smokers	Ex-smokers	Never smokers
1972	52	23	25	41	10	49
1974	51	23	25	41	11	49
1976	46	27	27	38	12	50
1978	45	27	29	37	14	49
1980	42	28	30	37	14	49
1982	38	30	32	33	16	51

Source: General Household Survey (OPCS, 1983).

The 1982 survey showed that smokers are now in the minority in every social group including male unskilled manual workers. However there remain large social class differences in smoking behaviour, as shown in Table 8.2. The ratio of the proportion of smokers in professional groups compared to unskilled manual groups is 1 : 2.5 for men, and 1 : 2 for women. Whilst a decline in most social groups for both sexes has been observed, this is not the case for women in the unskilled manual group. Here the proportion remains at about the same level as a decade previously.

When analysed by age, there has been a fall in prevalence of smokers in all age groups as shown in Table 8.3. An exception to this trend appears to be in young women aged 20–24 where a more detailed analysis shows that between 1980 and 1982 the proportion of smokers remained at 40%. It is clear then that in terms of smoking policy younger women and particularly those in social classes IV and V are an important target group.

Table 8.2   Prevalence of cigarette smoking by sex and socio-economic group amongst adults (16 years and over) in Great Britain 1972–1982

Socio-economic group		Percentage smoking cigarettes					
		1972	1974	1976	1978	1980	1982
Professional	male	33	29	25	25	21	20
	female	33	25	28	23	21	21
Unskilled	male	64	61	58	60	57	49
Manual	female	42	43	38	41	41	41

Source: General Household Survey (OPCS, 1983).

Table 8.3 Percentage of current, ex- and never-smokers of cigarettes by age amongst adults (16 years and over) in Great Britain 1972, 1982

Age Group	Year	Men Current Smokers	Ex-smokers	Never smokers	Women Current smokers	Ex-smokers	Never smokers
16–24	1972	49	7	44	44	6	50
	1982	36	7	57	35	8	57
25–34	1972	56	17	27	49	10	41
	1982	40	20	39	37	15	48
35–49	1972	55	23	22	48	11	41
	1982	40	32	28	38	15	47
50+	1972	50	33	17	33	10	57
	1982	36	44	20	29	20	52

Source: General Household Survey (OPCS, 1983).

A fall in smoking prevalence could be due to more smokers giving up (demonstrated by an increase in ex-smokers) or to fewer people starting to smoke (demonstrated by an increase in never-smokers). It can be seen from Table 8.1 that the proportion of ex-smokers and never-smokers have both risen over time indicating that both factors are operating. With men both contributions are about equal, but for women the rise in the percentage of ex-smokers has been far more significant than that of the never-smokers.

Analysis within the various age groups reveals that in all age groups in both sexes more people are both giving up and not starting than previously. The increase in those not starting to smoke are more amongst men than women, and more amongst younger people than older people. The increase in those giving up smoking are slightly more amongst men than women, but more amongst older people than young people. The difference between the sexes is likely to be largely attributable to the higher prevalence of smoking amongst men since there is more room for improvement. This may also be true for the older age groups.

However the most impressive finding is that a substantial proportion of older smokers can give up smoking. For example, in 1972 amongst men aged 35–49 55% were current smokers and 23% were ex-smokers. The same cohort when examined 10 years later comprised only 41% current smokers and 37% ex-smokers (OPCS, 1982). Thus a quarter of the smokers had given up, demonstrating the potential for action directed towards older smokers.

WHY DO PEOPLE SMOKE?

An understanding of why people start and continue to smoke is clearly important in framing policies for smoking control. Models seeking to explain smoking behaviour attempt to incorporate many influences acting throughout a complex process and not surprisingly no single explanation is entirely satisfactory.

A striking feature of the smoking story is the wide geographic variation in the prevalence of smoking and the consumption of tobacco per smoker (Cox & Marks, 1983). Table 8.4 describes prevalence data for 10 developed countries. The percentage of men smoking ranged from 73% (Japan) to 26% (Sweden) and for women from 37% (UK) to 15% (Japan). Given these differences and the wide availability of

Table 8.4 International comparisons of the prevalence of cigarette smoking amongst adults

Country	Date of survey	Percentage smoking cigarettes	
		male	female
Australia	1980	40	31
Austria	1981	33	22
Canada	1979	39	30
Finland	1981	36	19
W. Germany	1979	41	28
Japan	1979	73	15
New Zealand	1976	38	31
Sweden	1980	26	26
UK	1980	42	37
USA	1980	37	29

Source: Cox & Marks 1983.

cigarettes in these countries it would seem unlikely that smoking is an innate behaviour. Rather it appears that it is determined by the interplay of many factors.

When considering these influences, it is useful to divide the smoking 'career' into two stages, as the factors which initiate smoking are distinct from those which maintain it. The principal factors acting on the novice are the powerful psychosocial pressures from peer group and family influences. Low self esteem and poor achievement at school are both positively correlated to smoking behaviour in the young (Bynner, 1969; Bewley et al, 1973). Some may get sensorimotor rewards from handling, sucking and playing with cigarettes, while a few may have an indulgent motive, finding the taste of cigarette smoke pleasant (Russell et al, 1974). However, the majority when starting will experience physical side effects such as nausea, cramps and coughing. Despite these drawbacks the young experimenter will often persist under pressure from his peers. The aggressive, commercial marketing of the tobacco companies, commonly presenting an image of the smoker as mature, attractive and successful, reinforces and exploits those with feelings of low 'self-esteem'. However, it is still by no means clear why some children succumb to these influences whilst others do not.

As smoking behaviour becomes established, most explanatory models place increasing emphasis on the pharmacological and psychological effects of nicotine, in providing the basic motivation to smoke. This is viewed in two main ways. The addiction or dependence model sees the desire for nicotine as the need to prevent the aversive effects of nicotine withdrawal (Russell, 1971). The 'psychological tool' view differs in that it sees smoking as being rewarding in its own right, the smoker attempting to control mood through the stimulant and sedatory actions of nicotine within the central nervous system (Ashton & Stepney, 1982). It has been argued that smoking then becomes a learned dependence and is commonly acquired during adolescence with other learned behaviours (Marsh & Matheson, 1983). The importance of this is that it should be possible to 'unlearn' the smoking behaviour.

Although nicotine dependence, both physical and psychological, clearly plays a part in smoking behaviour, its relative importance is controversial (Raw, 1978). A straightforward addiction model fails to explain satisfactorily the absence of withdrawal symptoms in some abstainers, or why some smokers refrain from smoking for prolonged periods for practical or social reasons without apparent hardship. A large study of attitudes in some 2667 smokers and 1092 non-smokers and ex-smokers has recently been carried out on behalf of the DHSS and OPCS (Marsh & Matheson, 1983). In this survey 53% of ex-smokers reported that it was 'not at all difficult' to give up. Perhaps more interestingly 41% of ex-smokers recalled stopping as actually being easier than they expected. Giving up smoking certainly becomes harder as consumption increases. Of those smoking ten a day or less, three-quarters reported that they found it 'not at all difficult'. However, even among those giving up 30 cigarettes a day or more, 47% reported little difficulty. On the basis of an addiction model this level of consumption would be expected to produce unpleasant withdrawal symptoms.

More recent models of smoking behaviour have attempted to move away from a narrow behaviouristic approach, to recognise the wider social and economic influences in individual choice. Smokers are viewed as rational beings making a series of reasoned choices with both positive and negative consequences (Eiser & Sutton, 1977). This avoidance of placing the smoker in the 'sick role' and regarding the behaviour as a reasoned response to a set of prevailing circumstances both external and internal, has important implications for approaches to smoking cessation.

People may be continuing to smoke principally as a perceived response to the stress provoked by social and economic factors often beyond their influence. If this is true then policy aimed at helping people stop could be directed at providing alternative coping mechanisms or attempts to resolve the origins of stress. Some approaches to cessation now concentrate on the promotion of coping skills through experiential learning techniques particularly in self help groups such as Wessex's Operation Smokestop (Wessex Positive Health Team, 1982). The importance of social support in improving the chances of smoking withdrawal suggests that the social elements have been undervalued.

However, the overall importance of stress in initiating smoking is probably only minor; Marsh & Matheson (1983) found that high stress in smokers was no barrier to the resolve to give up. In certain circumstances a high level of stress, coupled with a reasonable sense of optimism for success in giving up actually increased the desire to quit. Nevertheless among the general public there is a widely held view, no matter how misplaced, that smoking is an understandable response to the stress of modern day life. To understand the origin of this belief, it is important to consider commercial influences and the politics of tobacco (Taylor, 1984).

The international tobacco industry is a multi-billion dollar business. In 1981 £5553 million was spent on buying tobacco in the UK (Social Trends, 1983). If the 15 million smokers in Great Britain were to decrease consumption by just one cigarette per day, expenditure on tobacco would drop by at least £250 million per year. It is not surprising therefore that tobacco interests pervade all levels of society, and the industry spends in excess of £100 million per year on advertising, sports and arts sponsorship, etc. Whilst accepting that many people think smoking is helpful in coping with stress, Cowley (1983) considers that the effect is chiefly a placebo one, 'the greatest con of the century'. He believes that by debunking the myth and restricting the promotion of tobacco considerably more people will not start smoking and many more will give up. Recent experience in Australia seems to bear this out.

In summary, a number of factors appear to influence the occurrence and maintenance of smoking. Physical and psychological dependence on nicotine is likely to be of relevance in the heavier smokers, but is not now considered to be the major force in the majority of smokers. Rather, smoking behaviour needs to be viewed in a wider context, as much an outcome of decision making as of habit. Attitudes, beliefs and values are clearly important and these explain why smoking behaviour is subject to change and large geographic and demographic variation.

WHY DO PEOPLE DECIDE TO STOP SMOKING?

Regular smokers have a very ambivalent attitude towards their habit. The Marsh & Matheson survey (1983) found that 70% of all current smokers have made at least one attempt to stop and half of these have made at least three attempts. Even amongst the youngest smokers 65% showed the same history of attempts to give up. Self-reported explanations for stopping need to be considered cautiously as reasons given with hindsight can be clouded by self justification and lack of insight. However there appear to be three main explanations — health reasons, economic reasons and social reasons.

In the above OPCS survey, 37% of smokers who had stopped gave expense as one of their reasons, 39% indicating that the presence of current illness, especially respiratory infections was partly responsible. A collection of social pressures, which centred on the influence of close friends and relatives, self perception and personal resolution, accounted for action in 38% of smokers. A fifth also consistently gave fear of future illness as a reason for trying to give up. About 10% of women gave pregnancy as their reason. No particular reason was associated more with success than any other. Those trying and those succeeding all gave the same ratio of expense, current illness and health fears, and social factors as reasons for stopping. However the complex processes which ultimately provide the motivation to stop are not likely to be determined solely through relatively superficial responses to survey questions. This is a still largely unresearched field.

An important influence in the desire to give up was the sense of achievement and respect from others. Thirty per cent of smokers said that they smoked without really enjoying it and there was very widespread expectation of greater self-esteem amongst smokers if they succeeded in giving up. However, many smokers were concerned about the supposed disadvantages of giving up (e.g. fewer feelings of wellbeing and more of depression and anxiety; and weight gain). These are largely unfounded as the study of ex-smokers showed. Only 6% felt ill-tempered after stopping and only 6% mentioned putting on weight. Confidence in the ability to stop did not have a bearing on the desire to stop.

The health professions justify their interest in promoting the avoidance of smoking on health grounds, although they may use the economic and social aspects to strengthen the effectiveness of programmes. Provision of information about the risks of smoking is mandatory in stop-smoking programmes so that people can make informed decisions about their lifestyles. Comparisons of the Marsh and Matheson survey (1983) with an earlier survey by McKennel & Thomas (1967) shows that over the period 1964–1981 smokers have become increasingly aware of the health risks. Smokers' acceptance of the general risk of heart disease has grown from about one-fifth to over half and for lung cancer from half to two-thirds. However many smokers consider that only the very heavy smokers are vulnerable, and do not consider themselves at risk. In 1981 only 14% of smokers thought that heart disease was more likely among smokers as a whole than non-smokers, and for lung cancer the proportion was 11%. However, there is almost universal acceptance among smokers and non-smokers that common respiratory problems are more likely in smokers.

Although a person may believe that smoking is harmful to health, his or her smoking decisions are not altered unless the individual accepts that to smoke is harmful to his or her own personal health (Ajzen & Fishbein, 1980). It would seem that what smokers believe about the probability of health problems in others often has little to do with their beliefs about their own behaviour. It is interesting to note here that several past surveys of the attitudes and behaviour of medical students, who might be expected to be well informed on health risks, were not markedly affected by health knowledge (Bynner, 1967; Knopf & Wakefield, 1974).

Many things in life are dangerous but few people, it seems, realise that smoking is *so* dangerous. The vast majority of smokers do not believe that the level at which they smoke is at all harmful, or that smokers would do themselves much good by giving up. Although most smokers appreciate that there are dangers associated with smoking, very few have a clear idea of the relative size of these risks, or the benefits to be gained by stopping. This needs to be remedied. As Peto has pointed out, we must transmit clear and comprehensible facts about the risks involved. 'Out of 1000 young smokers, one will be murdered, six will be killed on the roads and 250 will be killed before their time from smoking' (Peto, 1983).

WHY DO EX-SMOKERS RELAPSE?

It is essential that smoking cessation is viewed as a process of both stopping and maintaining abstinence. Many cessation techniques obtain high cessation rates but these changes often tend to be short-lived. The key difficulty is to sustain the behaviour change. Russell (1980) has suggested a two-dimensional model for smoking cessation. Outcome is related to the level of motivation generated and the degree of dependence that has to be overcome. He considers that inadequate attention to the latter is the reason why so many smokers fail in their attempts and relapse.

Hunt et al (1971) reviewed 87 studies which had used a wide range of cessation techniques and found a characteristic relapse pattern. Immediately following the end of an intervention, a steep fall in the proportion abstaining occurs. At three months only 35% of quitters are still abstinent and at six months months only 25%. The relapse rate then slows with some 5% falling away over the second six months leaving approximately 20% remaining abstinent at one year. A one year abstention is usually accepted as defining an ex-smoker for evaluation purposes. Such a set of results can be regarded as being well in excess of the spontaneous cessation rate.

It is difficult to determine precisely what represents the 'background' cessation rate. In one study of the effectiveness of general practitioners anti-smoking advice, the natural long term cessation rate in the non-intervention group was only 0.3% (Russell et al, 1979). Comparisons with, for example, self help approaches are difficult because undoubtedly the composition of populations of smokers who elect to give up in different ways varies. Withdrawal clinic or group attenders are in general more highly motivated but probably heavier, more dependent smokers. There is a scarcity of information about the 95% of smokers who try and sometimes succeed in stopping on their own.

A number of individual studies have suggested that men find it easier to give up smoking than women (Burns, 1969). However, in a large review of over 30 studies, Gritz (1978) concluded that in the majority of cases the male – female cessation rate differences were non-significant. However, where differences did occur men were consistently more successful than women.

Previous smoking history consistently predicts for success in smoking cessation. Those who succeed in stopping tend on average to have smoked fewer cigarettes (Gordon et al, 1974), to have smoked for a shorter time and are less likely to have inhaled (Friedman et al, 1979). This fits with Russell's belief that the more dependent heavy smoker is not receiving adequate support to combat the addictive element.

Several studies have linked success in stopping to the personality of the smoker. A greater measure of extraversion and emotional stability predicts for continued abstinence (Cherry & Kiernan, 1976). Several studies have linked relapse to feelings of frustration, anxiety and sadness and report the use of smoking behaviour to control 'negative affect' (Marlatt & Gordon, 1980). A greater frequency of 'negative affect' smoking was reported among women (Ikard et al, 1969) suggesting that cigarettes are being used more by women in an attempt to control mood and combat feelings of anger and anxiety.

However, the thesis that women smokers are tied to the smoking habit by the stresses and conflicts of modern domestic and working life (Jacobson, 1981) is not supported by recent self reported attitude data (Marsh & Matheson, 1983). Although women certainly scored higher on the stress scale than men (especially those groups of female manual workers who smoke heavily), higher levels of stress were associated with a greater resolve to give up smoking. If anything, more highly stressed women are more likely to be intending quitters than are highly stressed men. Of course, a reported intention does not mean an attempt to stop let alone a success in stopping, but the number of attempts does in general correlate to eventual success. Successful quitters are also reported to have more higher education and to consume less coffee and alcohol (Friedman et al, 1979).

The question of where and when a relapse might occur has been considered in several studies (Lichtenstein et al, 1977; Marlatt & Gordon, 1980). An important pattern which has emerged from the Lichtenstein survey is the importance of social environment in relapse. Other people are usually present (83%), they are often smoking (62%) and they are often the source of the cigarette. Alcohol consumption frequently precedes relapse. The importance of social support in maintaining abstinence is further suggested by the finding that the presence of a smoking spouse is related to relapse following intervention programmes (West et al, 1977).

Ultimate success in quitting is, not surprisingly, also found to be related to insight, self-esteem and confidence, and the extent to which individuals feel they are able to control and be responsible for changes in their lives (Condiotte & Lichtenstein, 1981). Feelings of frustration, anger, anxiety and depression often precede relapse and certain social settings favour recidivism. Those highly dependent on nicotine are particularly vulnerable unless a nicotine substitute is used. Cessation methods should try to develop the behavioural and cognitive skills required to cope with the precursors of relapse and to teach recognition of those social situations in which relapse is most likely.

HOW CAN SMOKERS BE MOTIVATED TO TRY TO STOP?

More positive attitudes towards the benefits of giving up smoking lead more smokers first to resolve and then to attempt to give up. Marsh & Matheson (1983) concluded from their large study of smokers and non-smokers that the attitudes most effective in this process concern the likelihood of positive health benefits from giving up. Those concerned with money and greater self-esteem are also effective. They found that, when these attitudes in smokers are combined with (i) a higher level of personal stress, (ii) some confidence in their likely success in giving up and (iii) the belief that they will not suffer too much emotional unease as a result, then the process is accelerated. Neither stress nor a record of past failure inhibits the resolve to give up but actually increases the likelihood that further attempts will be made.

Programmes using one or a combination of motivating forces leading to more positive attitudes can be personalised at the level of the individual. An example would be the doctor's straightforward advice to a patient about the benefits of stopping smoking. Alternatively action can be focused on groups of individuals or communities using mass media approaches, such as television, radio, newspapers, posters and leaflets. Such initiatives cannot be tailored in the same way as one to one contact. The decision to try to stop is ultimately made by an individual on the basis of available information, attitude and beliefs.

Educational approaches can be directive (e.g. 'In the interests of your health, stop smoking') — or non-directive (e.g. 'Here are the facts for and against smoking, it is up to you to decide what to do'). If there were no pressures to smoke or to continue smoking then the task of educators should on ethical grounds concern the latter; that is to give 'value-free' information about smoking and to devlop adequate decision-making skills so that individuals can make rational decisions about their health. This is clearly not the case in this country, as in addition to the addictive aspects of smoking there are still considerable social and commercial pressures which encourage smoking (Royal College of Physicians, 1983).

Many health promoters consider, therefore, that it is perfectly permissible to use a combination of approaches including directive means within smoking programmes. 'Value-fair' and 'value-laden' information, it is argued, will help to neutralise the propaganda methods used to promote smoking by the tobacco industry and other interested groups.

Mass media initiatives

The mass media, particularly television, are attractive to health educators and health promoters because of the efficiency and relative cheapness with which they can reach huge audiences. The earlier anti-smoking campaigns in the UK attempted principally to publicise the dangers of smoking and to create anti-smoking attitudes. In general they achieved an increase in the awareness of the health messages but little change in attitudes to smoking or smoking behaviour (Health Education Council, 1972).

The fact that so many smokers try several times to give up and that many dissonant smokers already have anti-smoking attitudes (Marsh & Matheson, 1983) suggests that the problem is not whether to stop but how to stop. In response to one single Granada TV's 'Reports Action' programme broadcast in 1977 which offered viewers a free anti-smoking kit some 500 000 people asked for the kit. This would seem to indicate that large numbers of people were motivated at least into asking for advice on how to stop (Raw & van der Plight, 1981).

In the United States better results have been reported. The more aggressive use of anti-smoking commercials over the period 1968–1970 has been estimated to have reduced US cigarette consumption by 17%. Warner (1977) argues that the cummulative effect of persistent publicity, supported by other public policies, held down the 1975 levels of consumption by 20 to 30%.

Failure of some mass media campaigns (Eiser et al, 1978; Raw & van der Plight, 1981) to achieve a sustained decline in cigarette smoking may be attributable not to the fact that they failed to motivate but that they failed to offer appropriate support in giving up. The more successful programmes using mass media usually have a community component, whereby personal help is available to those giving up, e.g. counselling from doctors, stop-smoking groups etc. The use of television in several of the community based heart disease prevention programmes has been found to have contributed to their success, e.g. the Stanford Heart Disease Prevention Programme (Farquhar et al, 1977) and the North Karelia project (Puska et al, 1979). In the Stanford study, two years after a combined media and community programme there was a net 5.5% reduction in smokers in the study town when compared to the control town.

More impressive results have recently been reported from South Australia (Cowley, 1983) and New South Wales, Australia (Egger et al, 1983). In the latter study a control town was compared with two neighbouring towns; one had been exposed to an anti-smoking mass media campaign, and the other to the campaign plus simultaneous supportive community programmes. Sophisticated marketing techniques were used which appealed to smokers 'emotional' fears about smoking. Two years after baseline measurements had been performed, the prevalence of smoking dropped in the control town by 2–5%, in the media only town by 6–11%, and in the media and community programme town by 6–15%. The differences were statistically significant, demonstrating that the appropriate use of the media can as well as motivating smokers to stop, actually achieve cessation in an appreciable number.

Despite the evidence from overseas, the role of the media remains controversial in this country (McCron & Budd, 1979). However, it is suggested that the reason, that mass media interventions in smoking have not been found to be particularly successful in the UK, is more a result of inappropriate design, delivery, and lack of integration with supporting programmes, rather than an inherent problem of efficacy.

Counselling by health professionals

There is a range of opportunities for health professionals such as doctors, nurses and health education officers to give advice on the importance of stopping smoking. Those already suffering the consequences of smoking, e.g. heart disease, are particularly susceptible to counselling (Croog & Richards, 1977). Raw (1976) found that advice to stop and simple information from a chest physician achieved a higher percentage reduction (39%) in smoking at 3 month follow up than those not receiving instructions.

In the study by Rose & Hamilton (1978), a group of men at high cardiorespiratory risk were randomly assigned to 'normal care' (control) or intervention group. The latter received advice on smoking risks and two information booklets on why and how to stop, together with follow-up consultations. Three years after screening, abstinence rates were 35.5% for the intervention group and 14.5% for the normal care/control group. At the 10 year follow up, the intervention group mortality was 18% lower than the control group from coronary heart disease and 23% lower from lung cancer (Rose et al, 1982).

Other studies have looked at the role of the general practitioner and the results have been mixed. In a randomised control trial, Porter & McLullough (1972) failed to show any differences with counselling after six months. However the intervention was of low input; the counselling was once only and consisted of smoking and disease information coupled with a leaflet. More favourable results have been reported in other studies (Russell et al; 1979, Handel, 1973). The Russell study showed that when GP's gave a simple but firm advice against smoking, together with a leaflet and warning of a follow-up, they achieved a one year success rate of 5.1% cessation compared with 0.3% in non-intervention controls. This activity might expect to yield approximately 25 long term abstainers per year per general practitioner. The potential effect of over 20 000 GPs acting in this way in Britain would be considerable. For example, if just 10% of GPs regularly advised their smoking patients to give up, there would be approximately 50 000 fewer smokers each year. But what activity do GPs take on smoking?

Jamrozik & Fowler (1982) reported that although 80% of smokers claimed that they would stop if advised to by their general practitioners, only 10% had been so advised. In their larger study Marsh & Matheson (1983) found that one-third of smokers had been encouraged by their doctors to stop smoking, and of these 57% had tried to do so. Of those smokers not advised to give up, 89% said that they would try to stop if encouraged. Older smokers and women smokers were more willing than others to follow such advice.

A recent survey in Wessex asked a random sample of 214 general practitioners to report on attitudes and behaviour to preventive medicine practice. Eighty-six per cent saw it as their role to discourage patients from smoking (Catford & Nutbeam, 1984). As regards the kind of help that would be offered to smokers, 65% would themselves offer 'specific' advice and 70% would prescribe nicotine chewing gum. Only 13% reported using the Health Education Council 'Give up Smoking' pack. Some 18% would refer patients to stop smoking groups but this must to a large extent reflect their availability in the area.

It is clear then that health professionals and particularly doctors, have an important role to play in counselling and motivating people to try to give up. Any smoking cessation programme must therefore consider the best way of utilising this potential.

Social and economic measures

In addition to specific mass media initiatives and advice from health professionals, there are other ways that smokers can be motivated. Life events, such as pregnancy, parenthood, a new relationship with a non-smoking partner or a change of working environment can precipitate action. Seasonal influences may operate, e.g. New Year's resolution, family holiday or National Don't Smoke Day. In New South Wales, Egger et al (1983), report that pressures from families and friends accounted for 13–15% of cessation attempts.

The cost of smoking is often given as a reason for stopping smoking (McKennell & Thomas, 1967; Marsh & Matheson, 1983), and in practice as prices go up, consumption falls and vice versa (Russell, 1973; Peto, 1974). As a consequence increased taxation is a measure widely proposed to reduce the habit (Royal College of Physicians, 1983). The tax on tabacco has always been high and at present the combination of tax and VAT account for almost two-thirds of the cost of a packet of cigarettes. However, despite substantial increases in tax, price rises have been less than increases in the retail price index (Atkinson & Townsend, 1977).

The elasticity of demand for a product is the percentage change in consumption that results from a 1% change in price. Estimates of the elasticity in demand for tobacco have varied widely from 0.12–0.65. These variations arise from differences in the other factors which are introduced to explain consumption and the econometric methods of estimation. Atkinson & Townsend (1977) considered that a price increase of around 56% would produce a fall of about 20%. They also argued that there might be disadvantages to massive price increases. As smoking is highly related to socio-economic status, the tax burden of substantial increases would fall heaviest on the low income groups who are the heaviest smokers. For heavy smokers unable to respond because of dependency, extra expenditure on cigarettes would cause hardship to the smoker and his family.

The view that increased tobacco taxation is regressive has recently been disputed and in fact the contrary case has been put forward. Over the last 20 to 30 years, as taxation has not kept pace with inflation cigarette prices have fallen relative to other goods. Townsend (1983) has argued that lower income groups have proved responsive to these changes and have increased their smoking levels. However, over the last two years there have been real price increases, which although not restoring prices to the levels of the 1950s, have greatly reduced working class smoking levels.

Although the total cost of smoking is certainly a motivating factor in producing the desire to stop, sudden increases in price do provide the catalyst to try to stop. The generally observed response to a rise in cigarette prices is an initial abrupt fall in total consumption. This comprises both an increase in cessation attempts as well as reduction in consumption per smoker. Rather than small piece-meal rises in tobacco taxes, it would be more effective if the Exchequer imposed infrequent large lump-sum increases in the interests of the public health. This would be with the proviso that they at least kept in line with increases in either disposable income or the retail price index, whichever brings about the greatest price rise.

HOW CAN SMOKERS BE HELPED IN THEIR ATTEMPTS TO GIVE UP?

About half of all smokers want and are resolved to try to give up. A whole range of approaches have now been developed to assist them to stop. They range from do-it-yourself instruction books to specific medical treatments, from television programmes to self-help groups. The West Midlands Health Authority have recently published (1982) a whole series of summary case-studies, presented in a humorous vein. The booklet demonstrates the wide range of options available. This section will discuss the principle approaches and present the results of evaluations where available. However, it should be emphasised that the majority of smokers that stop do so without outside help. In the New South Wales 'Quit for Life' programme, 88–99% of smokers quit by stopping suddenly or by slowly reducing without external help of any sort (Egger et al, 1983). A large American study reported that 95% stop without the aid of an organised cessation programme (US Department of Health, Education and Welfare, 1977). Marsh & Matheson (1983) also found that most ex-smokers gave up alone, 21% in concert with a spouse or friend.

Smokers interested in stopping often ask whether they should gradually reduce the number of cigarettes (tapering) or attempt to stop abruptly ('cold turkey'). Advice in this area is particularly important. It is necessary to distinguish between gradual reduction as an end in itself and as a preparation for total cessation. Most heavy smokers find it extremely difficult to reduce their consumption of cigarettes to less than about 10 per day. This is because, as the number of cigarettes smoked per day decreases, the reinforcing value of each remaining cigarette increases (Levinson, 1971). As tapering down occurs the total smoke intake does not necessarily decrease as inhalation per cigarette may increase to compensate. Furthermore, a reduction in the amount smoked is very difficult to maintain, and smokers who attempt to continue smoking, but at a reduced level, usually relapse back to their original levels (Dubren, 1977a). Similarly, prolonged tapering methods over two weeks generally tend to undermine the resolve to quit and merely increase the tendency to procrastinate. Thus a brief period of gradual reduction of about a week followed by abrupt and total cessation appears to be the best approach to stopping (Wynder & Hoffman, 1979). Tapering down is thus, at best, a preparation strategy (Flaxman, 1978).

Self-help leaflets and books
Approaches that encourage self-help are attractive because most smokers favour a procedure which they can use on their own and that does not require participation in an organised programme (Schwartz & Dubitzky, 1967). Furthermore, in practical terms, self-help approaches are much more likely to influence larger numbers of people than labour intensive specific individual or group interventions. For example if withdrawal clinics were the only means available, over one million clinics would be required to meet the needs of the 15 million smokers in the UK.

There are a variety of pamphlets, manuals and kits designed to help the individual through the stages of giving up. Evaluation of their effectiveness in isolation is sparse, but there have been some encouraging results reported. For example, Glasgow et al (1981), found a cessation rate of 7% at six month follow-up amongst a group of 41 heavy smokers given self-help literature. More recently in the New South Wales 'Quit for Life' programme there was a 17% abstinence rate at three months amongst 1500 smokers who had requested 'Quit' kits (Egger et al, 1983). However, some reviews suggest that when self-help manuals are used without guidance or appreciable input from a clinician or other leader, success is poor.

Self-help mass media programmes
A useful form of self-help assistance might be provided through use of the media, particularly television and radio. During 1981–1982 BBC Television broadcast on several occasions a series of six programmes, designed to support cessation attempts, entitled 'So you want to stop smoking'. The one year follow-up did not demonstrate a

measurable difference in the proportions smoking between viewers and non-viewers. However, many smokers who were trying to give up during this period had watched the series and were not smoking at the time of the one year follow-up survey. Dyer (1983) found that 65 000 smokers in Britain gave up at the time of the series and of these some 38 000 attributed their giving up at least partly to the series.

However, it cannot be emphasised too strongly that successful giving up usually requires motivation, initial help or advice on how best to stop, and longer term support. Interventions which offer only one of the stages are at a considerable disadvantage. Had there been for example a simultaneous initiative to motivate smokers to try to give up, linked to the parallel development of supportive community programmes, the results of the BBC series might have been much improved. It may be that future initiatives of this kind could best be operated on a more manageable regional basis. They might well then mirror the successful Stanford and North Karelia integrated smoking control programmes, mentioned earlier (Farquhar et al, 1977; Puska et al, 1979). Nevertheless, it is clear that self-help mass media programmes can be helpful in an integrated and comprehensive strategy.

General support from health professionals
In addition to motivating smokers to stop, health professionals can give general advice and support during the process of giving up. The Health Education Council has developed a 'Give Up Smoking' (GUS) pack for use by general practitioners. As well as providing instruction leaflets for the smoker, practice receptionist and general practitioner, regular follow-up of progress is recommended.

In Scotland when the GUS packs were first introduced considerable interest was shown by general practitioners. Some 25% requested further supplies of the pack on behalf of over 70% of all Scottish general practitioners (Ledwith, 1983). However, in Wessex the packs were used only by 13% of general practitioners (Catford & Nutbeam, 1984) but this may reflect inadequate promotion of the pack in England. In New South Wales, Egger (1983) reported a 48% abstinence rate amongst smokers who were supported by doctors using specially prepared kits. This method of intervention was found to be the most effective out of a range of community anti-smoking programmes and self-help approaches. The role of health professionals must therefore not be underestimated in smoking cessation programmes.

Specific treatment methods
A variety of specific techniques have been used to treat the dependent smoker. These include drug therapy, hypnosis, various types of aversion therapy, acupuncture and others. These treatments have been well reviewed by Raw (1978), however some brief comments will be made on their relative efficacy.

Broadly, drug treatments attempt either to treat withdrawal symptoms by use of a tranquilliser or to prevent the symptoms by substitution of nicotine (or the alkaloid lobeline which in some respects is pharmacologically similar). There is no evidence that tranquillisers can help people stop smoking. Several, including diazepam have been evaluated with negative results (Whitehead & Davies, 1964).

A recent review of the effectiveness of nicotine chewing gum has reported encouraging results (Raw, 1984). Abstinence rates at one year in 14 published studies ranged from 49% in a traditional clinic to 9% success in a general practice population.

In the studies where placebo controls were included, the treatment group consistently did better with only one exception — that of the British Thoracic Society. The average success rate for traditionally run clinic treatments using the gum was in the order of 35%. Clinic populations are clearly self-selected and biased towards the more dependent but motivated smoker; however, these results must be regarded as promising.

In the study by the British Thoracic Society (1983) nicotine gum failed to increase the success rate over either advice (with or without a supporting booklet) or placebo gum, in patients attending hospital with smoking related diseases. On average hospital physicians were able to encourage almost 10% of such patients to stop. However the populations studied were not supported or motivated by a traditional clinic structure and this may partly explain the apparent ineffectiveness of the gum. Another study by Raw et al (1980) found that the use of the gum gave rise to lower blood nicotine levels averaging less than half that of smoking values. The results suggest that the gum is much safer than continuing to smoke even in those smokers with cardiovascular disease. However, two patients (3%) became addicted to the gum. In addition, many smokers have found that the gum has an unpleasant taste. Finally, it is argued that the gum is cost effective on the professional's time as it takes only a few minutes to prescribe, explain its use and to follow up progress. However its use as part of a lay-group therapy approach is to some extent limited as it is controlled as a prescribed drug. Nevertheless, the clear advantage to those offered nicotine gum as an adjunct to general practitioners' advice confirms its value in a primary care setting (Russell et al, 1983).

High success rates have been claimed for hypnosis, acupuncture and other techniques, but these have usually come from poorly designed studies. When subjected to careful experimental control, hypnosis has been shown to be no better than other techniques or non-specific placebo treatment (Perry & Mullen, 1975). Forms of aversion therapy have been the most used treatment approach. These have included either electric or covert aversion therapy, or, rapid smoking or satiation techniques, which use excessive cigarette smoke as the aversive stimulus. Again there is little evidence that these aversion therapies have a specific effect over and above the benefits of general advice, support and attention of health professionals (Raw, 1978).

In general, abstinence rates of the order of 15–25% at one year follow-up should be expected for the well established specific treatment methods. As these techniques are normally directed at the nicotine dependent smokers, they certainly have a place, if only a limited one, in smoking cessation strategies. This is because such heavy smokers are particularly likely to suffer ill health and many are unlikely to stop unaided. The use of nicotine chewing gum appears to be the best and most cost effective specific treatment available to date, although it has the practical limitation that it has to be prescribed by a doctor.

Group therapy

All specific treatment approaches have the difficulty of forcing smokers to accept a 'sick' role. Whilst this may be acceptable to some, millions of smokers in the UK clearly do not consider themselves 'ill'. This is demonstrated by the observation that there have been only modest demands from the public for anti-smoking 'treatments'. Taylor & Batten (1983) argue that whereas smoking now represents deviant behaviour, which can be overcome, the majority of smokers do not accept the principle of smoking as deviancy. Rather than casting smokers as either 'sick' or 'childish' (commonly done by health professionals) interventions should de-emphasise the deviant status of smoking behaviour and this it is argued will have a greater appeal to smokers. They suggest that the most promising avenue seems to be a group setting where smokers and non-smokers can share an understanding of their experiences, and learn how to respond to situations without the use of tobacco. There has therefore been much interest recently in the group therapy approach.

Smoking withdrawal group clinics are usually distinguished from treatment clinics by the fact that specific treatment methods if used, take second place to the dissemination of health information coupled with advice on how to give up. Group discussion and support is an important element (Bernstein & McAllister, 1976). Some of the earliest groups reported began to form in the mid-1950s in Sweden (Ejrup, 1960). In Britain after the first Royal College of Physicians' report in 1962, experimental anti-smoking group clinics began to develop mainly organised by hospital chest physicians. The predominant pattern was a weekly attendance for six or seven weeks for health education and support.

Despite the suggestion that there is a place for anti-smoking group clinics (Royal College of Physicians, 1962, 1977), they have never occupied an important position in UK smoking prevention policy. The situation has been different in North America where, in recent years, there have been over 1000 smoking cessation programmes (Schwartz, 1980). The influence of psychologists with an interest in learning theory has been particularly important there.

A recent survey by Raw & Heller (1983) showed that in 1982 there were some 56 group clinics in Britain and Northern Ireland, covering a population of about 15 million smokers. Each Health Region had at least one clinic but there were no clinics in Eire apart from the five day plan courses run by the Seventh Day Adventists. Almost two thirds of these clinics were run by health education officers, the remainder by doctors, clinical psychologists, community nurses and representatives of the Seventh Day Adventist Church. Most clinics were funded from NHS health education budgets, staff running the clinics as part of their normal duties.

The survey, however, did not include an innovative smoking cessation programme in Wessex (Wessex Positive Health Team, 1982; Taylor & Batten, 1983). This consists of a network of stop-smoking groups across the region. The programme is based on self-help group therapy principles and utilises group leaders or facilitators, who receive a short training. A key objective is to help smokers to understand that non-smokers have the same needs for mood control, but that non-smokers find other ways of achieving it than through the perceived means of smoking. On this awareness can then be built the skills for identifying and coping with stress factors. In the two years following its inception in 1981, over 100 group facilitators were trained and became active. These comprised doctors, nurses, teachers, health education officers, health visitors, social workers, youth workers and volunteers. Preliminary results reveal an average 40% quit rate at the end of the six week courses. There were variations in the success rates for each group ranging from 0–73%. Full results are expected in 1984/85, including long term follow-up.

Assessing reports of the effectiveness of group clinics is difficult. The information collected is largely limited to immediate throughput data and the longer term follow-up required for outcome assessment is not usually available. Before it can be said that a procedure is beneficial, it is necessary to show that those smokers given help would not have done equally well without any intervention at all. The only way to do this is by randomly assigning some subject to a no-treatment group. Many studies have included 'attention placebo' controls. Very few have used 'no treatment' controls but in one such attempt Russell et al (1976) found that few smokers would be abstinent if they had not attended the clinics.

Success rates reported by different group clinics vary widely (Raw, 1978; Schwartz, 1978). Much of this can be explained by the differences in the populations studied. Not all studies reported drop out rates or included drop outs as failures; these ranged from 21% (Ross, 1967) to 76% (Mausner, 1966). Duration of follow-up has also varied widely and as success rates alter markedly with follow-up time, this is an important consideration when evaluating results.

Another point concerns the criteria for success. Some group clinics quote a reduction in cigarettes smoked as well as total abstinence as a measure of success. However, smoking reduction is not a reliable dependent variable as compensation for reduced numbers smoked can be made by increased inhaling. Unless a measure of carboxyhaemoglobin is available to measure grades of reduction, only total abstinence should be regarded as success. Validation of abstinence is also desirable in checking the truth of smokers' reports. Reported deception rates have reached 40% (Sillett et al, 1978). Estimation of carboxyhaemaglobin can now be done conveniently by measuring expired air carbon monoxide (Jarvis et al, 1980).

Irrespective of the methods used in group clinics, abstinence of 15–20% at one year follow-up are usual (Raw, 1978). These match the rates found with the specific treatment methods, with the possible exception of nicotine chewing gum. Because group clinics are less labour intensive than many of the personalised treatment methods, they are more cost effective.

Success rates of group clinics are generally higher than individual self-help approaches, but their use has to be considered carefully in view of the resource implications. As well as directly influencing attenders, there is often a considerable 'knock-on' effect in the community. Press interest is often raised and this in itself can stimulate other smokers to give up, or strengthen the resolve of those at present attempting to do so.

In summary then, it is suggested that a range of approaches have a place in an integrated strategy to help smokers in their attempts to give up. Self-help assistance is likely to be the most frequently used approach assisted by health professional counselling wherever possible. Nicotine chewing gum may be useful here for the dependent smoker. For a smaller population who need peer support, group therapy is indicated, and for the small minority of highly dependent smokers specific treatment techniques may be necessary to overcome the nicotine addiction. The next section discusses how ex-smokers can be helped to stay stopped, and avoid relapse.

HOW CAN EX-SMOKERS BE HELPED TO STAY STOPPED?

Relapse is a common feature of smoking cessation initiatives. Commonly, high quit rates are achieved at the end of programmes but the long term success rate is often much lower. Maintenance of cessation is therefore an important consideration when formulating stop smoking plans. A number of areas for action exist. These can be directed at helping the smoker to understand the types of situation that are likely to stimulate relapse so that avoidance tactics can be employed. Alternatively, action can concern minimising the risk of starting again by tackling the environmental influences that initiate or predispose to relapse.

Direct help

Support for ex-smokers can be provided by many types of health professionals. The more successful smoking-cessation packs for general practitioners stress the importance of medium term follow-up (6–12 months). Encouragement and praise can be given, and in so doing ex-smokers can feel that someone else is interested in their progress. They can also be specifically reassured about the transient nature of withdrawal effects. Only about 6% of ex-smokers report having any difficulties with ill-temperedness or weight gain (Marsh & Matheson, 1983). A few pilot programmes are also being run by psychologists, which attempt to equip ex-smokers with specific social skills to resist relapse (Taylor, 1983).

Many of the self help information packs contain a section on maintenance of cessation and describes the types of situations that predispose to relapse. For example, relaxing after the evening meal or meeting up with a group of smoking friends, often tempts the recent ex-smoker into relapsing. Ways of resisting the first cigarette that commonly triggers relapse are also discussed. Media approaches commonly use 'booster' messages designed to give the new ex-smoker continued support and encouragement during the first few months or so immediately after total cessation. Effective television commercials have been developed following careful market research in both the Southern Australian and New South Wales anti-smoking programmes (Cowley, 1983). Another approach in the United States uses taped telephone messages. Dubren (1977b) reported that in a pilot study, successful quitters who were given the telephone number were twice as likely to be abstinent one month after stopping than those who were not given access to these messages. Evaluation in this area is sparse.

Community programmes

Over and above direct help, general community programmes encouraging healthy lifestyles seem to be supportive in their own right in preventing relapse. If action is also directed at promoting exercise and healthy nutrition, an ethos seems to develop within neighbourhoods which considers health as a valuable community asset. Not only are giving-up attempts encouraged but maintenance of quitting is also provided. Those that begin to take regular exercise and eat healthily appear to be more likely to give up smoking and help others do the same.

As part of their multiple coronary risk factor reduction initiatives, Stanford and North Karelia have developed integrated programmes for smoking cessation (Farquhar et al, 1977; Koskela & Puska, 1982). They used a combination of techniques — individual counselling, group and mass media intervention. Sucess rates were increased when mass media programmes were linked to sustained community action on a number of topics. The power of continuing social support as an important component in cessation and maintenance strategies is also well demonstrated by the results of the Multiple Risk Factor Intervention Trial (MRFIT). Cessation rates for the 3103 male smokers, aged 35–37, who received an initial intensive 10-week intervention programme followed by maintenance were high. Forty-six per cent had given up at four year screening compared to 27% amongst the control (usual care) group (Hughes et al, 1981). Even though this was a special group of smokers at high cardiovascular risk, the high quit rates achieved were particularly encouraging.

Support at the workplace
Those trying to give up smoking commonly find difficulties arising in the workplace. There can be considerable peer pressure to continue smoking and the conditions and stresses of many occupations can promote the feeling of the need to smoke. However, much can be done in the workplace to aid smokers in giving up and to provide an environment which does not trigger relapse.

The importance of creating a working environment which discourages smoking has been emphasised by the Ulster Cancer Foundation (1980) and the Trades Union Congress. There are considerable economic advantages for employers to have a non-smoking workforce (Fielding, 1982). Benefits include reduced absenteeism for health reasons, better productivity, reduced fire risks, lower costs for cleaning fixtures and fittings and few personnel problems resulting from smokers annoying the non-smoking majority. If management and staff side accept that the workplace should be health promoting, smoking prevention initiatives can flourish. Organisational changes can provide more non-smoking areas, and stop-smoking groups can be organised by occupational health staff. In so doing a supporting environment can be extended into a large area of the smoker's life. The risk of relapse for the smoker wishing to stop is lessened and another element helping maintenance of cessation is added.

Studies of industrial schemes for smoking cessation have shown them to be very effective mainly because of their potential for recruitment and peer support (Danaher, 1980). In comparison with community stop-smoking groups, recruitment to work-place schemes is high. This must reflect the convenience of the service, the effectiveness with which it can be publicised and also encouragement from colleagues who provide a supporting environment.

However, the widespread adoption of stop-smoking schemes by employers in the UK has been disappointing. In one survey 94% of companies did not have any formal smoking policy other than for safety reasons, but 51% believed that employees smoking should be of concern to employers (Harris & Seymour, 1983). Forty-five per cent of the company respondents could not see any advantages in adopting a policy against smoking, and only 18% cited health as a reason for controlling smoking in designated areas. In comparison the approach of industry in the United States has been more vigorous. Fifteen per cent of major companies in one recent sample were offering smoking cessation programmes (National Inter Agency Council on Smoking and Health, 1980).

The evidence from the survey by Harris & Seymour (1983) suggested that British companies have a functional attitude towards smoking and that safety and conforming to regulations are more important than employees health. The existence of an occupational health department paradoxically seemed only to act as a reinforcement to this trend. However, one-third of companies expressed willingness to 'consider' introducing a stop-smoking programme.

In 1980/1981 another research group distributed two booklets to 158 companies. One suggested ways of organising occupational smoking cessation (East & Moreton, 1980) and the other describing a self-help cessation programme (East & Towers, 1979). At follow-up, only two companies had run and completed cessation programmes. Companies frequently supported the idea but failure to organise was attributed to lack of available personnel and the cost to the company especially in view of the recession (Moreton & East, 1982). There are clearly then considerable opportunities in the UK for work-based smoking cessation schemes.

Social and economic measures

Non-smoking as the normal way of behaving is useful not only in preventing the commencement of smoking but also in the maintenance of cessation (Royal College of Physicians, 1983). Others smoking in social situations are a common cause of relapse (Lichtenstein, 1977). In the UK at present smoking is banned or at least restricted to specific areas in many theatres, cinemas and shops. About two-thirds of British Rail carriages are now non-smoking although limitations on buses are more variable. There are very few non-smoking areas in restaurants and pubs.

Restrictions on smoking within NHS premises particularly hospitals not only reduce opportunities to smoke but they set a positive example for reinforcing the non-smoking norm. This exemplary role of the NHS as a 'shop window' for health has been recognised by the Department of Health and Social Security (DHSS, 1977). A recent study in Wessex reviewed the restrictions operating in 190 hospitals and health centres in the region (Catford & Nutbeam, 1983). The survey found that the levels of smoking restriction were high and that patients, visitors and staff complied well with the restrictions. However for ambulant patients the situation clearly favoured the smoker — for example, only 18% of acute hospitals could offer smoke-free day rooms to all non-smokers yet 92% could offer dayroom accommodation to all smokers. Cigarettes were also sold in a quarter of acute and maternity hospitals.

Marsh & Matheson (1983) found that both smokers and non-smokers generally agree that smoking should be restricted in public places. However, more specific outright bans on smoking divide smokers and non-smokers, particularly bans on buses and in restaurants. Twenty-five per cent of smokers and 53% of non-smokers (i.e. 40% overall) favoured a total ban on smoking in all public places. Twenty-nine per cent of non-smokers said they were 'frequently' bothered by cigarette smoke and 42% said occasionally. Twenty-four per cent of people reported that they 'let people know they are bothered' — a response which a decade ago would have been regarded as slightly eccentric.

Considerable scope for improvement seems to be possible in promoting non-smoking areas in public places as a means of minimising the risks of relapse amongst ex-smokers. Health education programmes promoting the rights of non-smokers and the risks associated with passive smoking (Shephard, 1982) could well be useful. The fact, for example, that smokers now represent a minority group is not common knowledge — about half of smokers and non-smokers still believe that at least two-thirds of the population smoke. Other measures may also be helpful, for example, further restriction of tobacco advertising and price increases (Royal College of Physicians, 1983). Marsh & Matheson (1983) found that people notice cigarette advertising and there was widespread support for further curbs. Twenty-three per cent of smokers and 44% of non-smokers still claimed to see cigarette advertising on television. This is perhaps an indication of the success of sports sponsorship which was opposed by 47% of non-smokers and 30% of smokers. Economic measures likely to maintain non-smoking include maintaining high prices for tobacco. Fifty-seven per cent of smokers believe that they can save money as a result of giving up. If this money is then committed, for example, by hiring video equipment (a common ploy), it may be very difficult economically for ex-smokers to start smoking again. Another potential financial incentive is the differential rates of life insurance offered to non-smokers by some insurance companies. Ex-smokers taking out these policies would know that they might not be eligible to benefit if they started smoking again.

CONCLUSIONS

More action directed at encouraging and supporting more smokers to give up smoking is justifiable for a number of reasons. Not only is smoking control the highest priority amongst action to improve the public health (Royal College of Physicians, 1977) but, as the previous sections have demonstrated, smoking cessation programmes can be very effective. The majority of smokers have already tried to give up and at least half want and are resolved to give up. Both smokers and non-smokers want the government to spend more on encouraging people to give up smoking (Marsh & Matheson, 1983). In times of financial constraint, another important consideration is that smoking cessation programmes are highly cost-beneficial (Kristein, 1977).

Atkinson & Townsend (1977) have estimated that the total net economic benefits of a proportionally larger non-smoking population would be significant in this country. Savings in NHS usage, sickness benefits and widows' pensions would considerably outweigh the extra costs of retirement pensions and the costs of the programmes concerned. Smoking cessation is likely to reduce not only the rate of premature deaths, but also the prevalence of long term handicap and disability principally from heart and lung disease. The latter clearly have major resource impacts on health and social services as well as social security. Atkinson & Townsend's cost benefit ratio may therefore be quite conservative.

Wynder & Hoffman (1979) are dismayed that the medical-care establishment has not come to grips with the purely economic, as well as the medical and humanitarian, aspects of the smoking and health issue. They say 'We are sometimes asked whether a one-year success rate of 20 or 25% indicates a worthwhile and cost-effective effort. Such a question is astonishing when one considers that the five-year survival rate among lung cancer is less than 10% and the hospital cost alone for lung-cancer therapy is several thousand dollars; we estimate the cost per person for a year long cessation programme to be about $80.'

An important start has been made in reducing the prevalence of smoking. But if tobacco-related diseases are to be largely eliminated, large scale smoking control programmes are required. These should concern not only preventing people from starting but also helping those who smoke to give up. Ambitious smoking-cessation programmes need to be mounted of varying types which are well co-ordinated and integrated. More attention needs to be paid to those who want to stop smoking but do not seek help. Community physicians in view of their special training and responsibilities are in a unique position to stimulate action within primary care teams, within health authorities, within the community and through the media (Catford & Woolaway, 1984).

Programmes should consist no longer of 'preaching' but rather of 'practising' smoking cessation. The majority of smokers now want to give up and the task is to help them to do this. Smoking is the greatest challenge currently in the field of public health. The history of the first public health revolution shows that considerable progress can be made against formidable obstacles providing there is commitment, application and resourcefulness. A second public health revolution — one spearheaded through smoking control — could be a reality by the year 2000 provided there is action now.

ACKNOWLEDGEMENTS

We thank Martin Raw and Don Nutbeam for their constructive comments and Marian Macdonald for her help in preparing this paper.

REFERENCES

Ajzen I, Fishbein M 1980 Understanding attitudes and predicting social behaviour. Englewood Cliffs, Prentice-Hall

Ashton H, Stepney R 1982 Smoking as a 'psychological tool'. In Smoking Psychology and Pharmacology. Tavistock Publications, London, Ch 5, p 91–119

Atkinson A B, Townsend J L 1977 Economic aspects of reduced smoking. Lancet ii: 492–494

Bernstein D A, McAlister A 1976 The modification of smoking behavior: progress and problems. Addictive Behaviors 1: 89–102

Bewley B R, Day I, Ide L 1973 Smoking by children in Great Britain. SSRC.MRC, London

British Thoracic Society 1983 Comparison of four methods of smoking withdrawal in patients with smoking related diseases. British Medical Journal 286: 595–597

Burns B H 1969 Chronic chest disease, personality and success in stopping cigarette smoking. British Journal of Preventive and Social Medicine 23: 23–27

Bynner J M 1967 Medical Students' Attitudes towards Smoking. HMSO, London

Bynner J M 1969 The Young Smoker, HMSO, London

Catford J C, Nutbeam D 1983 Smoking in Hospitals. Lancet July 9: 94–96

Catford J C, Nutbeam D 1984 Prevention in Practice: What Wessex General Practitioners are doing. British Medical Journal (in press)

Catford J C, Woolaway M C 1984 Quitting for life. The role of health authorities in smoking cessation. Health Education Journal (in press)

Cherry N, Kiernan K 1976 Personality scores and smoking behaviour. British Journal of Preventive and Social Medicine 30: 123–131

Condiotte M M, Lichtenstein E 1981 Self-efficacy and relapse in smoking cessation programs. Journal of Consulting and Clinical Psychology 49: 648–658

Cowley J 1983 Unpublished data Health Promotion Services. South Australia Health Commission

Cox H, Marks L 1983 Sales trends and survey findings: a study of smoking in 15 OECD countries. Health Trends 15: 48–52

Croog S H, Richards N P 1977 Health beliefs and smoking patterns in heart patients and their wives: a longitudinal study. American Journal of Public Health 67: 921–930

Danaher B G 1980 Smoking cessation programs in occupational settings. Public Health Reports 95(2): 149–157

Department of Health and Social Security 1977 HC(77)3 Health Services Management Non-Smoking in Health Premises

Dubren R 1977a Study of smoking intervention techniques. Project Report HSM–21–72–557 to the National Clearing House for Smoking and Health. Centre for Disease Control Atlanta

Dubren R 1977b Self-reinforcement by recorded telephone messages to maintain non-smoking behaviour. Journal of Consulting Clinical Psychology 45: 358–360

Dyer N 1983 So You Want to Stop Smoking — Results of a follow-up one year later. BBC Broadcasting Research Special Report London

East R, Towers B 1979 No smoke. Health Education Research Team. Kingston Polytechnic London

East R, Moreton W J 1980 Organiser's handbook for the occupational quit smoking programme. Health Education Research Team. Kingston Polytechnic London

Egger G, Fitzgerald W, Frape G et al 1983 Results of large scale media anti-smoking campaign in Australia: North Coast "Quit for Life" programme. British Medical Journal 287: 1125–1128

Eiser J R, Sutton S R 1977 Smoking as a subjectively rational choice. Addictive Behaviors 2: 129–134

Eiser J R, Sutton S R, Wober M 1978 Can television influence smoking? British Journal of Addiction 73(3): 215–219

Ejrup B 1960 Proposals for treatment of smokers with severe clinical symptoms brought about by their smoking habit. British Columbia Medical Journal 2: 441–453

Elkan W 1982 The economics of coronary heart disease. Lloyds Bank Review 146: 32–49

Farquhar J, Macoby N, Wood P et al 1977 Community education for cardiovascular health. Lancet 1: 1192–1195

Fielding J E 1982 Effectiveness of employee health improvement programs. Journal of Occupational Medicine 24(11): 907–916

Flaxman J 1978 Quitting smoking now or later: gradual abrupt, intermediate and delayed quitting. Behaviour Therapy 9: 260–270

Friedman G D, Siegelaub A B, Dales L G, Seltzer C C 1979 Characteristics predictive of coronary heart disease in ex-smokers before they stopped smoking: Comparison with persistent smokers and non-smokers. Journal of Chronic Diseases 32: 175–90

Glasgow R E, Schafer L, O'Neil H K 1981 Self help books and amount of therapist contact in smoking cessation programs. Journal of Consulting and Clinical Psychology 49(5): 659–667

Gordon T, Kannel W B, McGee G 1974 Death and coronary attacks in men after giving up cigarette smoking Lancet ii: 1345–1348

Gritz E R 1978 Women and Smoking. In: J L Schartz (ed) Progress in Smoking Cessation. American Cancer Society, New York/WHO

Handel S 1973 Change in smoking habits in a general practice. Journal of the Royal College of General Practitioners 23: 149

Harris J, Seymour L 1983 No smoking – still not a sign of the times at work. Occupational Health 35(7): 308–313

Health Education Council 1972 Anti-smoking TV campaign Research Bureau Ltd for HEC London

Hughes G H, Hymowitz N, Ockene J K, Simon N, Vogt T M 1981 The multiple risk factor intervention trial (MRFIT) V Intervention on smoking. Preventive Medicine 10(4): 476–500

Hunt W A, Barnett L W, Branch L G 1971 Relapse rates in Addiction Programs. Journal of Clinical Psychology 27: 455–456

Ikard F F, Green D E, Horn D 1969 A scale to differentiate between types of smoking as related to the management of affect. International Journal of the Addictions 4(4): 649–659

Jacobson B 1981 The Ladykillers Why smoking is a feminist issue. Pluto, London

Jamrozik K D, Fowler G H 1982 Anti-smoking education in Oxfordshire general practices. Journal of the Royal College of General Practitioners 32: 179–183

Jarvis M, Russell M A H, Saloojee Y 1980 Expired air carbon monoxide: a simple breath test of tobacco smoke intake. British Medical Journal 281: 484–485

Koskela K, Puska P 1982 An evaluation of a community-based anti-smoking programme as a part of a comprehensive cardiovascular programme (The North Karelia project) Eds Davies J K, Coltart C European Monographs in Health Education research 3

Kristein M M 1977 Economic issues in prevention. Preventive Medicine 6: 252–264

Knopf A, Wakefield J 1974 Effects of medical education on smoking behaviour. British Journal of Social and Preventive Medicine 28: 246–251

Ledwith F 1983 The readiness of general practitioners to give advice about smoking. Report to the Fifth World Conference on Smoking and Health. Winnipeg Canada

Levinson F L, Shapiro D, Schwartz G E et al 1971 Smoking elimination by gradual reduction. Behaviour Therapy 2: 477–487

Lichtenstein E, Antonuccio D O, Rainwater G 1977 Unkicking the habit: The resumption of cigarette smoking. Western Psychological Association. Seattle, Washington

Marlatt G A, Gordon J R 1980 Determinants of relapse. Implications for the maintenance of behaviour change. In: Davidson P O, Davidson S M (Eds) Behavioural Medicine: Changing Health Lifestyles New York, Brunner Mazel p 474

Marsh A, Matheson J 1983 Smoking attitudes and behaviour. An enquiry carried out on behalf of DHSS and OPCS. HMSO, London

Mausner B 1966 Report on a smoking clinic. American Psychologists 21: 251–255

McCron R, Budd J 1979 Mass communication and health education. In: Health Education: Perspectives and choices p. 199–216 ed. by I Sutherland. George Allen and Unwin, London

McKennel A, Thomas R 1967 Adults and Adolescents smoking habits and attitudes. HMSO, London

Moreton W J, East R 1982 Smoking cessation programmes in the workplace. A report prepared for the Health Education Council: Health Education Research Team Kingston Polytechnic London

National Interagency Council on Smoking and Health 1980 Smoking and the workplace: toward a healthier work force p 79. National Interagency Council on Smoking and Health, New York

Office of Population Censuses and Surveys 1982 Social Survey Division General Household Survey: unpublished data

Office of Population Censuses and Surveys 1983 OPCS Monitor GHS 83.3 Cigarette smoking: 1972 to 1982. London, HMSO

Olsen N D L, Roberts J, Castle P 1981 Smoking Prevention. A health promotion guide for the NHS. Action on Smoking and Health (Ash), London

Perry C, Mullen G 1975 The effects of hypnotic susceptibility on reducing smoking behaviour treated by an hypnotic technique. Journal of Clinical Psychology 31: 498–505

Peto J 1974 Price and consumption of cigarettes a case for intervention. British Journal of Preventive and Social Medicine 28: 241–245

Peto R 1983 The practicalities of the primary prevention of cancer. Paper presented to Conference on Prevention and Early Detection of Cancer. Faculty of Community Medicine 25th June London

Porter A M W, McCullough D M 1972 Counselling against cigarette smoking. A controlled study from General Practice. Practitioner 209: 686

Puska P, Koskela K, McAlister A, Pallonen U 1979 A comprehensive television smoking cessation programme in Finland. International Journal Health Education 1979 22(4) Oct–Dec suppl: 1–29

Raw M 1976 Persuading people to stop smoking. Behaviour Research and Therapy 14(2): 97–101

Raw M 1978 The treatment of cigarette dependence. In: Israel Y, Glaser F B, Kalant H, Popham R E, Schmidt W, Smart R G (eds) Research Advances in Alcohol and Drug Problems, Vol 4. Plenum Publishing Corporation, New York. p 441–485

Raw M, Jarvis M J, Feyerabend C, Russell M A H 1980 Comparison of nicotine chewing-gum and psychological treatments for dependent smokers. British Medical Journal 281: 481–482

Raw M, van der Plight 1981 Can television help people stop smoking? Health Education and the Media (Proceedings) Pergamon, Oxford

Raw M 1984 A review of the evidence for the effectiveness of nicotine gum as a smoking withdrawal aid. (manuscript in preparation)

Raw M, Heller J 1983 Smokers' clinics in Britain. A descriptive survey. Submitted for proceedings of the Fifth World Conference on Smoking and Health, Winnipeg, Canada

Rose G, Hamilton P J S 1978 A randomised controlled trial of the effect of middle-aged men of advice to stop smoking. Journal of Epidemiology and Community Health 32(4): 275–281

Rose G, Hamilton P J S, Colwell L, Shipley M J 1982 A randomised controlled trial of anti-smoking advice: 10 year results. Journal of Epidemiology and Community Health 36: 102–108

Ross C A 1967 Smoking withdrawal research clinics. (American Journal) Public Health 57: 677–681

Royal College of Physicians 1962 Smoking and Health. Pitman Publishing Co. London

Royal College of Physicians 1977 Smoking or Health. Pitman Publishing Co. London

Royal College of Physicians 1983 Health or Smoking? Pitman Publishing Co. London

Russell M A H 1971 Cigarette smoking: natural history of a dependence disorder. British Journal of Medical Psychology 44: 1–16

Russell M A H 1973 Changes in cigarette price and consumption by men in Britain, 1946–71: A preliminary analysis. British Journal of Preventive and Social Medicine 27: 1–7

Russell M A H 1980 The smoking withdrawal clinic. In: Smoking and Smoking related diseases Proceedings of a seminar held December 3rd–5th 1980. Harrogate Department of Community Medicine of Manchester

Russell M A H, Peto J, Patel U A 1974 The classification of smoking by factorial structure of motives. Journal Royal Statistical Society 137: 313–346

Russell M A H, Armstrong E, Patel U 1976 Temporal contiguity in electric aversion therapy for cigarette smoking. Behaviour Research and Therapy Volume 14: 103–123

Russell M A H, Wilson C, Taylor C, Baker C D 1979 Effect of general practitioners advice against smoking. British Medical Journal 2: 231–235

Russell M A H, Merriman R, Stapleton J, Taylor W 1983 Effect of nicotine chewing gum as an adjunct to general practitioners' advice against smoking. British Medical Journal 287: 1782–1785

Schwartz J L 1978 Helping smokers quit: state of the art. In Schwartz J L ed Progress in smoking cessation American Cancer Society p 32–65. New York

Schwartz J L 1980 The multistep process of stopping smoking: the multitude of intervention needs. In Ramstrom L M Ed. The smoking epidemic: a matter of worldwide concern. Alquist and Wiksell Stockholm, p 194–201

Schwartz J L, Dubitzky M 1967 Expressed willingness of smokers to try 10 smoking withdrawal methods. Public Health Reports 82(10): 855–861

Shephard R J 1982 The Risks of Passive Smoking. Croom Helm, London

Sillet R W, Wilson M B, Malcom R E, Ball K P 1978 Deception among smokers. British Medical Journal 1978 2: 1185–1186

Social Trends 1983 No. 13 Central Statistical Office. HMSO, London

Taylor D 1983 Unpublished data. Department of Psychology, University of Southampton

Taylor D, Batten L 1983 Evaluation of community anti-smoking groups in the Wessex region: Operation Smokestop Second Evaluation Report. Department of Psychology, University of Southampton

Taylor P 1984 Smoke Ring. The Politics of Tobacco. Bodley Head, London

Townsend J 1983 Cigarette tax and social class patterns of smoking in the United Kingdom. Report to the 5th World Conference on Smoking and Health. Winnipeg, Canada

US Department of Health, Education and Welfare 1977 The Smoking Digest. Progress Report and a Nation Kicking the Habit. US Department of Health, Education and Welfare Public Health Service, National Institute of Health, National Cancer Institute Office of Cancer Communications, p 127

Ulster Cancer Foundation 1980 Smoking and the workplace Proceedings of a Joint Seminar. Belfast

Warner K E 1977 The effects of the anti-smoking campaign on cigarette consumption. American Journal of Public Health 67: 645–649

Wells N 1982 Coronary heart disease, the scope for prevention. Office of Health Economics, London No. 73

Wessex Positive Health Team 1982 Smoking Prevention: Operation Smokestop Smoking cessation self-help groups in Wessex. Lifeline Report No. 5. Wessex Regional Health Authority, Winchester

West D W, Graham S, Swanson M, Wilkinson G 1977 Five year follow-up of a smoking withdrawal clinic population. American Journal of Public Health 67(6): 536–544

West Midlands Regional Health Authority 1982 The people say how they gave up smoking. Public Relations Division West Midlands Regional Health Authority, Birmingham

Whitehead R W, Davies J M A 1964 A study of methylphenidate and diazepam as possible smoking deterrents. Current Therapy Research Clinic Exp. 6: 363–367

Wynder E L, Hoffman D 1979 Tobacco and Health, a societal challenge. New England Journal of Medicine 300(16): 894–903

9. The control of endemic goitre and cretinism

P. O. D. Pharoah

THE GEOGRAPHICAL DISTRIBUTION OF GOITRE

Endemic goitre is a world wide problem and its geographical distribution has been well documented by a comprehensive review of the world literature (Kelly & Snedden, 1960). Almost no country is exempt and it was estimated that 200 million people are affected. However, the international picture will have been altered since the review with the implementation of preventive programmes in many countries.

Areas with a high prevalence are determined by certain geological features. They include the following.

(a) Mountainous regions, e.g. the Alps, the Andean Cordillera, the Himalayas and the mountain chain extending through south-east Asia and the countries of the South Pacific, e.g. Burma, Indonesia, Papua New Guinea, the Philippines.

(b) Alluvial plains that have recently been the site of quarternary glaciation, e.g. the Great Lakes basin of Canada and the USA, Finland and the low-lying Netherlands. Geochemists explain this on the leaching of iodine from the soil by glaciation or flooding in the last Ice Age with insufficient time having elapsed for replacement of the iodine from oceanic sources (Chilean Iodine Educational Bureau, 1956).

(c) Areas where water supplies permeate through limestone, e.g. the Peak District and the Cotswolds in England and in parts of Columbia.

THE AETIOLOGY OF GOITRE

(a) Iodine deficiency

References to goitre can be found in the Hindu and Chinese literature of 4000 years ago (Langer, 1960). Even in these times remedial measures included the Sargassum and Laminaria seaweeds and preparations of pig and deer thyroids. In 1811, Courtois isolated the element iodine from the seaweed Fucus vesiculosus when in the process of producing saltpetre for use in the Napoleonic wars. Previously Fucus vesiculosus had been used for the treatment of goitre and this prompted both Prout in 1816 and Coindet in 1820, independently to prescribe iodine for the treatment of goitre. Subsequently Coindet described iodism and the development of hyperthyroidism (later called Iod-Basedow disease) which he ascribed to excessive dosage. In spite of his warnings the remedy fell into disrepute because of the toxic effects resulting from the excessively large doses used (Langer, 1960). Fear of iodine-induced hyperthyroidism reach its zenith under the influence of Kocher and a review of the literature of that period indicated that up to 5000 times the optimum dosage of iodine was used (Matovinovic & Ramalingaswami, 1960).

Interest in iodine was rekindled following Baumann's observation that an acid hydrolysate of the thyroid gland contained 10% iodine. Subsequently Harington & Barger (1927) synthesised thyroxine and showed that iodine was an integral part of the active hormone.

It is now generally accepted that dietary iodine deficiency is the major cause of endemic goitre. Although Boussingault 150 years ago, advocated the use of iodised salt for goitre prevention (quoted by Kelly & Snedden, 1960) it was not until the trial by Marine & Kimball (1920) in Akron, Ohio in which sodium iodide supplements were given to schoolgirls that the prophylactic value of iodine was convincingly demonstrated. Since then, other evidence has been adduced in support of the iodine deficiency hypothesis. Endemic goitre occurs in areas of low soil iodine content and an inverse relationship can often be demonstrated between soil iodine and goitre prevalence (Roche & Lissitzky, 1960). Also urinary iodine excretion is low and thyroidal uptake is regularly elevated in areas of endemic goitre (Follis, 1964) and goitre may be produced experimentally in animals fed on a diet low in iodine (Axelrad et al, 1955).

However, some anomalies in the correlation between iodine deficiency and the prevalence of goitre were noted and adequate prophylaxis with iodine has not always been successful in eradicating endemic goitre. This suggested that factors other than iodine deficiency play a role in pathogenesis.

(b) Organic goitrogens
The development of goitre in rabbits fed on a diet of cabbages drew attention to the possibility of goitrogens being present in food (Webster & Chesney, 1930), an observation that subsequently led to the development of antithyroid drugs. Other dietary goitrogens have since been implicated, most of which are to be found in plants of the Brassica and Crucifera families.

There are two major groups of substances that are dietary goitrogens:

(1)   the thiocyanates which primarily inhibit the trapping of iodine by the thyroid and whose goitrogenic action can be overcome by administering iodine. Cassava or manioc is a tuberous plant that is widely used throughout Africa because it is relatively easily cultivated and has a high carbohydrate content. Various parts of the plant may be consumed and its toxic propensities have been reviewed (Nestel & MacIntyre, 1973). In particular, its goitrogenic action has been attributed to the glucoside, linemarin, which yields a thiocyanate on hydrolysis (Ermans et al, 1972). In a recent study in Zaire the variation in goitre prevalence rates and a recent increase in prevalence in one area could not be attributed solely to the degree of iodine deficiency observed but was related also to the level of urinary thiocyanate excretion which was attributed to cassava consumption (Ermans et al, 1980; Delange et al, 1982);

(2)   the thiourea or thionamide-like goitrogens which interfere with organification of iodine or the coupling of the iodotyrosines. Their goitrogenic potential can be countered by giving thyroid hormones but not iodine. This category of goitrogen has been incriminated in an area of endemic goitre in Western

Columbia which did not respond to a programme of iodine prophylaxis. This was thought to be due to at least three sulphur containing compounds with marked antithyroid activity which has been isolated from the water supply (Gaitan, 1973; Gaitan et al, 1973). A thionamide-like goitrogen in cassava has also been reported (Ekpechi, 1967; Ekpechi et al, 1966), in addition to the thiocyanate mentioned earlier.

Generally, goitrogens in plants exist in small quantities and either large amounts of the food must be consumed or the goitrogen must be concentrated at some stage in the food chain. This mechanism was thought to be responsible for the seasonal epidemics of goitre found among Tasmanian school children. It was hypothesised that the spring flush of weeds consumed by the cattle contained a goitrogen which was concentrated in the milk (Clements & Wishart, 1956). However, attempts to isolate the goitrogen were unsuccessful (Trikojus, 1974). A similar situation has also been described in Finland (Arstila et al, 1969).

(c) Bacterial contamination
McCarrison (1906), in the Himalayas, noted the increase in goitre prevalence in successive villages down river which he attributed to the progressive degree of pollution of the water. On the basis of this and other observations he concluded that a micro-organism was responsible. This mechanism has also been implicated in other areas of endemic goitre with E. Coli being incriminated as the causative organism (Malamos et al, 1971; Vought et al, 1967).

(d) Minerals
The greater predisposition to goitres in hard-water areas has long been appreciated. Prosser (1769) recognised that 'Derby neck' was associated with the hard-water of limestone regions and in 1810 it was noted that goitre was more frequent in institutions which used well-water of exceptional hardness for cooking (quoted by Kelly & Snedden, 1960). A Medical Research Council report of 1948 stated that a dietary iodine level which may be adequate in a soft water area is inadequate in areas of hard-water (Murray et al, 1948) and Day & Powell-Jackson (1972) found that the variation in goitre prevalence correlated not only with the degree of water hardness but also with the fluoride content of the water. Experimental support comes from the observation that calcium causes enhanced growth of the iodine-deprived rat thyroid (Taylor, 1954).

THE EPIDEMIOLOGY OF ENDEMIC GOITRE

In the past, comparison of goitre prevalence levels in different communities has been hampered by the lack of a consensus definition for the grading of goitre. A grading now commonly recognised was originally developed by Perez, Scrimshaw & Munoz (1960) and subsequently modified by the Pan American Health Organisation. It is as follows:

Grade 0a: no enlargement of the thyroid
Grade 0b: enlargement detectable by palpation but not visible even when the neck is fully extended

Grade 1:   gland palpable but only visible when the neck is fully extended
Grade 2:   gland visible when head is in normal position,
      :   palpation not needed for diagnosis
Grade 3:   very large gland which can be recognised from a distance

Even this classification is unnecessarily cumbersome and the distinction between Grades 0a, 0b and 1 on the one hand and between 2 and 3 on the other is subjective.

In addition to the above classification, each grade of enlargement may be subdivided according to whether the enlargement is diffuse or nodular.

Because iodine deficiency is the major determinant of endemic goitre, the highest goitre prevalence rates are to be found in those whose iodine requirements are greatest, i.e. women of child bearing age and, to a lesser degree, adolescent girls or boys. Goitres may increase in size with each pregnancy and regress when child bearing ceases. In order to assess the severity of the prevailing problem therefore it is important to determine age and sex prevalence rates of goitre (Clements, 1960). Surveys in the past have often covered certain groups only, e.g. school children or military recruits, thus yielding a distorted picture of the true prevalence. In severely affected areas the prevalence rate of goitre may approach 100% with even infants being affected.

Endemic cretinism

The syndrome of cretinism in most current textbooks is equated with hypothyroidism, either congenital or developing early in childhood. However, the clinical features of cretinism as described in the early literature are quite different and it is apparent that there are two distinct syndromes. It is necessary to examine the problem from the historical standpoint to clarify the problem that has arisen. The association between endemic cretinism and goitre was noted by Paracelsus in 1567 who wrote:

'but to speak of these creatures that they perchance also have defects of the body, that is they carry growths with them such as goitres and the like: this perhaps is not a characteristic of fools but also of others, however it fits most of them' (Major, 1945).

Although this recognition of an association between goitre and cretinism is often attributed to Paracelsus, it was implicit in the literature prior to that time e.g. the Reuner Musterbuch of 1215 depicts a figure with a large multilobed goitre, a stupid facial expression, brandishing a fool's staff in one hand and ear-trumpet in the other (Merke, 1960). In 1220, in the encyclopaedia of Jacques de Vitry, large goitres and deaf-mutism are both recorded as occurring in the Burgundy region and it was stated that 'ex mutis et surdis, muti et surdi infantes procreantur' (Merke, 1960).

The term 'cretin' first appeared in Diderot's encyclopaedia of 1754 and referred to 'an imbecile who was deaf and dumb with a goitre hanging down to the waist' (Cranfield, 1962). The derivation of the term was discussed by De Quervain & Wegelin (1936). The most likely origin is from 'Christianus' or 'Crestin' in the south-eastern French dialect, the afflicted persons being referred to as a 'pauvre chretien' because of their harmlessness or innocence. Other possible derivations include 'Cretira' from the Rhaeto-romanic language as a colloquialism for an unfortunate creature or from the Latin 'creta' in reference to the chalk-like pallor of the skin.

In 1847, Norris described the cretins in Chisleborough, Somerset, dividing them into four groups. These consisted of:

(a) Four perfect idiots
(b) Seventeen partial idiots, all quite unable to articulate so as to be understood and walking with an unsteady step and an unsteady waddling gait
(c) Five deaf and dumb
(d) A majority of the whole population viz. those with an obvious deficiency of intellect and, without a single exception, affected with bronchocoele (Norris, 1847).

At that time bronchocoele was the term used for goitre.
William Farr, the first Registrar-General and the father of vital statistics reporting on the 1851 census states:

'Cretins most of whom are deaf mutes. . . . The disease of cretinism is also accompanied by mental imbecility in a greater or less degree' (Farr, 1885).

In all these early descriptions of cretinism, mental retardation and deaf-mutism are invariably included and abnormalities of gait are frequently mentioned. Yet, apart from mental retardation, these clincial features are not associated with cretinism as it is seen today, i.e. sporadic cretinsim. The original description of sporadic cretinism was given by Thomas Curling in 1850 when he reported on two infants and noted:

In countries where cretinism and bronchocoele prevail, it was long supposed that there is some connection between the defective condition of the brain and the hypertrophy of the thyroid. . . . in the foregoing cases we have examples of an opposite condition viz. A defective brain or cretinism combined with an entire absence of the thyroid (Curling, 1850).

It is salutory to note that Curling was stressing the difference between his two cases and what were then the recognised signs of cretinism.
Fagge in 1871 described 4 further cases of sporadic cretinism and compared them with endemic cretinism. He also specifically drew attention to the comparative features of the two syndromes stating:

Sporadic and endemic cretinism are associated with a deficiency of the mental powers. Sporadic cretinism, instead of being associated with a goitre appears to be attended with a wasting or absence of the thyroid gland. Sporadic cretinism is not necessarily congenital (Fagge, 1871).

Endemic cretinism has disappeared from the developed world and is now largely confined to Third World countries. The declining prevalence has been recorded in several countries. In England, Norris wrote that the cretins of Chisleborough which he had described in an earlier publication had almost died out (Norris, 1847). This was later confirmed by Parker who stated 'one solitary cretin now survives of about 50 years of age, the march of civilisation having stamped out the disease' (Parker, 1896). A similar decline has been reported by several authors in Italy (Costa et al, 1964) and a steady downward trend can be observed in the statistics of the Sardinian Royal Commission of 1848.
These examples all relate to foci of the disease in Europe but the downward trend

has occurred in other countries also. The prevalence of deaf-mutism in the United Provinces of India decreased by a half between the censuses of 1881 and 1921 (Stott et al, 1939). Similarly census figures for Argentina show a steady decline in the number of deaf-mutes in all provinces between the years 1869, 1895 and 1914 (Greenwald, 1957). These declines predate knowledge about aetiology or any specific prophylactic measures.

Against this background of endemic cretinism disappearing from many countries are the increasingly numerous reports of sporadic cretinism and so, in time, the term cretinism has become synonymous with sporadic hypothyroidism. The endemic variety barely receives mention in Western textbooks of medicine which belies its importance as a clinical entity in many countries.

There were occasional voices warning that the distinction between the two forms of cretinism should not be blurred. Gordon in 1922 and again in 1938 was very specific in distinguishing between sporadic and endemic cretinism. He suggested that 'sporadic cretinism' be renamed 'childhood myxoedema' because 'cretinism as described in Europe is a clinically distinct entity from sporadic hypothyroidism' (Gordon, 1922, 1938).

The confusion over the two forms of cretinism, sporadic and endemic, has been intensified by the observation that the syndrome of endemic cretinism encompasses both a hypothyroid variety which is essentially the same as sporadic cretinism, and a syndrome of neurological impairment with deaf-mutism, cerebral diplegia, mental retardation and strabismus being the cardinal clinical features.

The subclassification of endemic cretinism into two types, namely, 'myxoedematous' and 'nervous' was initially made by McCarrison in 1908 as a result of his work in the Chitral and Gilgit valleys in the Himalayas (McCarrison, 1908). His description of the clinical features of the myxoedematous type was incomplete merely stating that 'it corresponds to that form of the affection met with in Europe and is described in any textbook of medicine'. His clinical description of nervous cretinism is more precise and remains a model of accuracy. The disability is described as pertaining more especially to the central nervous system. 'Deaf-mutism is as a rule complete, mentality is much disordered and there is a congenital diplegia with increased knee-jerks and a spastic rigidity more severely affecting the lower limbs with a characteristic gait'. A coarse nystagmus and internal strabismus were noted in some cases.

Two children with the nervous type of endemic cretinism are shown in Figures 9.1 and 9.2. Both are mentally retarded and deaf-mute. The child in Figure 9.1 also has strabismus and a characteristic position of adduction and internal rotation of the hips due to the spastic diplegia. Figure 9.2 is of a 10-year-old who was unable to walk and had upper motor neurone signs in the legs and arms. Note the kyphosis of the lumbar spine which is due to weakness of the para-spinal muscles.

The relative proportion of the two sub-types of endemic cretinism differs between countries. Reviews of the world literature indicate that the hypothyroid variety predominates in some African countries, while the nervous variety is more common in most other countries (Pharoah, 1976; Pharoah et al, 1980). Thus a classification of cretinism encompassing these variations would be as shown in Figure 9.3.

To encompass the clinical manifestations of both varieties of endemic cretinism, the Pan American Health Organisation arrived at the following definition (Pan American Health Organisation, 1963).

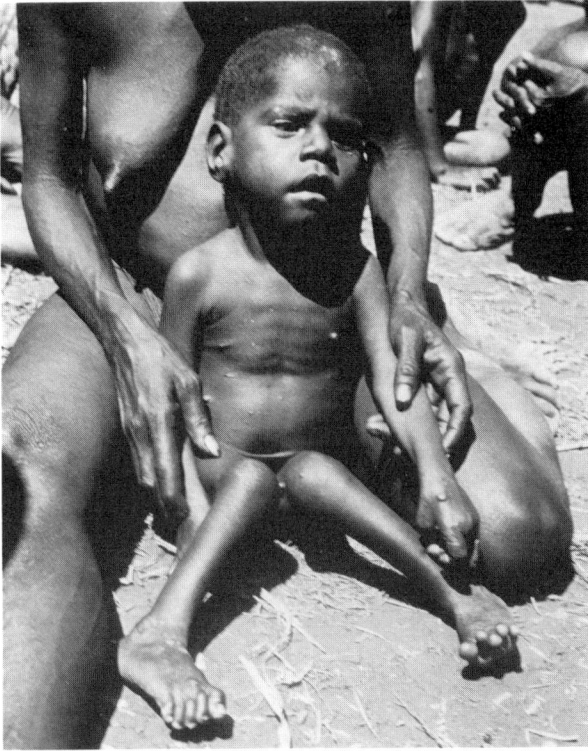

Fig. 9.1   Endemic cretinism showing diplegic adduction and internal rotation of the hip and strabismus.

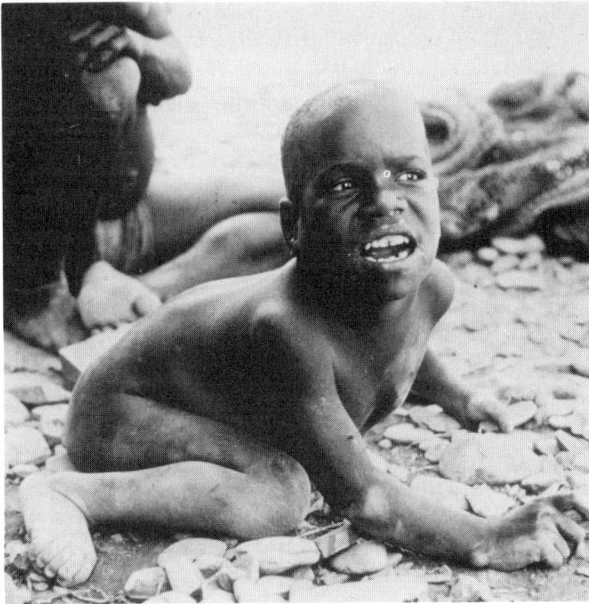

Fig. 9.2   Endemic cretin with severe spastic diplegia, unable to walk.

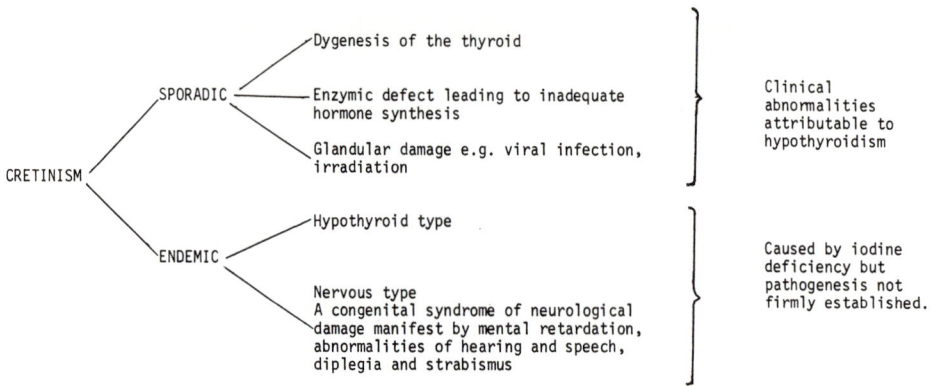

Fig. 9.3 Classification of cretinism.

'An individual with irreversible changes in mental development, born in an endemic goitre area and exhibiting a combination of some of the following characteristics not explained by other causes:

(a)   irreversible neuromuscular disorders
(b)   irreversible abnormalities in hearing and speech leading in certain cases to deaf-mutism
(c)   impairment of somatic development
(d)   hypothyroidism.'

More recently, in the light of a gathering momentum of interest and experience in endemic cretinism there has been redefinition of the syndrome which states:

The condition of endemic cretinism is defined by three major features:

(a)   Epidemiology. It is associated with endemic goitre and severe iodine deficiency.
(b)   Clinical manifestations. These comprise mental deficiency together with either:
(1)   A predominant neurological syndrome consisting of defects of hearing and speech, and with characteristic disorders of stance and gait of varying degree; or
(2)   Predominant hypothyroidism and stunted growth.
Although in some regions one of the two types may predominate, in other areas a mixture of the two syndromes will occur.
(c)   Prevention. In areas where adequate correction of iodine has been achieved, endemic cretinism has been prevented (Querido et al, 1974).

THE AETIOLOGY OF ENDEMIC CRETINISM

The importance of iodine deficiency as a cause of endemic goitre and the observation that endemic cretinism is only to be found in areas where goitre is endemic inevitably led to the suggestion that iodine deficiency is also responsible for endemic cretinism. Controversy over this last point centred round the fact that the prevalence of cretinism declined in several countries prior to any specific measure of iodine prophylaxis and that in some areas goitre was to be found without coexistent cretinism. A correlation between iodine prophylaxis and a decline in cretinism in Switzerland was shown by Wespi (1945). Iodination of salt was introduced independently in several Swiss cantons and the decline of deaf-mutism in each could be correlated with the extent of salt iodination. However, this correlation was only time related and other factors could have been held responsible. These deductions were subsequently criticised on the grounds that no cretins were born about the time that iodine prophylaxis was introduced, indeed, all the cretins were born at least 10 years previously (Koenig & Veraguth, 1961).

The controversy led to a double-blind controlled trial to assess the effectiveness of iodine as a prophylactic for endemic cretinism. A single intramuscular injection of iodinated oil had been shown to be an effective prophylactic for endemic goitre (McCullagh, 1959), and it had a long duration of action. Four years after a single 4.0 ml dose, a treated group had significantly higher serum protein-bound and urinary iodine excretion values and lower 24 hour radio-iodine uptake than an untreated control group (Clarke et al, 1960; Buttfield & Hetzel, 1967, 1971). This made the use of intramuscular iodinated oil an ideal vehicle for a controlled trial in relation to endemic cretinism. The trial was carried out in the Jimi valley in the highlands of Papua New Guinea, an area with a high prevalence of cretinism and goitre. On the occasion of a census, 16 500 people were enrolled in the trial and alternate families were injected with either iodinated oil or saline solution, each member receiving 4 ml if aged 12 years or over and 2 ml if under 12 years of age. Follow-up over the next 6 years found 6 cretins out of 687 children born to women who received iodinated oil; in 5 of the 6 cretins conception had occurred prior to the iodinated oil being given. The control group had 31 cretins among a total of 688 children; in 5 of these 31 cretins conception had occurred prior to the placebo injection of saline. From this it was concluded that iodinated oil is effective in preventing endemic cretinism provided it is given prior to conception. It indicated that maternal iodine deficiency during pregnancy leads to irreversible neurological damage to the developing fetus (Pharoah et al, 1971, 1972).

A trial using iodinated oil was also carried out in Ecuador. All the inhabitants of one village, Tocachi, were given iodinated oil and an adjacent village, La Esperanza, was used as the control. Subsequent follow-up of 217 children from Tocachi and 447 from La Esperanza found the former were more advanced in neuromuscular development but the results did not specifically report on cretinism (Ramirez et al, 1972; Fierro-Benitez et al, 1974).

A smaller study in Peru observed no significant difference in neuropsychiatric assessment between 46 children born to the oil injected mothers and 35 controls. However, this trial also did not specially mention cretinism (Pretell et al, 1972).

Further evidence on the importance of iodine in endemic cretinism arose from the observation that the disease was of recent onset in the Jimi valley of New Guinea. Following first contact with the European in 1953 there was sharp rise in the prevalence of cretinism from approximately 0.1% pre-1953 rising in the late 1950s and early 1960s and reaching a peak of 15% of the children born in 1965 (Fig. 9.4). This increase in prevalence was found to be due to an increase in incidence and was attributed to the substitution of locally produced salt by salt introduced by the European. The salt produced prior to European contact was from saline pools in a

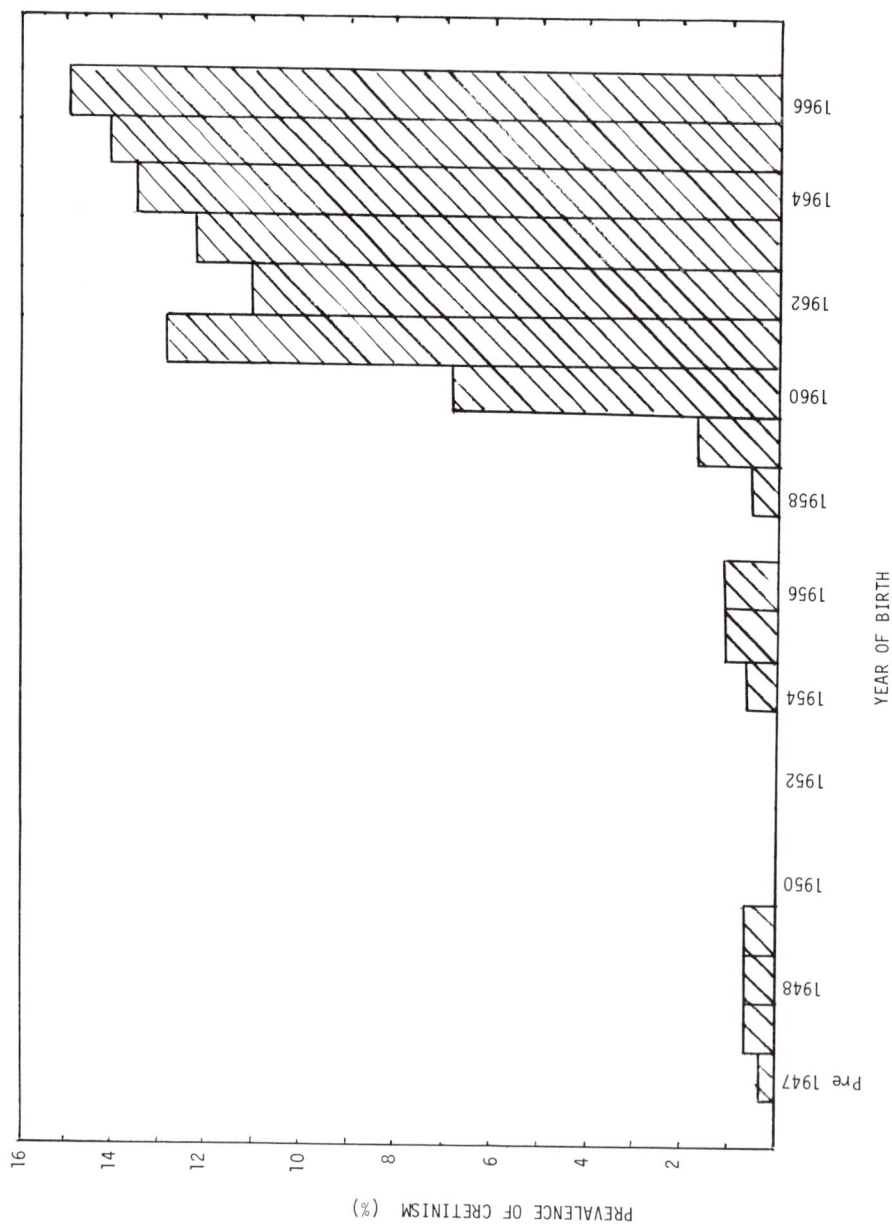

Fig. 9.4 Prevalence of cretinism by year of birth (reproduced by kind permission of the Editor, Lancet).

volcanic area, analysis of which revealed a very high iodine content (Pharoah & Hornabrook, 1973).

Thus the aetiology of the nervous form of endemic cretinism was strongly linked to iodine deficiency; giving iodine prevented the disease and withdrawing iodine precipitated an epidemic.

The above reports are concerned with trials where the 'nervous' type of cretinism predominates. Iodinated oil has also been assessed as a prophylactic for the 'myxoedematous' type of cretinism on Idjwi island in Lake Kivu in Central Africa (Thilly et al, 1974). The data on the effectiveness of iodine supplementation in preventing myxoedematous endemic cretinism is not quite so convincing. The Idjwi island trial found 4 myxoedematous cretins among 45 infants or mothers from the control villages but only 1 among 44 infants in the villages given intramuscular iodine. However, even this one case was to a mother who failed to receive iodinated oil because she was absent at the time (Delange et al, 1976). Subsequently, following the mass prophylaxis of all the inhabitants, there have been no further cases of cretinism found (Thilly et al, 1974). These several studies indicate that iodine is effective in preventing both forms of endemic cretinism.

Endemic cretinism shows a wide spectrum of severity of neurological deficit merging into normality. While it is now universally accepted that iodine given before conception can prevent the overt manifestations of the syndrome, more recently, interest has centred round the possibility that the effect of iodine may be of wider significance in preventing sub-clinical deficits of intellectual and motor performance and indeed, of shifting the frequency distribution of such measures in the whole population.

The use of Western based measures of intellectual ability such as the Stanford–Binet or the Gesell tests is fraught with difficulty when transferred to a totally different cultural environment. Nevertheless, within-culture comparisons have been made in several studies examining differences between children whose mothers had or had not received iodine.

The follow-up of the New Guinea controlled trial examined the children when they were aged 6–12 years (Connolly et al, 1979). Tests of grip strength, speed of movement, unimanual and bimanual accuracy and of motor impairment were performed. Even after exclusion of the cretins from the analysis, there were significant differences of speed/accuracy tests between the treated and control groups. The strength of this trial lay in the double-blind nature of the assessment of the children.

In the Ecuador trial the children followed-up were aged 2–9 years (Fierro-Benitez et al, 1974). These authors using the Stanford–Binet intelligence scale also observed a significant difference between the two groups of children, i.e. whose mothers had or had not received iodine. However, there were several methodological deficiencies — one village provided the test population and another the control so that the trial was not conducted blind; the number of children in the two groups was small and many were excluded from the assessment because they failed to co-operate or were suffering malnutrition.

The Peruvian trial used the Gesell, Stanford–Binet and Brunet–Lezine assessments on children up to five years of age (Pretell et al, 1972). Although the iodine treated group showed marginally higher IQ scores than the iodine deficient, the differences were not statistically significant.

In a double-blind trial in Zaire the Brunet–Lezine scale was used to assess children up to 2 years of age (Thilly et al, 1980). The treated group performed significantly better than the untreated.

The problem of comparison was addressed in a different manner in Java (Querido et al, 1978). Here the population of a village with a high goitre prevalence was compared with that of one with a low goitre prevalence. A battery of tests was used directed at measuring intelligence as well as non-intelligence (motor skill, concentration and perceptual capacity) factors. Although significant differences were observed in favour of the village with the low goitre prevalence, the presence of confounding variables detracted from the value of the study. For example, the village without goitre was closer to a major town, the main road and the primary school.

Although there may be criticism of the methodology of several of these studies, the overall indication is that there are subclinical deficits which can be ameliorated by iodine supplementation. Because of the wide spectrum of severity and of the different types of cretinism that are found world wide, it is suggested that the umbrella term Iodine Deficiency Disorders (IDD) be used to heighten awareness of the importance of iodine deficiency. The implications of this for a public health preventive programme are considerable because, while endemic cretinism may be relatively uncommon and therefore not worthy of a major preventive effort, an improvement in indices of psychomotor performance of the whole population may carry more weight in influencing a national policy decision.

THE PATHOGENESIS OF ENDEMIC CRETINISM

While lack of iodine has been shown to be the cause of both nervous and myxoedematous forms of endemic cretinism, the pathogenetic mechanism has not yet been determined.

In nervous cretinism the damage is considered to occur during fetal development probably in early pregnancy. Speculation has centred on the role played by thyroid hormones during this period.

The physiological response to iodine deficiency is for the serum thyroxine (T4) level to fall but for serum triiodothyronine (T3) level to be maintained constant (Pharoah et al, 1973; Greer et al, 1968) thus ensuring clinical euthyroidism. T3 requires less iodine than T4, weight-for-weight is physiologically much more active and it has a more rapid turnover. In the light of these hormonal changes consequent upon iodine deficiency, several hypotheses have been proposed to explain how iodine deficiency affects the developing fetus.

Trotter (1960) proposed that iodine deficiency-induced fetal hypothyroidism was responsible. However, comparisons between iodine deficient and control mothers in Peru found no significant differences in the T4 levels of their offspring in spite of T4 differences in the women themselves (Pretell & Stanbury, 1971). Also, the severest form of fetal hypothyroidism would be expected among children with congenital thyroid agenesis yet the clinical abnormalities found in such children constitute a different syndrome to that of nervous endemic cretinsim. Furthermore, the defect due to maternal iodine deficiency damages the fetus during early pregnancy at a time before the fetal thyroid is active. Follicle formation and the thyroidal accumulation of iodine in the fetus commences at about the 12th week of gestation (Hershman &

Hershman, 1972). Such evidence tends to negate fetal hypothyroidism as the pathogenic mechanism.

Maternal hypothyroidism is another possibility. Ideally, monitoring of maternal thyroid hormone levels should be carried out throughout pregnancy but under the conditions in which endemic cretinism is now seen such monitoring has not so far been possible. Evidence against the maternal hypothyroidism hypothesis is largely based on the finding that the thyroid hormones do not cross the placenta in significant quantities (Myant, 1958; Osorio & Myant, 1960; Fisher et al, 1970; Dussault et al, 1971). Also, it is unusual for hypothyroid women to conceive and a review of the literature of hypothyroid pregnancies showed an excess of congenital abnormalities among the offspring but no syndrome akin to that of endemic cretinism (Koenig, 1968).

Because neither maternal nor fetal hypothyroidism successfully explained the damage to the fetus consequent upon maternal iodine deficiency, it was suggested that, prior to the fetal thyroid becoming functional, elemental iodine was required for normal neurological development independent of its role in hormonogenesis (Pharoah et al, 1971). However, more recent experimental work shows that significant transplacental transfer of thyroid hormones does take place early in pregnancy (Ekins et al, 1983). The observation that very low maternal serum T4 levels are associated with an increased incidence of stillbirths, infant deaths and cretins (Pharoah et al, 1976) and that measures of infant motor performances correlate with the maternal T4 levels (Pharoah et al, 1981) must revive the hypothesis relating to maternal hypothyroidism and, in particular, to the role played by maternal thyroxine in fetal development.

THE TREATMENT OF ENDEMIC GOITRE AND CRETINISM

For the individual with a goitre as a result of iodine deficiency, the treatment of first choice is iodine. Lugol's iodine, which is iodine in a solution of potassium iodide, is most frequently used. The drawback to using Lugol's solution is that the dose must be repeated at frequent intervals and, in areas where goitre is now prevalent, this is not always easily achieved. An alternative to Lugol's iodine is the use of an intramuscular preparation of iodinated oil which provides a long-lasting depot of iodine and obviates the need for frequent treatment. More recently it has also been shown that iodinated oil given orally also has a long duration of effect (Kywe et al, 1978).

Many individuals having endemic goitre and given iodine will show a regression of the goitre. This is particularly likely to occur if the gland is diffusely enlarged and regression, therefore, most frequently occurs in adolescents and in young adult females. If the gland has become nodular with fibrosis and sometimes calcification also, regression is unlikely to occur.

In general, surgical removal of the enlarged gland is to be deprecated. The gland has enlarged as a physiological response to iodine deficiency and surgical removal is irrational. Yet it is surprising how frequently surgery is still being carried out, often under circumstances of great difficulty, with poor operating theatre facilities and lack of blood transfusion services. Figure 9.5 shows a young woman with gross enlargement of the thyroid gland, its vascularity is evident from the large blood vessel that is

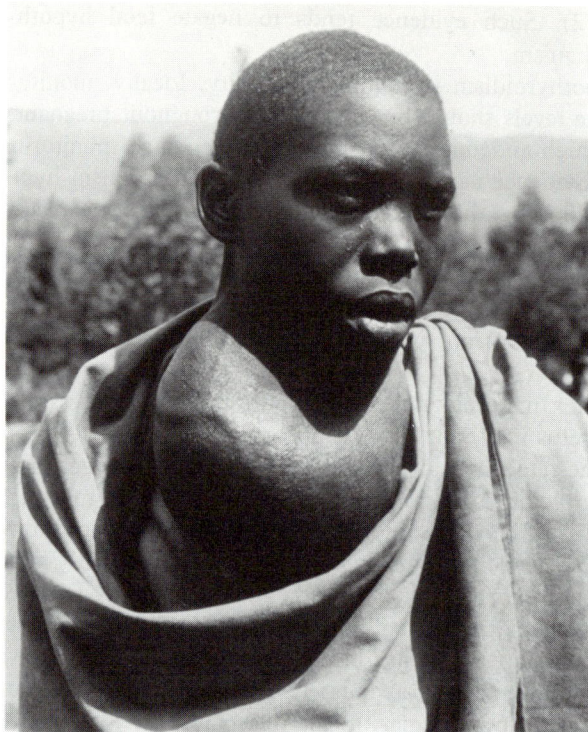

Fig. 9.5   Gross thyroid enlargement due to iodine deficiency.

visible on the surface which emphasises the difficulties of surgical removal. Surgical management is indicated when obstructive signs such as tracheal stridor develop. Yet, even in these cases, the administration of iodine should be the first line of treatment. If surgery is unavoidable the long-term follow up of the patient is imperative to ensure early recognition and treatment of hypothyroidism. Sometimes, the gland re-enlarges after surgery leading to a recurrence of obstructive signs and symptoms.

The nervous type of cretinism being a congenital abnormality is amenable to prevention only, management of the established syndrome is symptomatic.

THE PREVENTION OF ENDEMIC GOITRE AND CRETINISM

Goitre and cretinism are examples, *par excellence*, in which simple public health measures of iodine supplementation can eliminate the disease. The case for a public health preventive programme against goitre is not particularly strong. Apart from the occasional individual in whom obstructive symptoms develop, the goitre may be unsightly though otherwise symptomless. In some countries fullness of the neck in females caused by lesser degrees of thyroid enlargement is considered cosmetically attractive so that public acceptance of a preventive programme is not universal. However, the cretinism that normally accompanies a goitre endemic is of far greater seriousness and the case for a preventive programme cannot be denied.

Several different compounds of iodine have been used to supplement normal dietary sources. The generic term 'iodination' covers all forms of iodine supplementation. Strictly speaking 'iodisation' refers specifically to an iodide (usually potassium iodide) and 'iodation' to an iodate (usually potassium iodate) being the supplement but these terms have often been used interchangeably.

Estimates of the daily dietary requirement for iodine have generally been in the range of 50–150μg (Murray et al, 1948). The British Medical Association Committee on Nutrition recommended a daily minimum of 100 μg for adults with a higher level of 150 μg for children, adolescents and pregnant and nursing women (Report of the British Medical Association Committee on Nutrition, 1950). The Food and Nutrition Board of the National Research Council of the USA placed the optimum requirements at 150–300 μg daily for an adult and the Food and Agriculture Organisation of the United Nations recommended a daily allowance of 400 μg. It has been suggested that whether goitre alone is seen in an area or whether cretinism also occurs is a reflection of the severity of iodine deficiency; cretinism is observed when urinary iodine excretion levels fall below 20 μg per day (Querido, 1971).

Natural foods rich in dietary iodine are the various sea-foods. However, contrary to popular belief, sea salt is not particularly rich in iodine largely because the iodine tends to be lost in the manufacturing process.

A bibliography (Chilean Iodine Educational Bureau, 1952), covering the period 1825–1921 on the iodine content of food indicates that the iodine content is greater in animal than in vegetable products particularly if the latter come from areas of iodine deficiency. This differential in iodine content of various foodstuffs may explain the decline in cretinism in many countries that was observed prior to any formal measures of iodine prophylaxis. Hand-in-hand with socio-economic development there tends to be an increase in consumption of animal foods and therefore of iodine. The observation that cretinism is now largely confined to certain developing countries is probably due to the fact that a small proportion of their diet is of animal origin while the major component is vegetable.

METHODS FOR SUPPLEMENTING DIETARY IODINE

SALT IODINATION

Currently the method most widely applied is that of salt iodination. Nationally recommended levels show a 20 fold variation from 1 part potassium iodide per 10 000 parts salt to 1 per 200 000 parts salt (Matovinovic & Ramalingaswami, 1960). In adopting a specified level of salt iodination it is necessary to take into consideration such factors as salt consumption patterns, whether goitrogens may be enhancing the effects of iodine deficiency and the possibility of iodine loss dependent on the conditions under which the salt is stored and distributed.

Salt iodisation either with potassium or sodium iodide suffers from the disadvantage that the compounds are relatively unstable particularly in the presence of other impurities in the salt which leads to the gradual loss of iodine. Sodium iodide has the added disadvantage of being more hygroscopic than the potassium salt. Potassium iodate is now the compound of choice because of its greater stability. However, weight for weight it contains less iodine than potassium iodide, for which allowance must be made in meeting the iodine requirement. Large scale salt manufacture is either by the evaporation of sea-water or by the mining or quarrying of salt deposits. The type of salt, i.e. fine and free-running or coarse, and the proportion of impurities in it, is determined by the manufacturing process. Both these factors may influence the choice of iodine compound used.

Supplementation of the salt may be carried out by spray- or by dry-mixing the iodine compound with the salt or by the fortification of brine during the evaporation process. Dry-mixing is feasible with fine, free-running salt but this is often a luxury not usually affordable in countries where goitre is a problem. More commonly a coarse salt is consumed in which case spray-mixing is the process of choice. A spray-mixing system in which the components are simple, inexpensive and easy to operate has been developed by Hunnikin (1974).

Once salt has been iodinated other factors influence the level of iodine present before the product is consumed, e.g. the average length of time of storage, the humidity of the atmosphere, the degree of exposure to sunlight or heat, the acidity of the stored product due to the presence of impurities and the material used as salt containers. Thus any preventive programme of salt fortification must allow for quality control measures both during the manufacturing process and at the time of purchase for consumption. Major problems to implementing a preventive programme are:

(a) Lack of perception that iodine deficiency is a health problem. A goitre may not be undesirable; cretinism is frequently not recognised or, even if recognised, is not attributed to a lack of iodine. In countries where domestic cattle are an important aspect of the cultural milieu, goitre and the higher incidence of stillbirths in the animals could be used to heighten public awareness of the importance of salt iodination. (In one country recently visited, the author observed that salt imported for use as a cattle-lick was highly iodised while that for humans was not iodised.)

(b) Lack of finance. Countries where goitre and cretinism are serious problems are often those with the least financial resources and any form of iodine supplementation competes unfavourably with a host of other priorities. Nevertheless, the cost of iodine supplementation is extremely low and has been estimated in 1976–1977, to lie between US $0.0025–0.0052 per person per year (Demaeyer et al, 1979).

(c) Lack of technical expertise to ensure the continuous running of the iodination plant and to maintain adequate quality control of the programme.

(d) Marketing difficulties. In some countries there are numerous small manufacturers of salt and occasionally even individual villages may produce salt requisite to their own needs. Where this is so, there is no defined marketing network and iodine fortification of the salt is not logistically feasible.

IODINATED OIL

The use of iodinated poppy-seed oil as a prophylactic for endemic goitre was pioneered by McCullagh in Papua New Guinea (McCullagh, 1959). The oil is normally used as a contrast medium in radiography, marketed in the UK as Lipiodol ultrafluid by May & Baker Ltd, London; in France as Lipiodol ultrafluide by Andre Guerbet Laboratories, Paris and in the USA as Ethiodol by Savage Laboratories, Missouri City.

The oil contains approximately 475 mg of iodine per ml and it is used in doses of up to 5 ml for an adult. The duration of action of the oil is not clearly established; after injection the iodine is predominantly excreted in the urine. Following a dose of 2 ml it was found that urinary excretion of iodine fell to 50 μg per day after $3\frac{1}{2}$–5 years (Thilly et al, 1973). In the New Guinea controlled trial it was found that the serum thyroxine levels in women of child bearing age was still significantly higher following a single 4 ml dose of iodinated oil than in the control women 4–5 years later (Pharoah, 1972). On the basis of these results it is usually recommended that repeat injections be given every 5 years. The advantages of iodinated oil are that:

(a) it is suitable for use in areas where the salt marketing and distribution network is not well developed and, in particular, fails to penetrate more isolated areas
(b) the team members giving the injections do not require extensive training
(c) the oil is stable and does not require a cold chain to be maintained.

The disadvantages are:

(a) the necessity for maintaining a scrupulously sterile technique especially with multiple use of syringes and needles. These conditions may be difficult to attain in remote areas where a health service infra-structure may be very poorly developed or even non-existent
(b) the necessity of accurate recording of those injected to ensure that repeated doses are not given. This tends to occur because expectations are raised following the regression of goitre in many cases. Those whose goitres do not regress may request and receive further doses with the attendant possibility of iodine toxicity.

OTHER DIETARY IODINE SUPPLEMENTS

These include iodination of water supplies, of bread and the use of iodine containing tablets or sweets, however, they are unsuitable for use in those areas where goitre and cretinism are still a problem.

Iodination of water supplies was tried in the Netherlands but was later abandoned as uneconomic because only a small proportion of the water supply is used for domestic purposes of drinking or cooking.

The iodination of flour used in bread-making was introduced in Tasmania, following which there was an increased incidence of thyrotoxicosis which was attributed to the increased consumption of iodine. However, the thyrotoxicosis was largely limited to those over 50-years-old with multinodular goitres. Thyrotoxicosis has also been reported as a rare complication following prophylactic programmes using iodinated oil. The rarity of the condition is possibly related to the fact that, in those areas where iodinated oil has been used, the proportion of the population who survive to 50 years of age is relatively small.

The disappearance of endemic goitre from some areas, e.g. New Zealand has been attributed not to any specific prophylactic programme but to the use of iodophors as a disinfectant in the dairy industry with some of the compound finding its way into the milk.

EVALUATION OF PREVENTIVE PROGRAMMES OF IODINE SUPPLEMENTATION

Ideally population surveys in areas of known high prevalence of goitre and cretinism need to be carried out. Recommendations for surveillance include the following:

(a) Clinical examination for goitre and cretinism
(b) Biochemical examination
  (1) Urinary iodine excretion
  (2) Measures of thyroid function, e.g. Serum T4 and TSH (Schaefer et al, 1974).

Of these the urinary iodine is probably the most difficult in terms of collection and analysis of samples and in reliability. Measures of thyroid function have been extensively developed for mass use as a screening test for neonatal hypothyroidism. However, the expertise is not often available in those countries where goitre and cretinism are endemic.

Clinical surveys of goitre and cretinism prior to and following the introduction of iodine prophylaxis are eminently feasible and do not require highly trained observers. Furthermore, such surveys, because they are concerned with a small number of specific observations, are particularly appropriate as examples in the training of medical and paramedical personnel. They can be used to heighten awareness of the importance of prevention, to carry out population survey work and to inculcate the concept of evaluating any new health initiative be it preventive or curative.

SUMMARY

Endemic goitre and its more serious accompanying disorder, endemic cretinism, are still serious community health problems particularly in the poorest countries. They are diseases that are eminently preventable by simple and cheap preventive programmes. The evidence that the overt cretin is only the tip of the iceberg and that subclinical intellectual and motor deficits may also be the consequence of iodine deficiency serves to further underline the importance of prevention.

REFERENCES

Arstila A, Krusius F E, Peltola P 1969 Studies on the transfer of thio-oxazolidone-type goitrogens in cows milk in goitre endemic districts of Finland in experimental conditions. Acta Endocrinologica (Kbh) 60: 712–718
Axelrad A A, Leblond C, Isler H 1955 Role of iodine deficiency in the production of goiter by the Remington diet. Endocrinology 56: 387–403
Buttfield I H, Hetzel B S 1967 Endemic goitre in Eastern New Guinea. Bulletin of the World Health Organisation 36: 243–262
Buttfield I H, Hetzel B S 1971 Endemic cretinism in Eastern New Guinea: its relation to goitre and iodine deficiency. In: Endemic Cretinism. Hetzel B S, Pharoah P O D (eds) Institute of Human Biology, Papua New Guinea Monograph Series No 2: 55–69
Chilean Iodine Educational Bureau 1952 Iodine Content of Foods: Bibliography 1851–1921. London
Chilean Iodine Educational Bureau 1956 Geochemistry of Iodine. London
Clarke K H, McCullagh S F, Winikoff D 1960 The use of an intramuscular depot of iodised oil as a long-lasting source of iodine. Medical Journal of Australia 1: 89–92
Clements F W 1960 Health significance of endemic goitre and related conditions. In: Endemic Goitre, World Health Organisation Monograph Series 44: 235–260

Clements F W, Wishart J W 1956 A thyroid blocking agent in the etiology of endemic goiter. Metabolism 5: 623–639

Connolly K J, Pharoah P O D, Hetzel B S 1979 Fetal iodine deficiency and motor performance during childhood. Lancet 2: 1149–1151

Costa A, Cottino F, Mortara M, Vogliazzo U 1964 Endemic cretinism in Piedmont. Panminerva Medica 6: 250–259

Cranfield P F 1962 The discovery of cretinism. Bulletin of the History of Medicine 36: 489–511

Curling T 1850 Two cases of absence of the thyroid body and symmetrical swellings of fat tissue at the sides of the neck connected with defective cerebral development. Medico-chirugical Transactions, London 33 303

Day T K, Powell-Jackson P R 1972 Fluoride, water hardness and endemic goitre. Lancet 1: 1135–1138

Delange F, Iteke F B, Ermans A M (eds) 1982 Nutritional factors involved in the goitrogenic action of cassava. International Development Research Centre, Ottawa, Canada. IDRC 184e

Delange F M et al 1976 Evidence for fetal hypothyroidism in severe endemic goitre. In: Robbins J, Braveman L E (eds) Thyroid Research. Excerpta Medica, Amsterdam p 493

Demaeyer E M, Lowenstein F W, Thilly C H 1979 The control of endemic goitre. World Health Organization, Geneva

De Quervain F, Wegelin C 1936 Der endemische kretinismus. Verlag-Springer, Berlin

Dussault J H, Hobel C J, Fisher D A 1971 Maternal and fetal thyroxine secretion during pregnancy in the sheep. Endocrinology 88: 47–51

Ekins R P, Sinha A K, Woods R J, Connolly K, Pharoah P 1983 Placental transfer of thyroxine in early pregnancy. 13th Scientific Meeting of the Thyroid Club, London

Ekpechi O L 1967 Pathogenesis of endemic goiter in Eastern Nigeria. British Journal of Nutrition 21: 537–545

Ekpechi O L, Dimitriadou A, Fraser R 1966 Goitrogenic activity of cassava (a staple Nigerian food). Nature 210: 1137–1138

Ermans A M, Delange F, Van Der Belden M, Kinthaert K 1972 Possible role of cyanide and thiocyante in the etiology of endemic cretinism. Advances in Experimental Medicine and Biology 30: 455–486

Ermans A M, Mbulamoko N M, Delange F, Ahluwaliar R (eds) 1980 Role of cassava in the etiology of endemic goitre and cretinism. International Development Research Centre, Ottawa, Canada, IDRC 136e

Fagge C H 1871 Sporadic cretinism occurring in England. Medico-chirugical Transactions 55: 155–170

Farr W 1885 Vital Statistics: Memorial volume of selections from the reports and writings of William Farr. Offices of the Sanitary Institute, London p 57

Fierro-Benitez R, Ramirez I, Estrella E, Stanbury J B 1974 The role of iodine in intellectual development in an area of endemic goiter. In: Dunn T J, Medeiros-Neto G A (eds) Endemic Goiter and Cretinism: Continuing Threats to World Health. Pan American Health Organisation Scientific Publication No. 292 135–142

Fisher D A, Hobel C J, Garza R 1970 Thyroid function in the preterm fetus. Pediatrics 46: 208–216

Follis R 1964 Recent studies on iodine malnutrition and endemic goiter. Medical Clinics of North America 48: 1219–1238

Food and Agriculture Organisation of the United Nations 1954 Report on the 3rd conference on nutrition problems in Latin America. Food and Agriculture Organisation Nutrition Meetings Report Series No 8

Gaitan E 1973 Water-born goitrogens and their role in the etiology of endemic goiter. World Review of Nutrition and Dietetics 17: 53–90

Gaitan E, Merino H, Rodriguez G, Sanchez G, Meyer J D 1973 Environmental goitrogens. In: Scow R D (ed): Endocrinology, Excerpta Medica, Amsterdam p 1143–1149

Gordon M B 1922 Childhood myxedma or so-called sporadic cretinism in North America. Endocrinology 6: 225–254

Gordon M B 1938 Childhood myxedema (sporadic cretinism) in the United States. Transactions of the 3rd International Goiter Conference p 114–129

Greenwald I 1957 The history of goiter in the Inca Empire: Peru, Chile and the Argentine Republic. Texas Reports on Biology and Medicine 15: 874–889

Greer M A, Grimm Y, Struder H 1968 Qualitative changes in the secretion of thyroid hormones induced by iodine deficiency. Endocrinology 83: 1193–1198

Harington C R, Barger G 1927 Thyroxine III: Constitution and synthesis of thyroxine. Biochemical Journal 21: 169–183

Hershman J M, Hershman F K 1972 Development of the thyroid control system. Advances in Experimental Medicine and Biology 30: 417–428

Hunnikin C 1974 The spray method of iodating salt. In: Dunn J T, Medeiros- Neto G A (eds) Endemic Goiter and Cretinism: Continuing threats to world health. Pan American Health Organisation Scientific Publication No. 292: 184–190

Kelly F C, Snedden W W 1960 Prevalence and geographical distribution of endemic goitre. In: Endemic Goitre, World Health Organisation Monograph Series 44: 27–233

Koenig M P 1968 Die kongenitale hypothyreose und der endemische kretinismus. Springer-Verlag, Berlin

Koenig M P, Veraguth P 1961 Studies of thyroid function in endemic cretins. In: Pitt-Rivers R (ed) Advances in Thyroid Research. Pergamon Press, London

Kywe T, Tin T O, Khin M N, Wrench J, Buttfield I H 1978 Proceedings of the first Asia Oceania Thyroid Association. Singapore

Langer P 1960 History of goitre In: Endemic Goitre, World Health Organisation Monograph Series 44: 9–25

McCarrison R 1906 Observations on endemic goitre in the Chitral and Gilgit Valleys. Lancet 1: 1110–1111

McCarrison R 1908 Observations on endemic cretinism in the Chitral and Gilgit valleys. Lancet 2: 1275–1280

McCullagh S F 1959 Goitre control project. Papua New Guinea. Medical Journal 3: 43–47

Major R H 1945 Classic descriptions of disease. Thomas, Springfield, Illinois

Malamos B et al 1971 Endemic goiter in Greece: Some new epidemiological studies. Journal of Clinical Endocrinology and Metabolism 32: 130–139

Marine D, Kimball O P 1920 The prevention of simple goiter in man. Archives of Internal Medicine 25: 661–672

Matovinovic J, Ramalingaswami V 1960 Therapy and prophylaxis of endemic goitre. In: Endemic Goitre, World Health Organisation Monograph Series 44: 385–410

Merke F 1960 The history of endemic goitre and cretinism in the thirteenth to fifteenth centuries. Proceedings of Royal Society of Medicine 53: 995–1002

Murray M M, Ryle J A, Simpson B W, Wilson D C 1948 Thyroid enlargement and other changes related to the mineral content of drinking water (MRC memorandum no 18). HMSO, London

Myant N B 1958 Passage of thyroxine and triiodothyronine from mother to foetus in pregnant women. Clincial Science 17: 75–79

Nestel B, Macintyre R (eds) 1973 Chronic cassava toxicity. International Development Research Centre Ottawa, Canada, IDRC 010e

Norris H 1847 Notice of a remarkable disease analogous to cretinism existing in a small village in the west of England. Medical Times, London 17: 257–258

Osorio C, Myant N B 1960 The passage of thyroid hormone from mother to foetus and its relation to foetal development. British Medical Bulletin 16: 159–163

Pan American Health Organisation 1963 Report of the Scientific Group on Research in Endemic Goitre. Washington: Pan American Health Organisation

Pan American Health Organisation 1974 Report of the Technical Group on Endemic Goiter. Washington: Pan American Health Organisation

Parker W R 1896 An obsolescent variety of cretinism. British Medical Journal 2: 506–507

Perez C, Scrimshaw N S, Munoz H A 1960 Technique of endemic goiter surveys. In: Endemic Goitre, World Health Organisation Monograph Series 44: 369–384

Pharaoh P O D, Lawton N F, Ellis S M, Williams E S, Ekins R 1973 The role of triiodothyronine (T3) in the maintenance of euthyroidism in endemic goitre. Clinical Endocrinology 2: 193–199

Pharaoh P O D 1972 Endemic cretinism in the Jimi valley of New Guinea. MD thesis University of London

Pharaoh P O D 1976 Geographical variation in the clinical manifestations of endemic cretinism. Tropical and Geographical Medicine 28: 259–267

Pharaoh P O D, Buttfield I H, Hetzel B S 1971 Neurological damage to the fetus resulting from severe iodine deficiency during pregnancy. Lancet 1: 308–310

Pharaoh P O D, Buttfield I H, Hetzel B S 1972 The effect of iodine prophylaxis on the incidence of endemic cretinism. Advances in Experimental Medicine and Biology 30: 201–221

Pharaoh P, Connolly K J, Hetzel B S, Ekins R 1981 Maternal thyroid function and motor competence in the child. Developmental Medicine and Child Neurology 23: 76–82

Pharaoh P O D, Delange F, Fierro-Benitez R, Stanbury J B 1980 Endemic Cretinism. In: Stanbury J B, Hetzel B S (eds) Endemic Goiter and Endemic Cretinism. Wiley, New York. p 359–421

Pharaoh P O D, Ellis S M, Ekins R P, Williams E S 1976 Maternal thyroid function, iodine deficiency and fetal development. Clinical Endocrinology 5: 159–166

Pharaoh P O D, Hornabrook R W 1973 Endemic cretinism of recent onset in New Guinea. Lancet 2: 1038–1041

Pretell E, Stanbury J B 1971 Effect of chronic iodine deficiency on maternal and fetal thyroid hormone synthesis. In: Hetzel B S, Pharaoh P O D (eds) Endemic Cretinism. Institute of Human Biology. Papua New Guinea Monograph Series 2 117–124

Pretell E A, Torres T, Zenteno V, Cornejo M 1972 Prophylaxis of endemic goiter with iodized oil in rural Peru. Advances in Experimental Medicine and Biology 30: 249–265

Prosser T 1769 Account and method of cure of the bronchocele or Derby Neck. London

Querido A 1971 Epidemiology of Cretinism. In: Hetzel B S, Pharaoh P O D (eds) Endemic Cretinism. Institute of Human Biology, Papua New Guinea Monograph Series No 2: 9–18

Querido A, Bleichdrodt N, Djokomoeljanto R 1978 Thyroid hormones and human mental development.

In: Corner M A, Baker R E, Van De Pol N E, Swaab D F, Uylings H B M (eds) Maturation of the nervous system. Progress in brain research Vol 48. Elsevier Amsterdam p 337–344

Querido A et al 1974 Definitions of endemic goiter and cretinism, classification of goiter size and severity of endemics and survey techniques. In: Dunn J T, Medeiros-Neto G A (eds) Endemic goiter and cretinism: continuing threats to world health. Pan American Health Organisation Scientific Publication No. 292 267–272

Ramirez I et al 1972 The results of prophylaxis of endemic cretinism. Advances in Experimental Medicine and Biology 30: 223–237

Report of British Medical Association Committee on Nutrition 1950. London

Roche J, Lissitzky S 1960 Etiology of endemic goitre. In: Endemic goitre. World Health Organisation Monograph Series 44: 351–368

Sardinian Royal Commission Rapport de la commission cree pa son majestie le roi de Sardaigne pour etudier le cretinisme, Imprimerie Royale, Turin, 1848

Schaefer A, Slavaneschi J, Summons J, Tavera J, Wilson D 1974 Surveillance of iodine prophylaxis. In: Dunn J A, Mederios-Neto G A (eds) Endemic goiter and cretinism: continuing threats to world health. Pan American Health Organisation Scientific Publication No. 292; 282–283

Stewart J C, Vidor G I, Buttfield I H, Hetzel B S 1971 Epidemic thyrotoxicosis in Northern Tasmania: Studies of clinical features and iodine nutrition. Australian and New Zealand Journal of Medicine 3: 203–211

Stott H, Bhatia B B, Lal R S, Rai K C 1939 The distribution and cause of endemic goitre in the United Provinces. Indian Journal of Medical Research 18: 1059–1085

Taylor S 1954 Calcium as a goitrogen. Journal of Clinical Endocrinology and Metabolism 14: 1412–1422

Thilly C H, Delange F M, Camus M, Berquist H, Ermans A M 1974 Fetal hypothyroidism in endemic goiter: the probable pathogenic mechanism of endemic cretinism. In: Dunn T J, Medeiros-Neto G A (eds): Endemic goiter and Cretinism: Continuing Threats to World Health. Pan American Health Organisation Scientific Publication 292: 121–128

Thilly C H, Delange F, Goldstein-Golaire J 1973 Endemic goiter prevention by iodised oil: a reassessment. Journal of Clinical Endocrinology and Metabolism 36: 1196–1204

Thilly C H et al 1980 Fetomaternal relationship, fetal hypothyroidism and psychmotor retardation. In: Ermans A M, Mbulamoko N M, Delange F, Ahluwalia R (eds) Role of cassava in the etiology of endemic goitre and cretinism. International Development Research Centre, Ottawa, Canada IDRC 136e

Trikojus V M 1974 Some observations on endemic goitre in Tasmania and Southern Queensland. New Zealand Medical Journal 80: 491–492

Trotter W R 1960 The association of deafness with thyroid dysfunction. British Medical Bulletin 16: 92–98

Vought R L, London W T, Stebbing G E T 1967 Endemic goiter in Northern Virginia. Journal of Clinical Endocrinology and Metabolism 27: 1381–1389

Webster B, Chesney A M 1930 Studies in the etiology of simple goiter. American Journal of Pathology 6: 275–284

Wespi H J 1945 Abnahme der taubstummheit in der Schweiz als volge der kropfprophylaxe mit jordiertem kochsalz. Schwiezerische Medizinische Wochenschrift 28: 625–629

10. Infectious disease and human travel

N. S. Galbraith

INTRODUCTION

The problems of infectious disease in travellers have long been recognized (Maegraith, 1965; Dorolle, 1968) and the present concern arises because of the continuing increase in world travel, principally by air, in the past few years. This chapter reviews recent trends in infectious diseases associated with human travel with particular reference to experience in the United Kingdom (UK). Detailed up-to-date advice on prevention of these infections was published recently by Walker & Williams (1983) and will not, therefore, be considered here. A list of authorities providing advice on infectious diseases in travellers and their prevention is given in Table 10.1.

AIR TRAVEL

The first fare-paying passenger flight in the world took place on 15th July 1919; Major, later Colonel, Norman Pilkington of the famous glass firm in St Helens, Lancashire, made an urgent business trip to the continent flying from Hendon aerodrome, London's first airport (Fig. 10.1) to Paris — Le Bourget. In 1945, the first

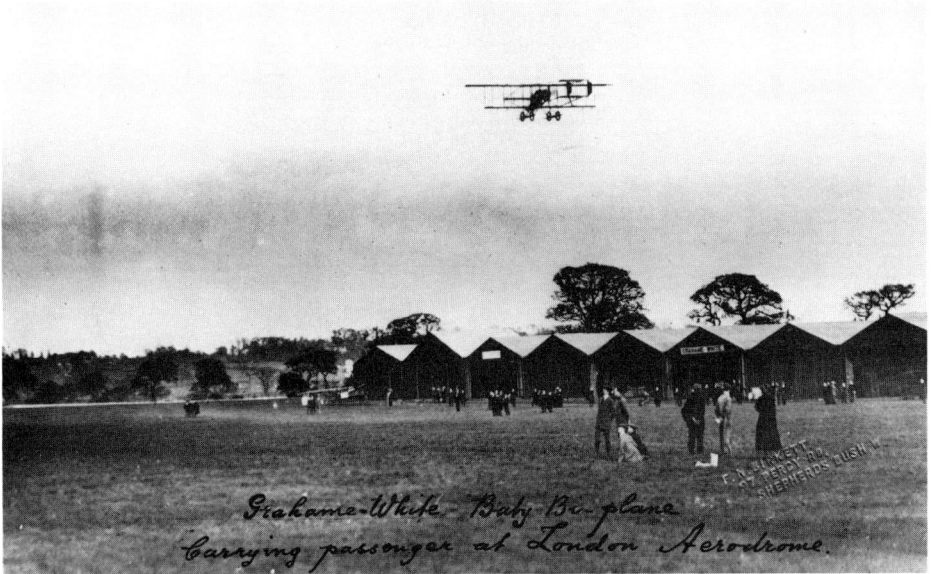

Grahame-White Baby Bi-plane
Carrying passenger at London Aerodrome.

Fig. 10.1 Hendon, London, in the 1920s. Reproduced by permission of The Royal Air Force Museum, Hendon.

Table 10.1 Health of the traveller

City	Centres providing advice on immunisation, malarial prophylaxis and other aspects of health protection
London	Department of Health and Social Security Alexander Fleming House Elephant & Castle LONDON SE1 6BY Telephone: 01–407 5522 Ross Institute London School of Hygiene & Tropical Medicine Keppel Street LONDON WC1 Telephone: 01–636 8636 British Airways Immunisation Centre 75 Regent Street LONDON W1R 7HG Telephone: 01–439 9584 PHLS Communicable Disease Surveillance Centre 61 Colindale Avenue LONDON NW9 5EQ Telephone: 01–200 6868
Birmingham	Department of Communicable & Tropical Diseases East Birmingham Hospital Bordesley Green BIRMINGHAM B9 5ST Telephone: 021–772 4311
Liverpool	Liverpool School of Tropical Medicine Pembroke Place LIVERPOOL L3 5QA Telephone: 051–708 9393
Glasgow	Communicable Diseases (Scotland) Unit Ruchill Hospital GLASGOW G20 9NB Telephone: 041–946 7120

Also Public Health Laboratories in England and Wales

year for which passenger statistics were available, just over 9 million passengers travelled on world scheduled air services (excluding the Union of Soviet Socialist Republics), a figure which increased over 70 fold to 639 million in 1981. Statistics on distances travelled were available earlier and in 1929, 170 million passenger kilometres were flown, this increased to 8000 million in 1945 and to 945 000 million in 1981, over a 100 fold increase from 1945 to 1981 (Fig. 10.2). This rise in distances travelled was most notable from the mid 1960s, when many areas of the tropics became easily accessible from the UK; for example, between 1962 and 1981 there was a 9.6 fold increase in passenger traffic to and from the Indian Subcontinent and an 8.7 fold increase to and from Commonwealth West Africa.

London—Heathrow became London's main airport at the end of the Second World War and in 1947 just over 63 000 passengers passed through to all destinations:

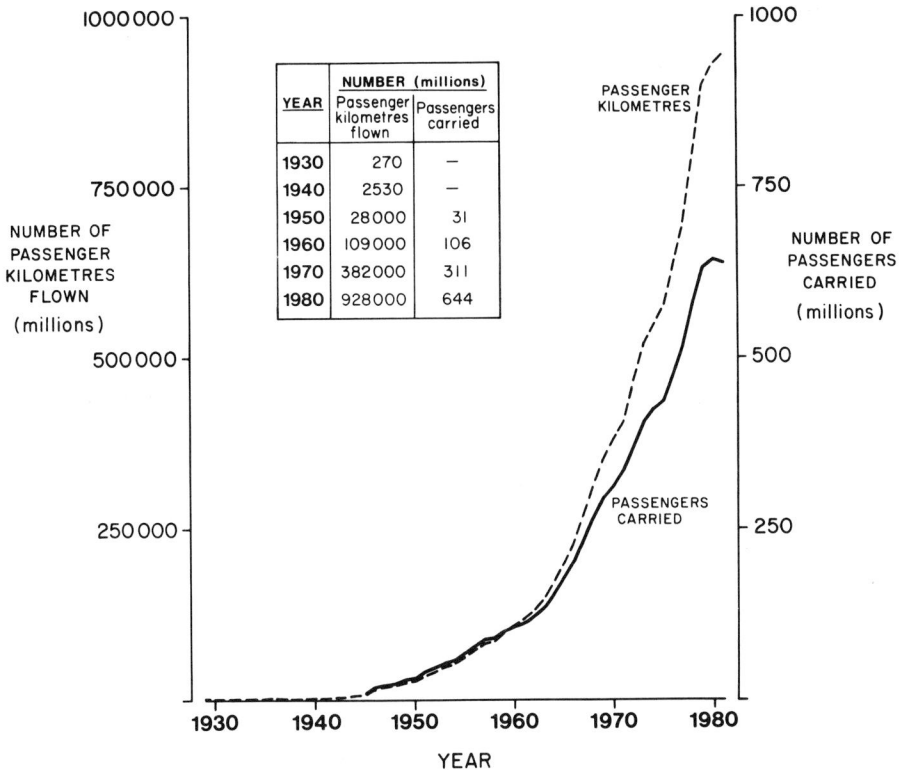

| YEAR | NUMBER (millions) | |
	Passenger kilometres flown	Passengers carried
1930	270	—
1940	2530	—
1950	28000	31
1960	109000	106
1970	382000	311
1980	928000	644

Fig. 10.2 Scheduled world air travel (excluding USSR) 1929–1981. From civil aviation statistics, Civil Aviation Authority, London.

by 1982, including other airports serving London, this had increased to about 40 million passengers. In 1977, the PHLS Communicable Disease Surveillance Centre was set up in England and Wales (Galbraith & Young, 1980) with one of its functions to detect and control imported disease which resulted from travel; the centre was sited in Colindale, North London, by a curious coincidence only a few hundred yards from the site of Hendon aerodrome where air passenger services began 58 years earlier.

SURVEILLANCE

The increased speed and volume of human travel rendered ineffective and obsolete the concept of quarantine as a means of controlling the international spread of infection. In the early 1950s this was replaced by a more active method of disease control termed surveillance (Langmuir, 1963), which comprises the early detection and reporting of infections and the rapid implementation of control measures to prevent their spread. The principles of communicable disease surveillance and the methods used in England and Wales were described in the previous volume in this series (Galbraith, 1982).

The routine information systems in the UK which are particularly relevant to the surveillance of infections associated with travel are (i) statutory notifications of infectious disease, (ii) laboratory reporting of microbiological data, and (iii) hospital data, including hospital discharges and deaths and clinic returns of sexually transmitted diseases. These routine information systems provide valuable data about trends in the major infectious diseases associated with travel which can be expressed as rates per 1000 travellers. The data do not, however, provide an accurate measure of imported disease because on the one hand, some travel-associated infections are more likely to be investigated and reported than the same infections when not associated with travel and on the other hand mild illness in travellers may escape recognition. To overcome these deficiencies special surveys have been undertaken. For example, in Scotland, Reid (1982) found that between 1977 and 1980 package holidaymakers reported most illness, nearly half of them had symptoms, and that minor alimentary disorders were the commonest complaint accounting for 80% of all illness. These illnesses were of clinical significance to the individual, and their frequency and clinical importance demand routine enquiry about travel in all febrile patients. However, many of the illnesses were probably of little public health importance in Scotland; for example Sharp (1982) studied the spread of infection from 2081 imported infections in Scotland between 1975 and 1981; these included 829 cases of salmonellosis, 345 of bacillary dysentery, 236 of malaria, 219 of campylobacter enteritis, 125 of giardiasis, 82 of enteric fever, 74 of viral hepatitis, 27 of tuberculosis and cases of brucellosis, measles, Legionnaires' disease and worm infestation. Secondary spread took place in less than 3% of cases and then was almost invariably confined to the household.

TRAVELLERS' DIARRHOEA

Gastro-intestinal infections have always been by far the commonest cause of illness in travellers from Westernised countries (Turner, 1975) and this was confirmed again by the Scottish surveys quoted above and by studies in the United States of America (USA) (Gangarosa et al, 1980). Most frequent amongst these infections is travellers' diarrhoea. This is usually an acute self-limiting disease occurring during or soon after travel and commonly associated with travel from North America, Europe and Australasia to parts of the world with lower standards of hygiene and sanitation. The disease, originally called 'Gyppy tummy' by British troops serving in Egypt before the First World War, has many other geographical names such as 'Delhi belly', 'Rangoon runs' and in Mexico 'turista'. It was ascribed to changes in diet and of climate until just over a decade ago when Rowe et al (1970) in a study of British soldiers in Aden, showed that it was due to an entero-toxigenic strain of *Escherichia coli*; confirmation of its aetiological role was obtained when a laboratory assistant in England unwittingly became infected with the organism and developed typical symptoms of travellers' diarrhoea. However, since the early 1970s, it has been shown that the syndrome is of diverse aetiology and that the causative organisms vary from place to place and at different times; *Salmonella* sp., *Shigella* sp. and *Giardia lamblia* cause a proportion of cases and recently *Campylobacter* sp. and rotaviruses have also been implicated (Nye, 1979).

GASTROINTESTINAL ILLNESS ON PASSENGER CRUISE LINERS

On 14th January 1970 the SS Oronsay, a cruise liner which had left Southampton on 16th December 1969, sailed into Vancouver harbour with 83 suspected cases of typhoid fever amongst the 1600 passengers and crew; 55 of these were subsequently confirmed by culture or serology. Investigations showed that the outbreak was probably waterborne (Davies et al, 1972). This episode led to the establishment of a surveillance system of gastrointestinal illness on cruise liners using American ports. Between 1975 and 1978, 25 outbreaks occurred on 5115 cruises and 12 of them were investigated by the Center for Disease Control, Atlanta, USA; bacterial pathogens were identified in 4, *Vibrio parahaemolyticus*, enterotoxigenic *E. coli*, *Shigella* sp. and *Salmonella* sp. but in the other eight no bacteria were isolated and it was thought they were probably of viral aetiology (Dannenberg et al, 1982); in one of them the virus was subsequently shown to be Norwalk virus (Gunn et al, 1980). Of the 12 outbreaks investigated four were considered to be waterborne, two foodborne and two due to person-to-person spread; in four the method of spread remained unknown. This surveillance programme accompanied by a programme of hygiene inspections appeared to be successful in reducing the incidence of gastrointestinal illness on cruise liners in the USA.

Similar problems have been experienced on cruise liners in Britain, a recent notable example of which was an outbreak of typhoid fever, dysentery and other diarrhoeal illness in passengers on a Russian cruiseliner on a North African cruise from Tilbury in 1978. Diarrhoeal illness was reported to the Port Medical Officer who ascertained that about 150 of 238 passengers were affected. Subsequently, routine national surveillance systems detected typhoid fever and dysentery in passengers widely dispersed in England, the Channel Islands and the Netherlands (Fig. 10.3). Investigations suggested that the outbreak was probably waterborne. This and other episodes indicate the need for a surveillance system and hygiene programme in the UK similar to that established in the USA.

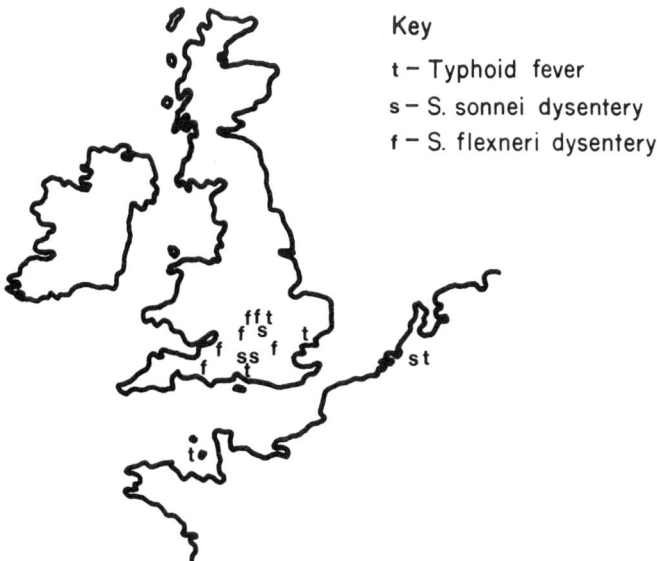

Key

t – Typhoid fever
s – S. sonnei dysentery
f – S. flexneri dysentery

Fig. 10.3   Typhoid and dysentery on a cruise liner. Geographical distribution of cases.

FOOD POISONING

In 1982, the Office of Population Censuses and Surveys collected information about the likely place of infection of food poisoning, formally notified or ascertained by other means, in order to obtain information about imported disease. Between 9 and 10% were infected abroad, a figure which may exaggerate the proportion of imported cases because the disease in travellers may be more likely to come to notice. The findings of the Scottish study (Sharp, 1982) suggested that salmonellas were the commonest cause of food poisoning acquired abroad. In England and Wales most imported cases of salmonellosis reported by laboratories in the decade 1973 to 1982 appeared to be sporadic cases but some outbreaks associated with particular cruise liners or hotels and resorts abroad were identified. For example, in March 1980 over 37 passengers on a particular liner on which cases of food poisoning had occurred in the past, developed *S. montevideo* infection; detailed investigation suggested frozen chicken as a possible source of infection although this was not confirmed. In another outbreak, 17 cases of *S. oranienberg* infection were identified in persons returning from the same hotel in Spain and this information was passed to the Spanish health authorities for investigation. Outbreaks associated with aircraft have also been reported; in 1976, a large outbreak of *S. brandenburg* infection took place in passengers and crews on scheduled air services from Paris between April 6th and 11th; investigation showed contamination of cold dishes from one supplier (World Health Organization, 1976).

Staphylococcal food poisoning, because of its shorter incubation period of only a few hours, often presents in travellers more dramatically than salmonella infections.

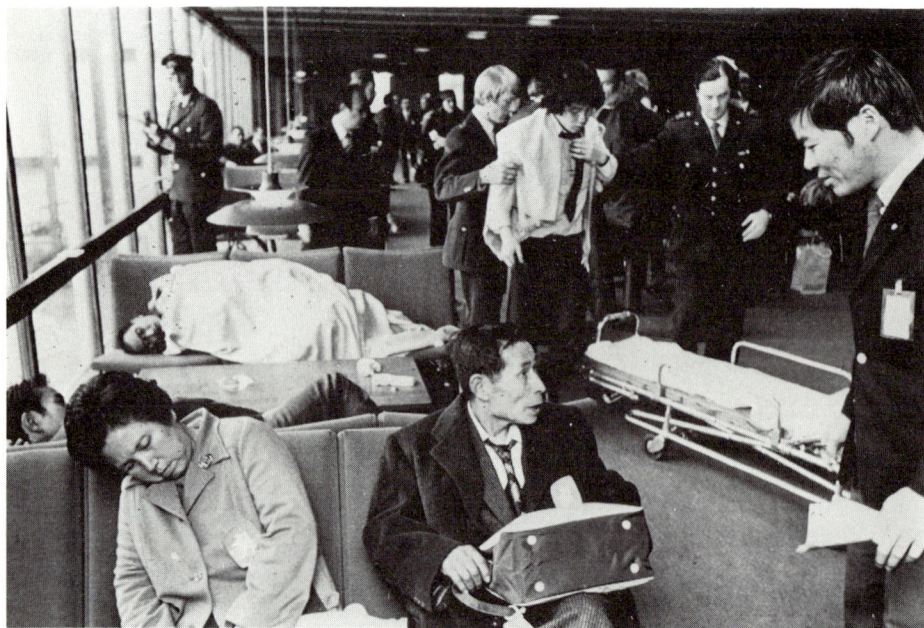

Fig. 10.4 Staphylococcal food poisoning aboard an aircraft. Sick passengers arriving at Copenhagen Airport, February 2, 1975. Reproduced by permission of Associated Press Ltd.

On 2nd February 1975, 196 of 343 passengers and 1 of 20 crew on an aircraft which arrived in Copenhagen from Tokyo developed acute gastroenteritis shortly before landing (Fig. 10.4); 143 passengers and the one crew member were admitted to hospital. Investigation showed the outbreak was due to staphylococcal food poisoning caused by ham contaminated by a food handler with an inflamed finger, and it demonstrated the importance of serving air crew different meals from the passengers and from each other (Center for Disease Control, 1975). Similar episodes have taken place on trains and on coach trips; an outbreak of over 20 cases, 12 of whom were admitted to hospital, was reported on a trans-Canada train (Chernenkoff et al, 1971) and an outbreak on a coach trip in Lincolnshire in September 1981 affected 64 of 102 old age pensioners, all of whom were admitted to hospital.

Vibrio parahaemolyticus is a marine organism of warm climates and gives rise to food poisoning associated with raw seafood or cross-contaminated cooked products. In-flight outbreaks have been reported associated with seafood; Peffers et al (1973), described an outbreak due to crab meat affecting passengers arriving in London from Bangkok and Desmarchelier (1978) reported a similar outbreak in 1976 due to seafood cocktail in passengers arriving in Sydney from Bombay. Imported infections in Britain have been increasingly recognised in the past decade; between 1972 and 1982, 77 cases were reported in England and Wales, 68 of which were imported.

Clostridium perfringens food poisoning is infrequently reported in travellers, although a large outbreak associated with turkey affecting nearly 200 passengers on a special train in the USA was probably due to this organism (Hart et al, 1960). Another outbreak amongst passengers and crews of eight flights leaving Atlanta in November 1970 was also due to turkey (Center for Disease Control, 1971).

TYPHOID AND PARATYPHOID FEVERS

In the winter of 1963 a large waterborne outbreak of typhoid fever took place in Zermatt, a Swiss skiing resort, giving rise to cases amongst returning tourists in many European countries and North America. Altogether there were 437 cases; 177 in local inhabitants, and national surveillance detected a further 260 cases comprising 77 Swiss tourists from other parts of Switzerland and 33 tourists from Germany, 37 from France, 78 from Britain, 14 from the USA and 21 from other countries (Bernard, 1965). Following this episode the surveillance of typhoid and paratyphoid fevers in England and Wales was revised, first in 1967 by making specific enquiries about travel in all notified cases and second in 1973 by national integration of notifications with laboratory reports; this enabled the identification of non-notified cases and the distinction of paratyphoid A fever from paratyphoid B fever.

In the decade 1973–1982 there were between 150 and 268 cases of typhoid fever in England and Wales each year and over these years the proportion infected abroad increased from less than 80% to nearly 90% (Fig. 10.5). Paratyphoid A fever varied between 24 and 55 cases per year, nearly all of which were infected overseas, and paratyphoid B fever decreased from 82 cases in 1973 to 49 in 1982 with an increasing proportion infected abroad. Most of the imported cases of typhoid and paratyphoid A fevers were infected in the Indian subcontinent and most cases of paratyphoid B fever in the Mediterranean area (Table 10.2). Spread of the disease in England and Wales was unusual. In the five years 1978–82 14 cases (not including

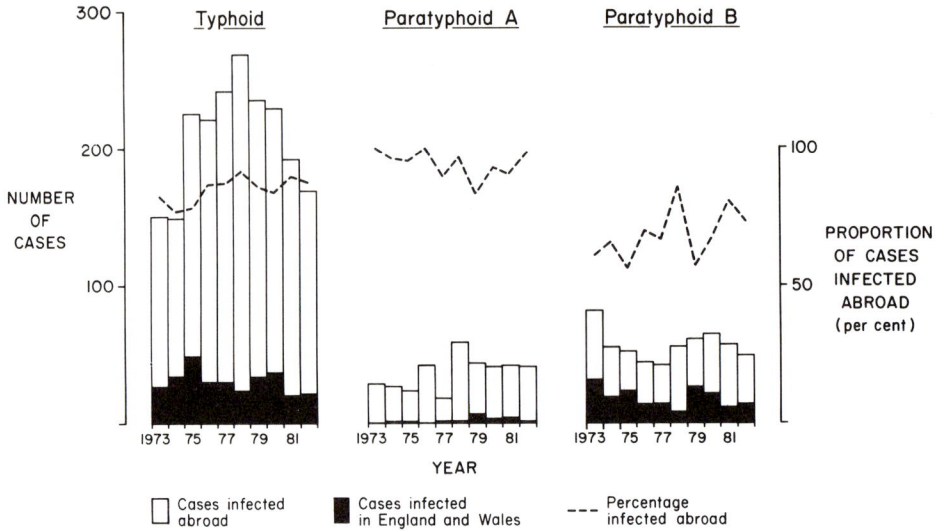

Fig. 10.5 Typhoid and paratyphoid fevers in England and Wales 1973–1982 showing indigenous and imported infections. Notifications and laboratory reports.

Table 10.2 Typhoid and paratyphoid fevers England and Wales 1973–1982 (place of infection)

Place of infection	Notifications and laboratory reports Number and percentage		
	Typhoid	Paratyphoid A	Paratyphoid B
Indian sub-continent	1175 (56.6)	279 (73.6)	40 (7.1)
Mediterranean	288 (13.8)	10 (2.7)	197 (35.0)
Middle East	100 (4.8)	25 (6.6)	106 (18.8)
West Africa	89 (4.3)	5 (1.3)	— —
Other	120 (5.8)	38 (10.0)	45 (8.0)
United Kingdom	305 (14.7)	22 (5.8)	175 (31.1)
Total	2077 (100.0)	379 (100.0)	563 (100.0)

symptomless infections), five of typhoid fever, three of paratyphoid A fever and six of paratyphoid B fever, were infected by imported cases; 11 were family members and three were health service staff.

The best protection for the traveller against enteric infection is to ensure safe drinking water and to avoid eating potentially contaminated foods. Typhoid vaccination is usually recommended for travellers outside North West Europe, North America and Australasia but this is difficult to justify in the Mediterranean area and in developed urban areas with high standards of hygiene and sanitation in other parts of the world. In the five years 1978–1982 the average annual number of UK travellers returning from the Mediterranean was 9 827 400, of whom on average 30 developed typhoid fever, an infection rate of 0.3 per 100 000 travellers per year; this is a very small risk and does not justify the annual vaccination of nearly 10 million travellers. The corresponding average annual infection rate in UK travellers returning from the Indian sub-continent was 82.48 per 100 000 travellers and from West Africa 29.9 per 100 000; vaccination might, therefore, be considered for UK travellers to rural areas of both these parts of the world.

CHOLERA

Classical cholera first became pandemic in the early part of the last century reaching the UK in the 1830s. The present pandemic due to the eltor biotype began in 1961 reaching Europe in 1971 (Barua, 1972) and the international spread up until 1981 was documented by Jusatz (1982) (Fig. 10.6).

The last indigenous case of classical cholera in the UK was reported in 1893 but there were imported cases until 1909. No further cases were recorded until 1970 when the eltor biotype reached the country. Between 1970 and 1982, 33 cases and four symptomless excreters were reported in England and Wales; all except one were infected abroad (Table 10.3). The indigenous infection was in a symptomless excreter, the wife of an airline pilot infected in India, who nursed her husband at home. No other spread took place in this country.

In Australia in 1972 an outbreak of 25 cases and 22 excreters was due to food served in flight on an international aircraft from London to Sydney; one patient died. The outbreak was caused by contaminated hors d'oeuvres taken on at Bahrain. The two UK cases in 1972 (Table 10.3) were in persons on a flight from Bahrain to London which was also revictualled in Bahrain and left only two hours before the Sydney flight (Sutton, 1974).

Cholera usually spreads by water or food so the main method of prevention in travellers is scrupulous care over drinking water and food. Vaccination is often recommended for travellers to Africa, Asia, the Middle East and other areas where the disease exists, but in a study of European travellers Morger et al (1983) considered vaccination unnecessary for the ordinary tourist.

Table 10.3   Cholera England and Wales 1970–1982

Year	Numbers of cases	excreters	Place of infection
1970	1	—	North Africa (1)
1971	3	—	Spain (3)
1972	2	—	Bahrain (2)
1973	5	2	Tunisia (5)
			India (1), UK (1)
1974	3	—	Portugal (2)
			Pakistan (1)
1975	1	—	Iraq (1)
1976	1	—	Nigeria (1)
1977	2	—	Iraq (1)
			Turkey (1)
1978	—	—	—
1979	—	—	—
1980	4	2	India (3), Tanzania (1)
			Indonesia (2)
1981	10	—	Tunisia (5)
			Pakistan (3)
			India (1), Iraq (1)
1982	1	—	Tunisia (1)
Total			
1970–1982	33	4	Africa (14), Asia (11),
			Middle East (5),
			Europe (7)

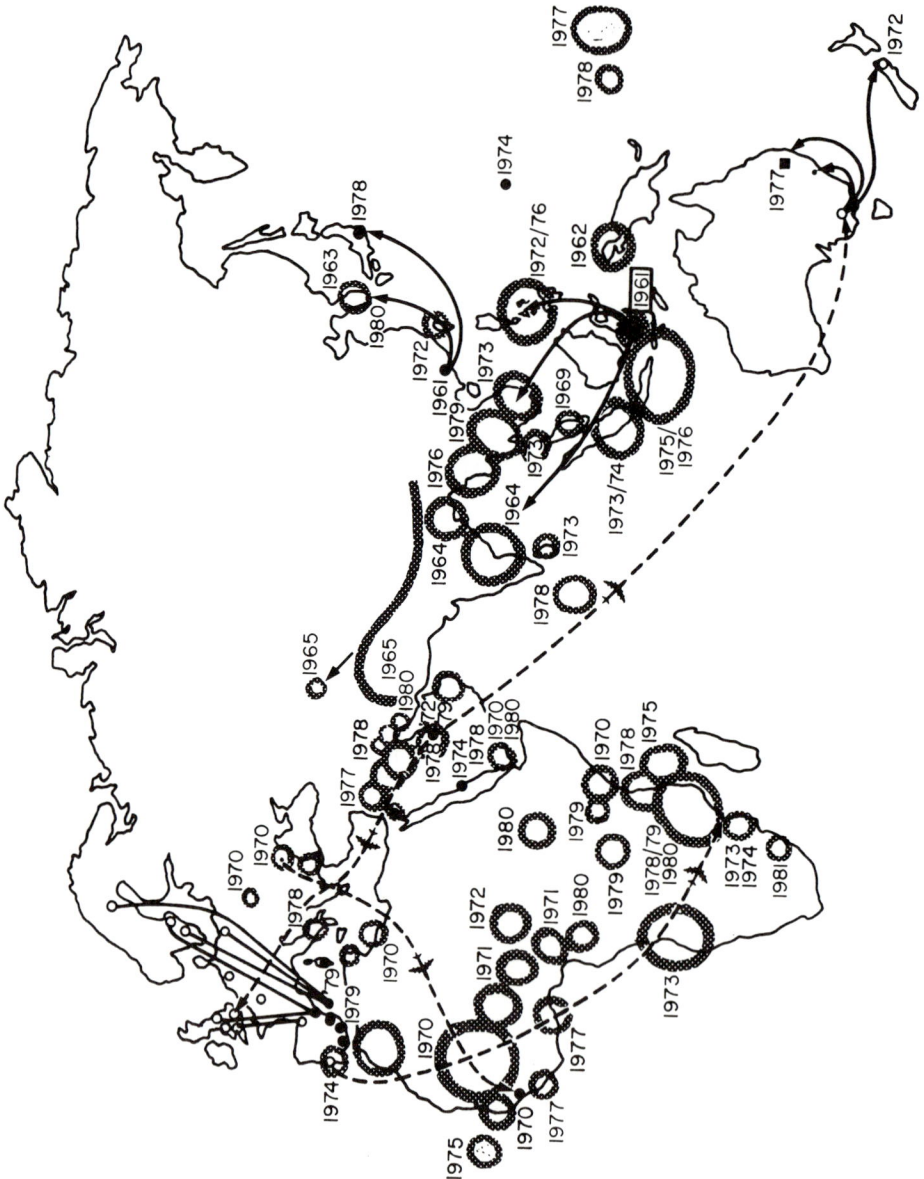

Fig. 10.6 World spread of cholera biotype eltor, 1961–1981. From: Jusatz 1982 International Journal of Microbiology and Hygiene. I. Abteilung Originale A 252: 257–267.

DYSENTERY

Both bacillary and amoebic dysentery are endemic in areas of the world with poor standards of hygiene and sanitation, where person-to-person spread is common in all age groups and where waterborne and foodborne outbreaks occur which may involve the traveller (Keusch, 1979).

In England and Wales bacillary dysentery due to *S. sonnei* is the commonest form of dysentery, usually spread by the faecal-oral route in young children; the trends in notifications reflect trends in the incidence of this infection (Fig. 10.7). Notifications reached the lowest recorded figure of 2709 in 1980 but increased in 1981, as did laboratory reports of *S. sonnei*. In contrast laboratory reports of other types of bacillary dysentery showed an increase between 1971 and 1982 which has been attributed to imported infection (Gross et al, 1979).

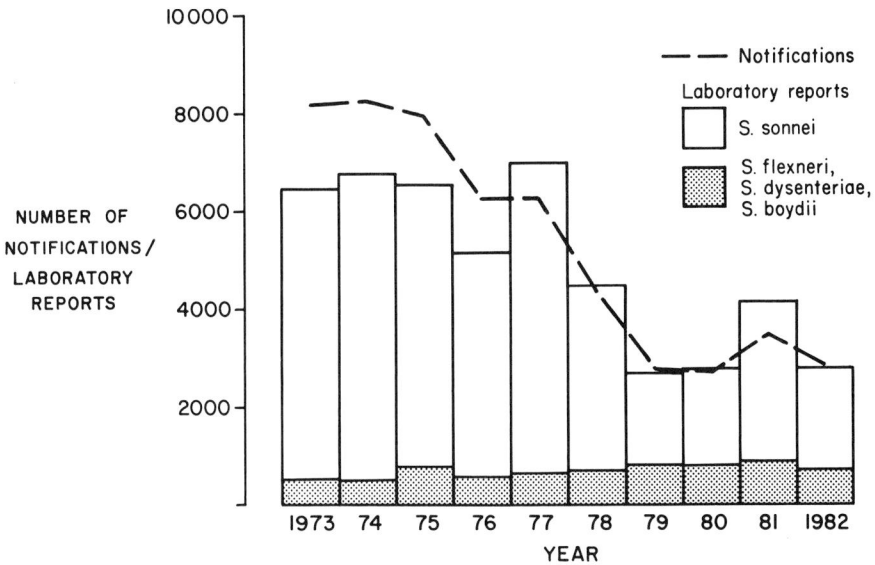

Fig. 10.7   Dysentery in England and Wales 1973–1982. Notifications and laboratory reports.

There are no reliable data on amoebic dysentery in England and Wales but data on amoebiasis from the Hospital In-patient Enquiry and from death certificates indicated about 190 cases and three deaths per year between 1962 and 1970 (Stamm, 1975). In the period 1973 to 1979 these figures declined to about 130 cases and two deaths each year. This decline may reflect improvements in domiciliary treatment of amoebic dysentery and therefore less hospitalisation and fewer deaths, rather than a decline in the incidence of the disease. Although a few cases have been reported in which the infection was acquired in England and Wales (McKendrick et al, 1981), it is likely that almost all of the cases were infected abroad.

HEPATITIS A

Hepatitis A is a worldwide infection commonest in areas of poor hygiene and sanitation. The infection is frequently asymptomatic in young children amongst whom spread is usually by the faecal-oral route, but common source outbreaks occur affecting adults, especially travellers from areas of low incidence such as North West Europe and North America. These adults are non-immune because they escape infection at an earlier age and are therefore 'at risk' when travelling to areas of high endemicity where sanitation is primitive.

An increase in the incidence of notified infective jaundice in England and Wales began in 1979. This was attributed mainly to an increase in hepatitis A in children, but the disease also increased in adults amongst whom outbreaks of shellfish-associated infection took place (O'Mahony et al, 1983). However, some of the increase may have been due to imported infection but because travel histories of notified cases are not usually available it is not possible to obtain a reliable estimate of the proportion of cases infected abroad. Laboratory reports between 1979 and 1982 showed that 1105 (11.4%) of 9653 cases were travel associated but these data are difficult to interpret because in only 40% of reports was a travel history given.

The most important preventive measure, as with other gastrointestinal infections, is care over water and food; shellfish are a common mode of spread of hepatitis A and should be avoided. Normal human immunoglobulin is recommended as a prophylactic for travellers who intend to visit areas of poor sanitation in parts of the world where the infection is common. A single dose of 750 mgm British immunoglobulin given to 1079 travellers between 1964 and 1967 was protective for up to 6 months (Pollock & Reid, 1969), but British immunoglobulin in the 1980s may be less protective because the proportion of the donor population who are immune to hepatitis A has declined (Mortimer & Parry, 1981). Reliance should therefore be placed mainly on simple hygienic measures of prevention.

INFLUENZA

Although respiratory infections are among the main causes of mortality and morbidity throughout the world (Miller, 1982) they are less commonly reported in association with travel than gastrointestinal infections. However, influenza gives rise to frequent epidemics and to pandemics every 10 to 20 years, which are usually due to the appearance of a new subtype of the virus; for example, in February 1957 the H_1N_1 (Asian) virus strain appeared in China and spread via Hong Kong to Australasia, Europe and America by August of the same year (Beveridge, 1977). Although this rapid world-wide spread of influenza is facilitated by air travel, outbreaks associated with the aircraft themselves are unusual; this may be partly due to difficulty in detecting such episodes but probably mainly because of the physical characteristics and ventilation of the aircraft cabin which tend to prevent the spread of droplet infection (Perin, 1976). However, an outbreak of influenza affecting the passengers on an aircraft in Alaska was reported in 1977 which followed a delay of $4\frac{1}{2}$ hours in take-off during which time many of them remained in the passenger cabin with the ventilation switched off. The index case was a lady who became ill with cough and fever shortly after boarding the aircraft; of the 53 passengers and crew, 38 subsequently became ill, the attack rate being highest in those who remained longest in the unventilated aircraft (Moser et al, 1979).

Spread of influenza A at sea is probably common but not often documented. In an outbreak in the remote island of Lewis in the Outer Hebrides in 1969–1970 this was clearly demonstrated; the virus was probably introduced by the crews of Spanish fishing vessels sailing out of San Sebastian, Northern Spain, where an outbreak was already in progress (Buchan & Reid, 1972). Subsequent spread to Scottish mainland ports and Norwegian ports took place.

MEASLES

Measles, unlike influenza, does not cause pandemics, but large outbreaks have occurred affecting a wide age range when the disease has been introduced by travellers into isolated non-immune communities (Christie, 1980). Because of the great increase in travel such isolated communities are unlikely to be found in the future but the probable eradication of measles by vaccination in some countries means that measles in travellers will assume importance as a method of reintroducing measles into these countries. Indeed, outbreaks of measles in the USA following importation of the disease has already been reported (Centers for Disease Control, 1981). Vaccination of travellers to prevent such introductions has not been recommended but all children in the UK should be vaccinated routinely as part of the childhood schedule at 15 months or at school entry.

DIPHTHERIA

Diphtheria has been virtually eliminated from North West Europe, North America and Australasia but remains common in other parts of the world. It is not surprising, therefore, that from time to time the disease is re-introduced into these areas by travellers. In England and Wales, for example, there were 35 notifications and two deaths between 1973 and 1982; 11 of the cases were in 1975 when an outbreak took place in Birmingham and London, which was traced to the recent arrival of two children from Bangladesh who were found to be pharyngeal carriers of *Corynebacterium diphtheriae* of the same type (Chattopadhyay et al, 1977). Immunisation of travellers is not necessary but all children in the UK should be immunised during the first year of life as part of the routine childhood schedule and should have a reinforcing dose at school entry.

TUBERCULOSIS

Because of the long incubation period of tuberculosis it is difficult to ascribe the disease to travel. However, it seems likely that susceptible travellers from countries where the disease is uncommon may acquire the infection when visiting other parts of the world where it is prevalent. For example, young Asians resident in the UK who were born in this country sometimes develop tuberculosis within six months of return from holiday on the Indian sub-continent and probably acquire the disease there. BCG vaccination of all travellers is unnecessary but vaccination of children going to areas where the disease is common is recommended.

LEGIONNAIRES' DISEASE

Legionnaires' disease, the principal feature of which is pneumonia, has been widely recognised since the identification of the causative bacterium in 1977. It is an ubiquitous organism often found in piped water systems and the cooling towers of air-conditioning systems. Outbreaks in travellers have been associated with these sources but there have also been many sporadic cases. The first reported outbreak in travellers was identified retrospectively in Scottish tourists returning from a hotel in Spain in 1973 (Reid et al, 1978); further cases associated with the same hotel took place during the following seven years until 1980 when an explosive outbreak occurred. Investigation then showed that contamination of the hotel piped water supply with *Legionella pneumophila* was the probable source of infection. This was confirmed when after the introduction of continuous chlorination no further cases were reported (Bartlett et al, 1983).

Altogether, between 1979 and 1982, there were 588 reported cases of Legionnaires' disease in England and Wales, 248 (42%) of which acquired the disease abroad (Table 10.4). Although nearly half of these cases, 115, had visited mainland Spain or the Balearic Islands, this was a reflection of the large number of tourists from Britain who visit Spain rather than an indication of high risk; for example, the rate per 100 000 visits by UK residents 1979–1982 was less than half that for Portugal (Table 10.4).

Table 10.4   Legionnaires' disease and travel England and Wales 1979–1982

| | Cases and travel in 4 year period 1979–1982 | | | |
Country visited	Cases number	Cases percentage	Visits by UK residents	Cases per 100 000 visits
Overseas travel				
Spain	115	19.6	11 996 000	0.96
Portugal	31	5.3	1 510 000	2.05
Italy	30	5.1	4 210 000	0.71
France	17	2.9	16 567 000	0.10
Greece	13	2.2	3 403 000	0.38
Germany	2	0.3	4 227 000	0.05
Holland	2	0.3	2 920 000	0.07
Other Europe	11	1.9	Not available	
Outside Europe	27	4.6	Not available	
Total overseas travel	248	42.2	—	—
UK travel	17	2.9	Not available	
No history of travel	323	54.9		
Grand total	588	100.0		

MALARIA

Malaria in travellers greatly increased during the 1970s following the resurgence of the disease, particularly in Asia, and the rise in international air traffic (Bruce-Chwatt, 1982a), and prophylaxis became complicated by the appearance of chloroquine resistant *Plasmodium falciparum*, in the Far East, South America and East Africa (Bruce-Chwatt, 1982b). Resistant parasites have subsequently been reported in many other parts of the world (Fig. 10.8) (Malaria Reference Laboratory, 1983).

The increase of the disease in travellers was particularly evident in those returning to Europe, and the highest figures were reported in the UK. Surveillance of malaria in the UK, maintained by the PHLS Malaria Reference Laboratory, was based on notifications, routine laboratory reports and reports to the reference laboratory. These

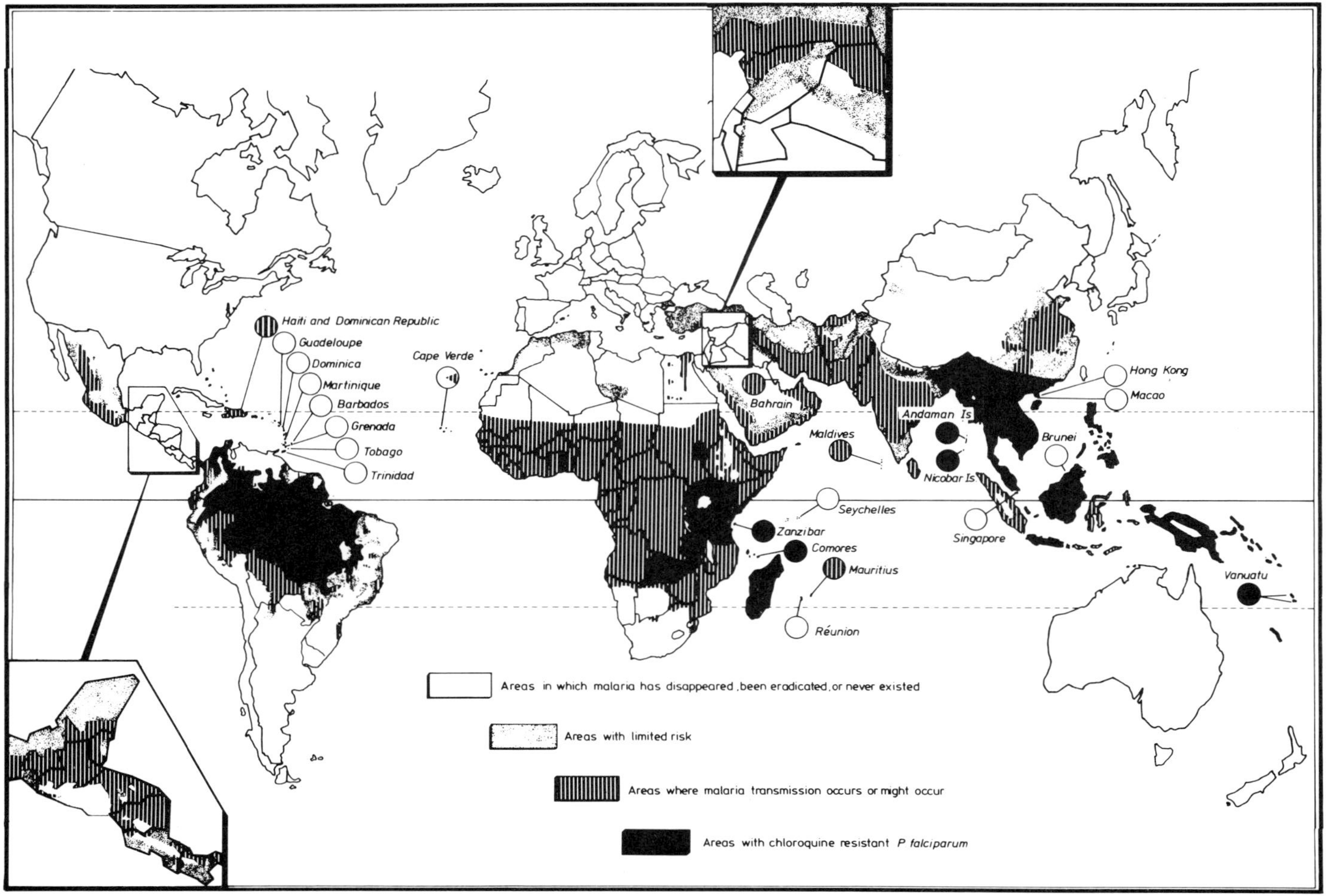

Fig. 10.8 Areas with reported falciparum malaria. Epidemiological assessment of malaria, June 1982. From: Malaria Reference Laboratory 1983 British Medical Journal 286: 787–789.

Legend:

- Areas in which malaria has disappeared, been eradicated, or never existed
- Areas with limited risk
- Areas where malaria transmission occurs or might occur
- Areas with chloroquine resistant *P falciparum*

Map labels: Hong Kong, Macao, Brunei, Andaman Is, Nicobar Is, Singapore, Vanuatu, Maldives, Bahrain, Seychelles, Zanzibar, Comores, Mauritius, Réunion, Cape Verde, Haiti and Dominican Republic, Guadeloupe, Dominica, Martinique, Barbados, Grenada, Tobago, Trinidad data related to the whole of the UK and provided information about the causative parasite. There was an increase from 541 reports in 1973 to a peak of 2053 in 1979 followed by a decline to 1471 in 1982. These overall changes were due to a rise in reported malaria caused by *P. vivax* followed by a fall after 1979 which obscured a continuing rise in *P. falciparum* (Fig. 10.9). Most of the *P. vivax* infections were acquired in the Indian sub-continent, and many were in immigrants who had settled in the UK but returned to their countries of origin for holidays with their families without appreciating that the incidence of the disease in their homeland had greatly increased and that prophylaxis was necessary; the recent decline has been partly attributed to the national health education programme in Britain about the need for prophylaxis. Most *P. falciparum* infections were acquired in Africa, mainly West Africa although the increase was greatest in East Africa, and some of these were in short term visitors. Altogether there were 45 deaths 1973–1982, almost all of them due to *P. falciparum* malaria in persons returning from West or East Africa; most of these deaths were a consequence of missed or late diagnosis together with lack of or incorrect chemoprophylaxis.

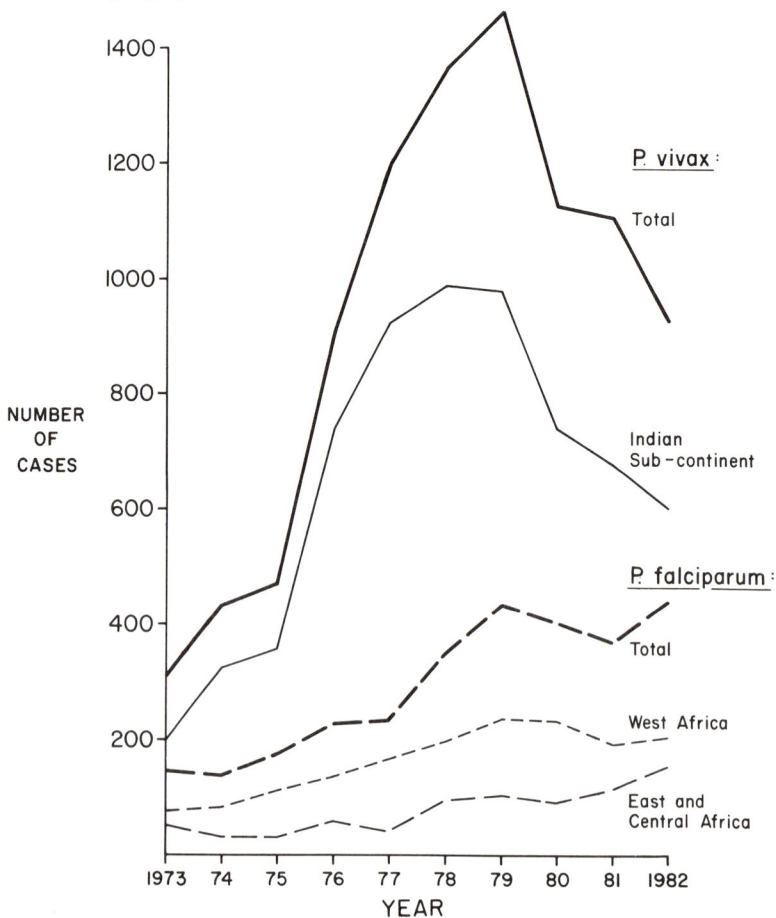

Fig. 10.9   Malaria in the United Kingdom 1973–1982. Causative parasites in cases from Africa and the Indian subcontinent. PHLS Malaria Reference Laboratory Data.

POLIOMYELITIS

Poliomyelitis was almost eliminated from Northern Europe, North America and Australasia in the 1960s, but because infection remains common and widespread in many other parts of the world unimmunised travellers may contract the disease. Gregory & Spalding (1972), for example, described two young businessmen who had not been immunised who acquired the disease on brief trips to the Middle East and Africa and both were severely paralysed. Immunisation is essential for all travellers to endemic areas and a reinforcing dose should be given if the last dose was more than five years earlier.

Sometimes poliovirus spreads to non-endemic areas causing disease in the unimmunised. Between 1976 and 1978 there were cases in gypsies in France and Britain and a large outbreak in a religious sect in Holland whose members refused vaccination and which also involved members of the same sect in Canada (Bijkerk et al, 1979). The episode showed that wild poliovirus could apparently spread in well vaccinated populations and cause paralytic disease in the unimmunised and once again emphasised the need to achieve and maintain high levels of infant immunisation throughout the community.

SEXUALLY TRANSMITTED DISEASE

The worldwide increase in travel is considered to have played a part in the rise in the incidence of sexually transmitted disease in many countries (Catterall, 1975).

Syphilis and gonorrhoea
Since 1964 information has been collected from sexually transmitted disease clinics in England and Wales concerning infections contracted abroad. Between 1964 and 1981, of new cases of gonorrhoea attending the clinics about 5% of males and 1% of females were infected abroad. Of new cases of syphilis about 15% males and 5% females were infected abroad. The proportion of males varied little over the period but the proportion of imported cases of syphilis in females rose from 3.2% 1964–1972 to 6.7% 1973–1981.

Beta-lactamase producing strains of *Neisseria gonorrhoeae* were first reported in West Africa and South-East Asia early in 1976, and by October 1977 cases infected with this organism had been reported in 13 other countries (World Health Organization, 1977). In the UK over half of the infections reported up until 1980 were contracted abroad, but by 1981 the infection became established in this country and in 1981 and 1982 most of the infections were contracted at home (Anonymous, 1983).

Acquired immune deficiency syndrome
This apparently new syndrome manifested by Kaposi's sarcoma and severe opportunistic infections was reported in homosexual males in the USA in 1981 (Waterson, 1983). The first cases occurred in 1979 and there was a rapid increase so that by mid-June 1984 4371 cases and 2074 deaths had been reported. During 1982–1984 the syndrome spread to many other countries in which most of the cases were in homosexuals who had had sexual contact with American nationals. In the UK, for example, 48 cases were reported up until the end of June 1984. In France and

Belgium, however, the experience differed because cases were also reported in heterosexuals most of whom were travellers recently arrived from Zaire or Haiti. This finding together with the hypothesis that the syndrome might be due to a transmissible agent has led to the suggestion that the disease may have originated in Central Africa (Fig. 10.10). An acute form of Kaposi's sarcoma in young males was recognised in Central Africa in the 1930s and there were reports of the recent appearance of the disease in Haiti; in both these areas the possible existence of severe opportunistic infections would be difficult to detect because of the lack of laboratory facilities but sick well-to-do inhabitants would be likely to travel to France or Belgium for diagnosis and treatment. Haiti is a holiday island frequented by American homosexuals where they could have acquired the disease; the subsequent rapid spread in the homosexual communities in the USA may have been facilitated by group sexual practices and extreme promiscuity which are believed to have recently become common.

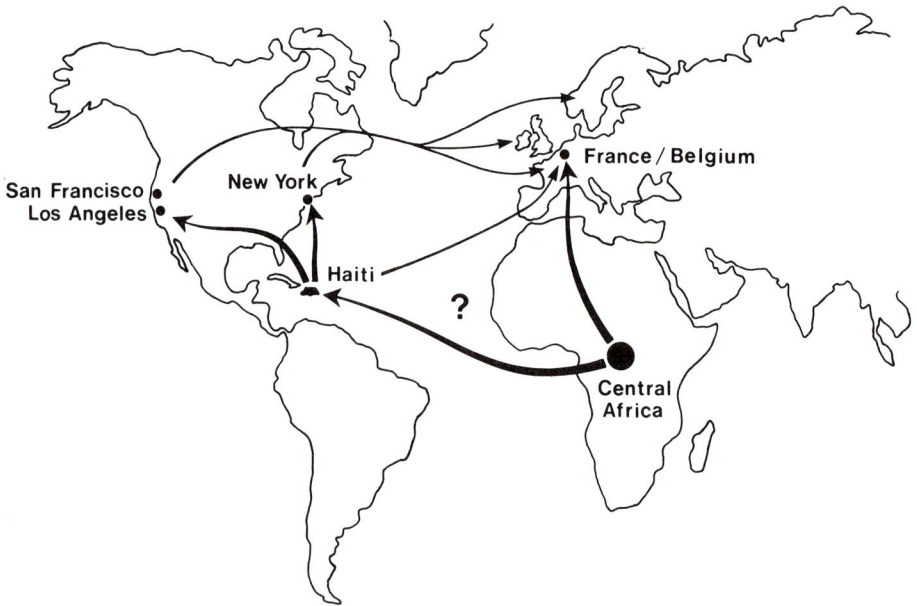

Fig. 10.10   Acquired immune deficiency syndrome. Hypothesis of spread from Central Africa.

ZOONOSES

Several important zoonoses are associated with travel, notably the recently described African viral haemorrhagic fevers, rabies and brucellosis.

African viral haemorrhagic fevers

Lassa fever was first recognised in a hospital outbreak in Nigeria in 1969. Subsequently hospital and community cases were reported in West Africa and the disease was shown to be a zoonosis, the animal host being the multimammate rat (Galbraith et al, 1978). Between 1969 and 1982, 11 cases were reported in persons who had travelled outside West Africa, eight of them to the UK. The first patient was a sick nurse flown home to the United States for investigation and treatment and from whom the virus was originally isolated; there were two secondary cases in laboratory workers. No spread of infection took place from the other 10 cases. In six of the cases information on surveillance was available; nearly 1500 contacts were followed up and none developed Lassa fever; 192 of them were examined serologically and remained sero-negative for Lassa antibody. This experience and the demonstration of control of spread in hospitals in Africa by strict barrier nursing have led to the view that the disease is rarely spread by the airborne route.

Marburg disease was described in an outbreak in the cities of Marburg, Frankfurt and Belgrade in 1967 in persons working with a consignment of African green monkeys from Uganda, although the definitive host of the virus remains unknown. Ebola virus, antigenically distinct from Marburg virus, causes a similar disease and was described in a large outbreak in the Sudan and Zaire in 1976; a single case in a laboratory worker in Britain occurred in the same year, when he pricked his finger whilst examining specimens from the Sudan (Simpson, 1977); again, the animal host is not yet known. Three subsequent episodes of Marburg disease and two of Ebola virus disease have been reported, one of which occurred outside tropical Africa in Johannesburg, South Africa. A hitch-hiker who travelled from Zimbabwe developed the disease and there were two secondary cases, his travelling companion and a nurse who cared for him in Johannesburg.

These viral haemorrhagic fevers are a hazard to the traveller in tropical Africa where endemic foci of the diseases are present (Fig. 10.11). Outside these endemic areas human to human spread may occur principally through infected blood, urine, secretions and body fluids contaminating broken skin or mucous membranes (Department of Health and Social Security, 1976). The risk of infection in the UK, though small, is therefore greatest in hospital and laboratory personnel caring for febrile patients recently arrived from the endemic areas. Spread outside hospitals and laboratories is very unlikely to take place except to persons attending sick patients and exposed to their blood, urine or secretions.

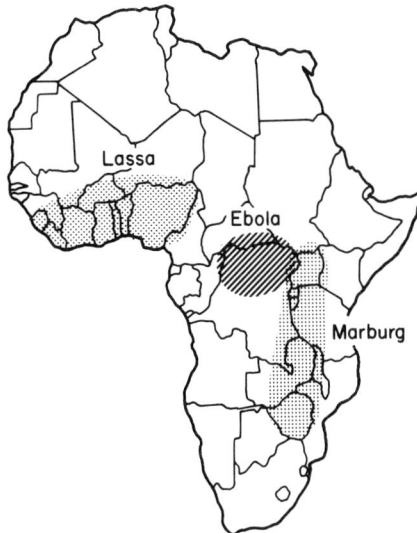

Fig. 10.11 Known approximate endemic foci of African viral haemorrhagic fevers.

Rabies

A disease of wild carnivores and bats in many parts of the world transmitted periodically to domestic animals, particularly dogs and cats, which may then infect man (Kaplan, 1977). Canine rabies was prevalent in the UK in the last century but the country has been rabies free since 1923. The last indigenous case of human rabies was in 1902.

Animal rabies in dogs and cats remains common in Africa and Asia where many human cases occur; for this reason travellers to remote areas of these continents or whose work may expose them to the risk of infection should be vaccinated before embarking on their journey. Post-exposure wound treatment and vaccination should be given immediately following a bite, lick or scratch from an animal which is suspected of being rabid (Department of Health and Social Security, 1977). However, ready access to this therapy is not always available and it is not surprising, therefore, that with the great increase in human travel imported cases of human rabies have become more frequent in the UK (Table 10.5). Of the 15 reported cases since 1946, 13 acquired the disease in Asia, 11 of them on the Indian sub-continent; seven of them occurred in the 12 years 1970–1982 compared with eight in the previous 30 years.

Table 10.5   Human rabies United Kingdom 1946–1982

Year	Number of cases	Place of infection
1946	1	Greece
1947	1	Pakistan
1955	1	Pakistan
1956	1	India
1963	1	Pakistan
1964	1	Indonesia
1967	1	India
1969	1	India
1975	2	Gambia (1), India (1)
1976	1	Bangladesh
1977	2	India (1), Pakistan (1)
1978	1	India
1981	1	India
Total	15	Asia (13), Africa (1), Europe (1)

Brucellosis

In England and Wales brucellosis eradication in cattle began in 1972 when nearly 300 human infections were reported by laboratories (Anonymous, 1980); in 1982 only 16 cases were reported. Between 1978 and 1982 135 cases were reported in England and Wales, in 36 of which the infection was acquired abroad, 22 of them in the Mediterranean area and usually attributed to the consumption of cheese or raw milk; 15 cases were due to *Brucella melitensis* and 21 to *Br. abortus* (Table 10.6).

CONCLUSION

This review of infectious disease and human travel illustrates the importance of surveillance in the detection and control of the spread of infection and in the

Table 10.6   Brucellosis acquired abroad, laboratory reports England and Wales 1973–1982

Brucella melitensis		Brucella abortus			
		Europe			
Spain	3	Malta	3	Ireland	2
Portugal	1	Italy	2	Spain ⎤	
Cyprus	1	France	1	Majorca ⎦	2
		Yugoslavia	1	Germany	1
		Africa			
Egypt	1	Kenya	1		
Sudan	1	Uganda	1		
		Asia			
Turkey	1	Israel	2	Middle East	1
Iraq	4	Iraq	2		
Arabia	1	Pakistan	1		
Oman	1	Yemen	1		
Total	14	Total	21		

monitoring of preventive programmes in travellers. As Carter (1982) has pointed out, the efficacy of this surveillance activity is dependent upon the rapid and frank exchange of information derived from it with national epidemiologists in other countries and with the World Health Organization. This requires personal contact between the nationally responsible epidemiologists and the regular production and distribution of information. The Weekly Epidemiological Record of the World Health Organization provides information worldwide, and in the UK both the Communicable Diseases (Scotland) Unit and the Communicable Disease Surveillance Centre issue weekly bulletins containing mainly national information, both of which are available free of charge on request for persons concerned with communicable disease control in the UK and overseas.

REFERENCES

Anonymous 1980 Human and bovine brucellosis in Britain. British Medical Journal 280: 1458
Anonymous 1983 Penicillinase-producing *Neisseria gonorrhoeae* in Britain 1982. British Medical Journal 286: 1628–1629
Bartlett C L R, Swann R A, Casal I, Canada Rovo L, Taylor A G 1983 Recurrent Legionnaires' disease from a hotel water system. Proceedings of the Second International Symposium on Legionella, June 1983, Washington DC, USA
Barua D 1972 The global epidemiology of cholera in recent years. Proceedings of the Royal Society of Medicine 62: 423–428
Bernard R P 1965 The Zermatt typhoid outbreak in 1963. Journal of Hygiene Cambridge 63: 537–563
Beveridge W I B 1977 Influenza. The last great plague. Heinemann, London
Bijkerk H, Draaisma F J, Van Der Gugten A C, Van Os M 1979 De poliomyelitis-epidemie in 1978. Nederlands Tijdschrift voor Geneeskunde 123: 1700–1714
Bruce-Chwatt L J 1982a Imported Malaria: an uninvited guest. British Medical Bulletin 38: 179–185
Bruce-Chwatt L J 1982b Chemoprophylaxis of malaria in Africa: the spent 'magic bullet'. British Medical Journal 285: 674–676
Buchan K A, Reid D 1972 Epidemiological aspects of influenza in Lewis. Health Bulletin Edinburgh 30: 183–186
Carter I D 1982 Communication and disease. Proceedings of the Royal Society of Edinburgh 82B: 101–115
Catterall R D 1975 Sexually transmitted diseases and the mobility explosion. Postgraduate Medical Journal 51: 838–842
Center for Disease Control 1971 Gastroenteritis aboard planes. Morbidity and Mortality Weekly Report 20: 67

Center for Disease Control 1975 Outbreak of staphylococcal food poisoning aboard an aircraft. Morbidity and Mortality Weekly Report 24: 57–59

Centers for Disease Control 1981 Multiple measles importations New York. Morbidity and Mortality Weekly Report 30: 288–290

Chattopadhyay B, Fellner I W, Mollison M D, Nicol W, Williams G R 1977 Diphtheria in London and Birmingham, 1975. Public Health London 91: 169–174

Chernenkoff W, Jellard C H, Toshach S, Jones S, Robertson H E, Chaudhry S, et al 1971 Outbreak of staphylococcus food poisoning on a trans-Canada train. Epidemiological Bulletin 15: 57–58

Christie A B 1980 Infectious diseases: epidemiology and clinical practice. Churchill Livingstone, London: 366–369.

Dannenberg A L, Yashuk J C, Feldman R A 1982 Gastrointestinal illness on passenger cruise ships 1975–1978. American Journal of Public Health 72: 484–488

Davies J W, Cox K G, Simon W R, Bowmer E J, Mallory A 1972 Typhoid at sea: Epidemic aboard an ocean liner. Canadian Medical Association Journal 106: 877–883

Department of Health and Social Security 1976 Memorandum on Lassa Fever. HMSO, London

Department of Health and Social Security 1977 Memorandum on Rabies. HMSO, London

Desmarchelier P 1978 Vibrio outbreaks from airline food and water. Food Technology in Australia 30: 477–481

Dorolle P 1968 Old plagues in the jet age. International aspects of present and future control of communicable disease. British Medical Journal 4: 789–792

Galbraith N S 1982 Communicable Disease Surveillance. In: Recent Advances in Community Medicine 2. Edited by Alwyn Smith. Churchill Livingstone, London

Galbraith N S, Berrie J R H, Forbes P, Young S E J 1978 Public health aspects of viral haemorrhagic fevers in Britain. The Royal Society of Health Journal 98: 152–161

Galbraith N S, Young S E J 1980 Communicable Disease Control: the development of a laboratory associated national epidemiological service in England and Wales. Community Medicine 2: 135–143

Gangarosa E J, Kendrick M A, Loewenstein M S, Merson M H, Mosley J W 1980 Global Travel and Travellers' Health. Aviation, Space and Environmental Medicine 51: 265–270

Gregory M C and Spalding J M K 1972 Poliomyelitis in Adults. Lancet i: 155

Gross R J, Thomas L V, Rowe B 1979 *Shigella dysenteriae, Sh. flexneri,* and *Sh. boydii* infections in England and Wales: the importance of foreign travel. British Medical Journal 2: 744

Gunn R A, Terranova W A, Greenberg H B, Yashuk J, Gary G W, Wells J G et al 1980 Norwalk virus gastroenteritis aboard a cruise ship: an outbreak on five consecutive cruises. American Journal of Epidemiology 112: 820–827

Hart C J, Sherwood W W, Wilson E 1960 A food poisoning outbreak aboard a common carrier. Public Health Reports Washington 75: 527–531

Jusatz H J 1982 150 years Pandemics of Asiatic Cholera 1831–1981. International Journal of Microbiology and Hygiene, I. Abteilung Originale A 252: 257–267

Kaplan C (ed) 1977 Rabies: The facts. Oxford University Press, Oxford

Keusch G T 1979 Shigella infections. Clinics in Gastroenterology 8: 645–662

Langmuir A D 1963 The surveillance of communicable diseases of national importance. New England Journal of Medicine 268: 182–192

McKendrick M W, Fothergill J, Geddes A M 1981 Amoebic liver abscess probably acquired in Birmingham, England. Scandinavian Journal of Infectious Disease 13: 80–82

Maegraith B G 1965 Exotic diseases in Practice. Heinemann, London

Malaria Reference Laboratory 1983 Malaria prophylaxis. British Medical Journal 286: 787–789

Miller D L 1982 Acute Respiratory Infections. In: Epidemiology of Diseases edited by Miller D L and Farmer R D T. Blackwell, Oxford

Moser M R, Bender T R, Margolis H S, Noble G R, Kendal A P, Ritter D G 1979 An outbreak of influenza aboard a commercial airliner. American Journal of Epidemiology 110: 1–6

Morger H, Steffen R, Schär M 1983 Epidemiology of cholera in travellers, and conclusions for vaccination recommendations. British Medical Journal 286: 184–186

Mortimer P P, Parry J V 1981 Anti-hepatitis-A-virus potency of immunoglobulin. Lancet i: 1364–1365

Nye F J 1979 Traveller's Diarrhoea. Clinics in Gastroenterology 8: 767–781

O'Mahony M C, Gooch C D, Smyth D A, Thrussell A J, Bartlett C L R, Noah N D 1983 Epidemic hepatitis A from cockles. Lancet i: 518–520

Peffers A S R, Bailey J, Barrow G I, Hobbs B C 1973 *Vibrio parahaemolyticus* gastroenteritis and international air travel. Lancet i: 143–145

Perin M 1976 Transportation in commercial aircraft of passengers having contagious diseases. Aviation, Space and Environmental Medicine 47: 1109–1113

Pollock T M, Reid D 1969 Immunoglobulin for the prevention of Infectious Hepatitis in persons working overseas. Lancet i: 281–283

Reid D 1982 Tourism and illness. Proceedings of the Royal Society of Edinburgh 82B: 23–35

Reid D, Grist N R, Najera R 1978 Illness associated with 'package tours': a combined Spanish–Scottish study. Bulletin of the World Health Organization 56: 117–122

Rowe B, Taylor J, Bettelheim K A 1970 An investigation of travellers' diarrhoea. Lancet i: 1–5

Sharp J C M 1982 Recent examples of travelling infection. Proceedings of the Royal Society of Edinburgh 82B: 97–99

Simpson D I H 1977 Marburg and Ebola virus infections. World Health Organization, Offset Publication 36, Geneva

Stamm W P 1975 Amoebiasis in England and Wales. British Medical Journal 2: 452–453

Sutton R G A 1974 An outbreak of cholera in Australia due to food served in flight on an international aircraft. Journal of Hygiene Cambridge 72: 441–451

Turner A C 1975 Travel Medicine. Churchill Livingstone, Edinburgh

Walker E, Williams G 1983 ABC of Healthy Travel. British Medical Association, London

Waterson A P 1983 Acquired immune deficiency syndrome. British Medical Journal 286: 743–746

World Health Organization 1976 Foodborne salmonella infections contracted on aircraft. Weekly Epidemiological Record 51: 265–266

World Health Organization 1977 Neisseria gonorrhoeae producing β-lactamase (pencillinase). Weekly Epidemiological Record 52: 357–359

11. Recent advances in zoonoses control

S. R. Palmer   J. C. Bell

INTRODUCTION

The zoonoses have been defined by the World Health Organization as 'Those diseases and infections (the agents of) which are naturally transmitted between (other) vertebrate animals and man' (World Health Organization, 1959). More than 150 infectious diseases are recognised zoonoses (Steele, 1979, 1980, 1981a, b). In developing countries they are of major economic importance through loss of animal production, as well as accounting directly for a considerable burden of human morbidity and mortality (World Health Organization, 1982). In developed countries, particularly Britain, the internationally important zoonoses such as bovine tuberculosis, brucellosis and anthrax have been successfully controlled and the few new human infections that do occur are almost invariably imported (Galbraith et al, 1980). Even so the zoonoses are still important. The zoonoses that are included in the statutorily notifiable infectious diseases of man in England and Wales in 1982 are shown in Table 11.1.

Table 11.1 Notifiable infectious diseases in humans in England and Wales 1982

Anthrax*	Paratyphoid & typhoid fever
Cholera	Plague
Diphtheria	Poliomyelitis
Dysentery	Rabies
Acute encephalitis	Relapsing Fever
Food poisoning (due to *Salmonella*)	Scarlet fever
Infective jaundice	Smallpox
Lassa Fever	Tetanus
Leptospirosis	Tuberculosis (due to *Mycobacterium bovis*)
Malaria	Typhus fever (murine typhus)
Marburg Disease	Viral haemorrhagic disease
Measles	Whooping Cough
Acute meningitis	Yellow fever
Ophthalmia neonatorum	

*Infections which are underlined are those which may be acquired from animals.

Zoonoses are a heterogeneous group of infections with varying modes of transmission and demanding widely differing control methods. However, their consideration as a specific group of diseases is useful since it draws attention to an area where interprofessional collaboration is essential and therefore where community physicians can play a leading role. For formulating successful policies for the management of zoonoses liaison is essential not only amongst doctors, veterinarians and environmental health officers but also between the agriculture and food industries and the lay public.

Zoonoses make up a considerable proportion of the burden of infectious diseases in Britain. For example, of the six major microbial causes of gastroenteritis reported to the Communicable Disease Surveillance Centre by Public Health and hospital laboratories, campylobacter and salmonella are established zoonoses and account for 68% of the total number of such infections (Table 11.2). Other zoonoses, whilst numerically less important, may cause severe disease. For example 6% of the infective endocarditides reported to CDSC between 1975 and 1980 were attributed to *Chlamydia psittaci* and *Coxiella burnetii* infections (CDSC unpublished); toxoplasmosis is an important cause of congenital defects (Hall, 1983). The zoonoses which may

Table 11.2   Principal microbial causes of gastroenteritis reported to CDSC

Agent	Number of infections reported in 1982
Campylobacter	12 822
Entamoeba histolytica	528
Giardia	4 089
Rotavirus	4 132
Salmonella (food poisoning serotypes)	12 051
Shigella	2 954

Table 11.3   Commoner zoonoses which may be acquired in Britain

Agent	Disease	Main animal reservoirs	Usual mode of transmission	Laboratory diagnoses reported to CDSC 1980–1982 (including infections required abroad)
Campylobacter sp.	Enteritis	Widespread but particularly poultry, cattle, wild birds, household pets	Unknown possibly food, water and direct contact	34 824
Chlamydia psittaci	Ornithosis/ Psittacosis	Wild and domestic birds and poultry	Airborne	1 039
Coxiella burnetii	Acute and chronic Q Fever	Cattle, sheep, goats	Airborne	447
Leptospira sp.	Weil's disease, canicola fever	Rodents, domestic and wild animals	Direct contact with urine	119
Listeria sp.	Septicaemia, Meningitis	Cattle, sheep.	Unknown possibly foodborne	452
Microsporum and *Trichophyton*	Animal ring worm	Cats, dogs, cattle	Direct contact	1 453
Orf/Cowpox/ paravaccinia	Skin nodules	Sheep, goats, cattle	Direct contact	144
Pasteurella sp.	Local abscess	Dogs, cats	Bites, scratches	895
Salmonella sp.	Gastroenteritis	Widespread but particularly poultry, cattle, pigs	Foodborne	33 351
Toxoplasma gondii	'Glandular fever' abortion, stillbirth, severe congenital infection	Cats	Ingestion	2 335
Yersinia enterocolitica, pseudotuberculosis	Enterocolitis, mesenteric lymphadenitis	Pigs, wild animals and birds	Foodborne direct contact	504

be acquired in the United Kingdom are summarised in Tables 11.3 and 11.4. Total laboratory reports to CDSC are given to provide a guide to the relative importance of individual infections. The animal reservoirs and modes of transmission refer to what is usual in Britain. Internationally the picture may be quite different.

In recent years, and set against the changing patterns of infectious disease in Britain, the zoonoses have gained a new emphasis. This has arisen in part from growing public awareness of the possibility of infections from pets and food but there have also been significant epidemiological, clinical and microbiological developments. Important developments include the following:

1. New human infections with animal reservoirs have been discovered. In Britain *Campylobacter jejuni* has been shown to be the single commonest cause of bacterial enteritis (Skirrow, 1982). In the United States of America, waterborne outbreaks of giardiasis have been attributed to fecal pollution by wild animals, particularly beavers (Craun, 1979).

In Africa Lassa fever has been shown to be endemic in the human population exposed to the excreta of the multimammate rat, *Mastomys natalensis* (Casals & Buckley, 1981). The elimination of smallpox has revealed the existence of human infection by monkeypox virus (WHO, 1979). More recently, in the USA, outbreaks of a newly recognised form of haemorrhagic colitis were shown to be caused by *Escherichia coli* serogroup 0157, H7. The vehicle of infection was hamburgers prepared at fast food restaurants and the organism was isolated from raw meat suggesting that it might have originated from cattle (Riley et al, 1983). Indeed whenever a new human infection is discovered the possibility of an animal source has always to be considered. The current search for the putative agent of Acquired

Table 11.4   Less common zoonoses which may be acquired in Britain

Agent	Disease	Main animal reservoirs	Usual mode of transmission	Laboratory diagnoses reported to CDSC 1980–1982 (including infections acquired abroad)
Bacillus anthracis	Anthrax	Imported animal products	Direct contact	0
Brucella sp.	Acute and chronic brucellosis	Cattle	Milk, dairy products	62
Corynebacterium ulcerans	Throat infection	Cattle	Milk	15
Cryptosporidium	Enterocolitis	Calves	Ingestion	0
Echinococcus granulosus	Hydatid disease	Dogs	Ingestion	21
Mycobacterium bovis	Intestinal and disseminated tuberculosis	Cattle	Milk	84
Streptobacillus moniliformis	Haverhill fever/ rat bite fever	Rats	Bites, milk, water	2
Streptococcus suis	Meningitis, arthritis	Pigs	Direct contact	5
Taenia saginata, solium	Taeniasis, cystercercosis	Cattle, pigs	Ingestion	8
Toxocara	Visceral and ocular larva migrans	Dogs, cats	Ingestion	16

Immune Deficiency Syndrome (AIDS) has included a search for animal disease agents (London et al, 1983; Hendrickson et al, 1983; Teas, 1983).

2. Infections which were previously thought to be confined to animals have been found to affect man e.g. *Streptococcus suis* infection of pigs (Chattopadhyay, 1979). Several infections fall into the category of 'emerging zoonoses'. Most recently cryptosporidiosis has been shown to be transmissible from calves to humans, and is one of the opportunist infections seen in patients with AIDS (MMWR, 1982a). Prediction of which animal disease agents will become pathogenic for man is difficult as was shown by the swine influenza vaccine story in the USA (Langmuir, 1979) and therefore national and international surveillance is of great importance.

3. Disturbing developments have occurred amongst the established zoonoses such as the discovery of transferable multiple drug resistance amongst enteric bacteria (Akiba et al, 1960) and the entry of multiply-resistant clones of *Salmonella typhimurium* into the human food chain (Rowe & Threlfall, 1981). The use of antibiotics in animal production has been blamed for this and it has been suggested that virulent clones of multi-resistant *Salmonella typhimurium* might evolve causing typhoid-like disease for which effective chemotherapy might not be available. In the UK outbreaks of ornithosis (Palmer, 1982), Q fever (Salmon et al, 1982; Hall et al, 1982), listeriosis (CDSC, unpublished) and Haverhill fever (CDSC unpublished) have occurred in the last three years emphasising the need for continuous vigilance and medico-veterinary collaboration.

4. Changes in animal husbandry and changing patterns of meat consumption have resulted in an increasing incidence of salmonella food poisoning (Fig. 11.1) and a shift in the prevalent salmonella serotypes (McCoy, 1975). Factory production of broilers and turkeys infected with salmonella has produced an epidemic of salmonella food

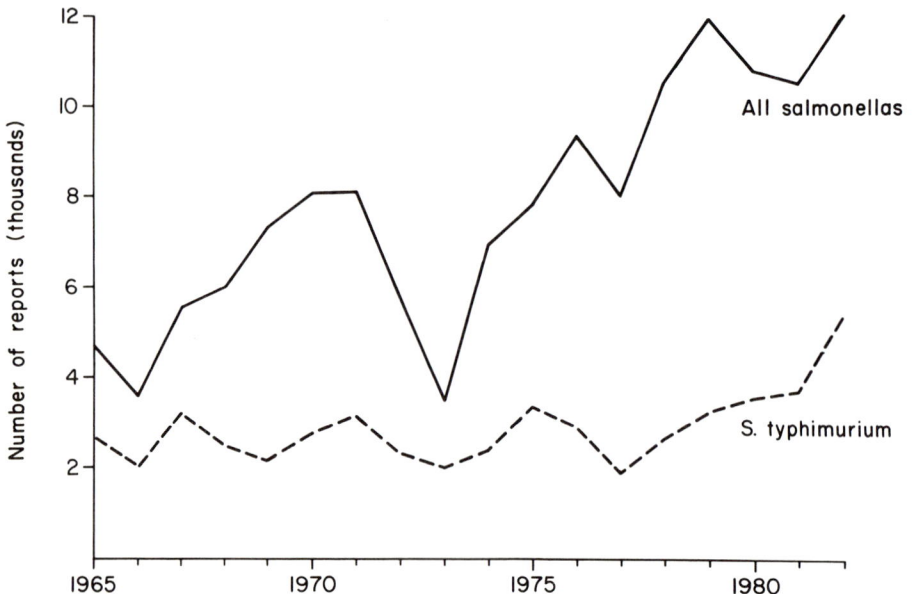

Fig. 11.1   Trends in *Salmonella* infections in England and Wales reported by Public Health and hospital laboratories, 1965–1982 (PHLS Communicable Disease Surveillance Centre).

poisoning in Britain (Rowe et al, 1980) and may also contribute significantly to the incidence of campylobacter infection. To these trends should be added the growing interest in natural foods which has highlighted well-known problems of infection from raw milk (Galbraith et al, 1982) and the popularity of health foods which may provide ideal vehicles for infection e.g. yersiniosis in soybean curd (MMWR, 1982b).

Zoonoses may be transmitted by direct contact with infected animals (e.g. rabies, orf) or indirectly through food and water contamination (e.g. salmonellosis, campylobacteriosis) by fomites (e.g. Q fever, psittacosis) and by arthropods (e.g. plague). Many zoonoses can be transmitted by several pathways. A knowledge of these epidemiological parameters is essential if successful control measures are to be developed. This review therefore includes recent advances in the understanding of the epidemiology of zoonoses, as well as advances in the implementation of controls.

RECENT ADVANCES IN CONTROL

Anthrax
In Britain anthrax in man is a hazard mainly to those working with wool or hides imported from countries where the disease is endemic in the animal population. The incidence of anthrax in humans in the UK declined four-fold from 1961 when it became a notifiable disease under the Public Health Acts to 1980. The decline in occupational infections has been attributed to the introduction of vaccination against anthrax in 1965 (CDSC, 1982a).

Brucellosis
The decline in human cases of brucellosis in UK can be directly attributed to veterinary efforts to eradicate the infection in cattle (CDSC, 1980). In 1951–1952 more than 18% of bulk milk samples contained brucella (Stableforth, 1954) and in 1960–1961 over 30% of dairy herds were infected (Leech et al, 1964). In 1967 voluntary schemes were introduced for testing and removing reactors from individual herds and in 1971 an eradication programme began. In November 1979 the whole of Great Britain became subject to compulsory eradication measures for brucellosis in cattle and was declared to be almost free of brucellosis by 1982 (Report, 1983). In that year there were only 15 reports of *Br. abortus* infection in humans in England and Wales, compared with over 250 in 1972 (CDSC, 1980). It should be noted that the main impetus for this highly successful eradication scheme was the substantial economic loss resulting from bovine abortions, infertility and the loss of milk yield, rather than risks to human health.

Hydatid disease
Echinococcus granulosus eggs ingested by humans produce fluid-filled hydatid cysts usually in liver, lungs and brain. The tape worm eggs are excreted by dogs infested after eating hydatid cysts in raw sheep offal. Sheep farmers and their families break into the sheep-dog cycle by ingesting eggs after handling affected dogs. Mid-Wales is an endemic focus of hydatid disease (Walters, 1978) and is reputed to have the highest incidence in Western Europe. Although the population at risk is small the health consequences of infestation are great. From 1975 to 1980, 28 deaths in England and Wales were attributed to hydatid disease (OPCS, 1977–1982).

The development of an anthelmintic drug, praziquantel, effective against mature and immature stages of *E. granulosus*, has facilitated a veterinary control programme involving treating the dog population in a defined area at regular intervals. In 1983 an eradication programme was started by the Welsh Office and the Ministry of Agriculture Fisheries and Food, beginning in South Powys. In the scheme the dog population of a defined geographical area is enumerated, the prevalence of *E. granulosus* infestation measured and regular treatment of the dogs undertaken. It is hoped that this project will measurably reduce the incidence of human disease.

Rabies

In recent years rabies in Europe has spread closer to the channel coast of France and the possibility of rabid pets being illegally brought into the UK demands continued vigilance (DHSS, 1977). The six months quarantine imposed on imported carnivores is unpopular and prosecution for illegal landings are necessary every year. There are frequent publicity campaigns. Contingency plans have been drawn up in case wildlife in urban areas becomes infected (Report, 1983). The disease was eradicated from Britain in 1922 and there have been no cases in animals outside quarantine since 1970 when a dog died nine months after importation (Report, 1971). The previous year a dog showed symptoms soon after completing six months quarantine (Report, 1970). Such prolonged incubation periods have been too unusual to justify prolonging the quarantine period.

The main risk to humans in Britain is from animal bites received in other countries. However, post-exposure active immunisation has become much less hazardous and painful with the introduction of the new human diploid cell vaccine in 1976. Since 1976 over 40 000 doses of HDCV have been used in Britain (Gardner, 1983). The number of enquiries and requests to the PHLS rose ten-fold in 1981 after a traveller who had recently returned from India died of rabies. Post-exposure vaccination should be considered as one aspect of the management of animal bites which will also include the evaluation of risk, tracing and surveillance of the animal and consideration of the need for passive immunisation with human anti-rabies immunoglobulin. Pre-exposure active immunisation is available from the National Health Service to those at special occupational risk of exposure such as quarantine station workers and veterinarians.

Salmonellosis

Salmonellosis is the most important zoonosis in Britain because of the serious loss of animal production it can cause, the high incidence of human infection and the threat of multiple antibiotic resistant clones entering the human food chains. In Britain, human infection is usually attributed to poultry and other meats and to unpasteurised milk (CDSC, 1982b). Reluctance to address the animal origins of the human infection has been due to the problems of dealing with subclinical infection in food animals, cross-contamination and multiplication during meat and poultry processing and because it is possible to prevent human infection by proper food preparation and storage and good kitchen hygiene. However a number of new statutes have created a new initiative in investigation and control of salmonellosis.

The Zoonoses Order (1975)

This Order was based on proposals of the Swann Committee set up in 1968 to examine the use of antibiotics in animal husbandry and veterinary medicine (Lowes, 1975). The Committee recognised that officers of the State Veterinary Service had no powers to investigate outbreaks of salmonellosis in animals and the powers and training of the Medical Officers of Health did not extend to living animals (Report, 1969). Outbreaks could therefore occur which might threaten human health but which could not be officially investigated. The Committee recommendations included the following:

(1) that a system of data collection and evaluation should be established so that problems might be recognised and defined;
(2) that veterinary equivalents of the then Medical Officer of Health should be established, to be concerned with all outbreaks of infectious disease in animals which might threaten human health;
(3) that those nominated veterinary officers should be given powers of control including rights of entry and investigation.

The following year an outbreak of *Salmonella paratyphi B* in people and dairy cattle in Yorkshire occurred (George et al, 1972). The cows had been infected from a stream which had been polluted by sewage effluent from a village where a human carrier lived. Farm workers were infected by drinking raw milk. A broken drain from the cess pit of one of the affected farm workers contaminated the water supply of several villages putting over 8000 people at risk. Nearly 100 people were clinically ill. This outbreak emphasised the lack of statutory powers noted by the Swann Committee and these powers were granted in the Zoonoses Order (1975) (MAFF, 1975).

The Zoonoses Order states that the presence in animals or birds of organisms of the genera brucella or salmonella is a risk to human health. This allows appropriate provisions of the Animal Health Act 1981 and of Section 1 of the Agriculture (Miscellaneous Provisions) Act 1972 to be applied when these organisms are found or suspected in animals or birds. There are provisions for a compulsory reporting procedure, the investigation of cases and emergency measures to protect human health.

Emergency powers are provided in case of an exceptionally serious risk to human health. They may be applied to 'any kind of mammal, except man, and any kind of four-footed beast which is not a mammal' and to 'a bird of any species'. There are provisions for a veterinary inspector to enter premises, require information and assistance and take samples. He may serve a notice declaring the premises to be an Infected Place and require it to be cleaned and disinfected. Animals and birds and their carcasses or products (including milk, eggs, wool, meat, offal, dung and used bedding) may only be moved onto or off an Infected Place under licence.

The compulsory reporting procedure applies only to cattle, sheep, goats, pigs, rabbits, fowls, turkeys, geese, ducks, guinea fowls, pheasants, partridges and quails. If, as a result of a laboratory isolation, it is suspected that salmonella or brucella is present in one of the listed species a veterinary inspector of the Ministry of Agriculture, Fisheries and Food (MAFF) or the Department of Agriculture and Fisheries for Scotland (DAFS) must be informed. The veterinary inspector responsible for receiving reports in a defined territory is called the Nominated Officer. He should keep Medical Officers for Environmental Health and Chief Environmental

Health Officers informed of infection in food animals in their territories. He also decides whether a report should be investigated by a visit to the affected premises to take samples, gather information and give advice.

The Zoonoses Order has therefore led to the creation of an effective surveillance system to assist in the epidemiological investigation of outbreaks of animal salmonellosis and human food poisoning (Bell et al, 1981). It has also increased communication amongst veterinary, medical and environmental health services.

The Diseases of Animals (Protein Processing) Order 1981 and the Importation of Processed Animal Protein Order 1981

The reservoir of salmonella infection in Britain which is most important in human disease is that in food animals, and an important factor in maintaining this reservoir is believed to be the regular re-introduction of salmonellae into flocks and herds via animal feeds (McCoy, 1975). The introduction of new salmonella serotypes into Britain in recent years has been attributed to imported contaminated fish meal and other feeds. In addition recycling of poultry waste and offal, in animal feeds, which is often contaminated, is believed to have intensified the problem.

In 1982 an important step was taken towards reducing this reservoir of salmonella infection when two new Orders came into effect.

These Orders require home produced and imported animal protein intended for use in animal feeds to be free of salmonellae. There are provisions for the sampling and testing of products and penalties for producers or importers who fail to comply. It is too early yet to assess the impact of these orders on the incidence of human and animal salmonellosis.

Milk-borne infection

The food value of raw cows' milk is offset by the considerable risk of acquiring a variety of infections from the milk. In Britain today these infections include salmonellosis, campylobacteriosis, and a variety of rarer diseases (Galbraith et al, 1982). In England and Wales between 1951 and 1980 at least 233 outbreaks of communicable disease involving 10 000 people were attributed to infected milk. Despite the fact that the proportion of pasteurised milk consumed in Britain has increased to over 95% in recent years there was no indication up to 1982 that the frequency of outbreaks was decreasing. In Scotland in 1981 and 1982 there were 11 general community outbreaks of salmonellosis involving almost 1000 people, as well as six outbreaks amongst farm workers and their families (Reilly et al, 1983).

In 1983 an important step in reducing the public health risk from raw milk was taken in Scotland when the Milk (Special Designations) (Scotland) Order 1980 was brought into effect. Surveillance data particularly relating to milk-borne salmonellosis collated at the Communicable Diseases (Scotland) Unit (Sharp et al, 1980) played a major part by highlighting the public health risks and was used effectively to promote the introduction of the Scottish legislation. A cost benefit study of one of the milk-borne salmonella outbreaks in Scotland has also shown the economic benefits of pasteurisation (Cohen et al, 1983).

Under the Order the retail sale of unpasteurised milk is banned throughout Scotland with the exception of a few Scottish islands where pasteurised milk is not yet available. Also exempted is goats' milk which is not included in the definition of 'milk' in the legislation.

NEW EPIDEMIOLOGICAL INSIGHTS

Campylobacter

In 1977 Skirrow highlighted campylobacter as an important human pathogen when he developed a selective culture medium. Since then campylobacter has become the most commonly reported bacterial enteric pathogen in the UK (Skirrow, 1982). Infection may cause diarrhoea, colitis, severe abdominal pain and fever.

Investigation of animals and environment has shown the organism to be ubiquitous in the faeces of birds, domestic and wild animals and in surface waters (Newell, 1982). The most well established route of infection in humans is via raw milk contaminated with bovine faeces (Robinson & Jones, 1981). Large outbreaks have occurred. In Luton in 1979 over 3000 people, mainly children, were affected after failure of pasteurisation at the dairy supplying school milk (Jones et al, 1981).

Most human infections in UK however are not associated with raw milk. Some are associated with infected pets, particularly puppies, but food and water may also be important vehicles of infection. Only a small number of well documented food-borne outbreaks have occurred and campylobacters have not been shown to multiply in foods. It is unlikely therefore that the bulk of infection is directly foodborne. Perhaps the most significant observation is that most poultry carcasses are contaminated with campylobacter strains which are also prevalent in the human population (Abbott et al, 1983). It is probable that campylobacters are introduced into the kitchen via raw poultry and are then spread to other foods during food preparation. The infective dose of campylobacter is low (Robinson, 1981) and does not depend upon multiplication of the organism in the food. Therefore reducing the contamination of raw poultry meat is probably more important in the prevention of campylobacter enteritis than in salmonella food poisoning.

In any outbreak of campylobacter enteritis the possibility of waterborne infection should be considered. In 1981 a large outbreak affected pupils and staff at an English public school (Palmer et al, 1983). The school was supplied with unchlorinated water from a private bore hole and the water was stored in an open-topped tank before distribution to most of the school houses. A survey of pupils showed that the attack rates in the school houses were closely associated with the distribution of this water; there was a significant association between water consumption and illness in staff and on one occasion campylobacter was isolated from the holding tank water. It is probable that the water supply was contaminated in the holding tank by wild birds.

Further work on the epidemiology of campylobacter infections is needed to establish modes of transmission so that preventive measures can be devised. Among the features which must be explained are the striking seasonal incidence of infection with the peak of infection occurring in the third quarter of the year (Fig. 11.2) and the predominance of reported infections in young adults.

Leptospirosis

Leptospires are excreted in urine by many species of animals. Occupationally exposed people may be infected by direct contact. Two new occupational groups at risk have

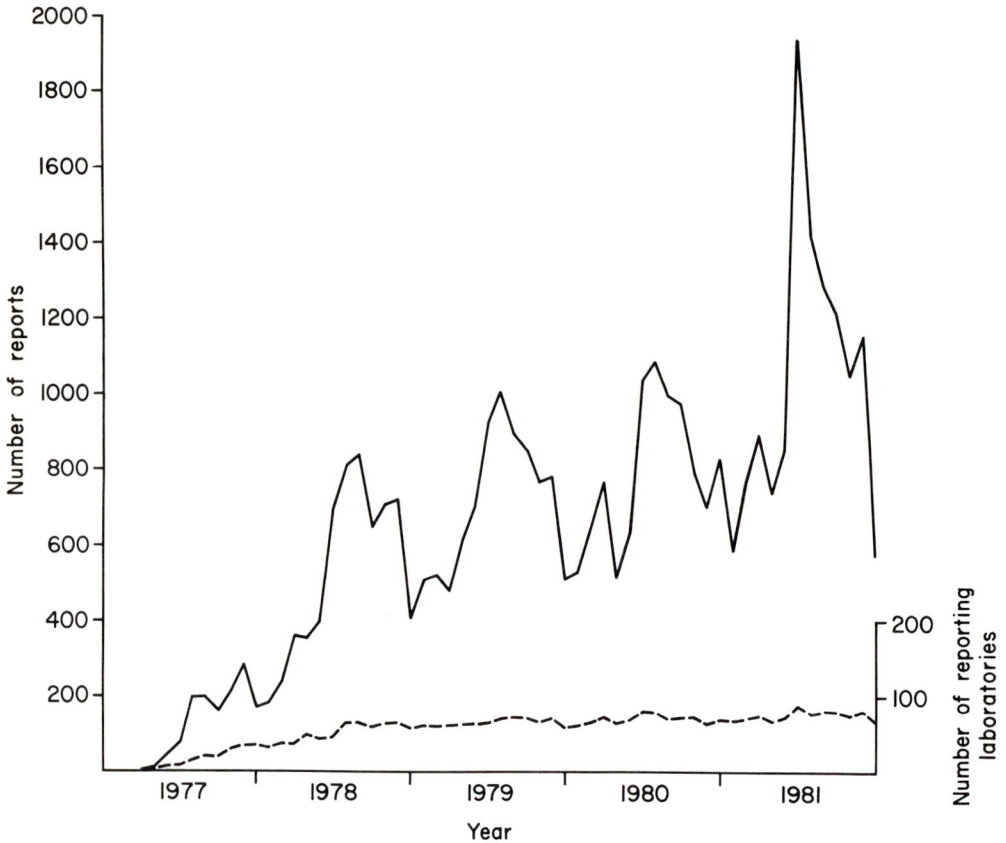

Fig. 11.2   Seasonal incidence of *Campylobacter* infections in England and Wales reported to the PHLS Communicable Disease Surveillance Centre, 1977–1981.

recently been defined. Workers in the fish farming industry have been shown to be at increased risk of infection from *Leptospira* serogroup *icterohaemorrhagiae*, the cause of Weil's disease (Gill, 1983) possibly when fish feed is contaminated by rat urine (Robertson et al, 1981). The risk to farm workers may also have increased in recent years as milking parlours have progressively replaced cowsheds. In milking parlours the milker stands at a lower level than the cows and is more exposed to urine. Recent surveys have shown that *L. hardjo* is endemic in the cattle population and leptospirosis, which often presents as a flu-like illness without jaundice, is increasingly being recognised as an occupational hazard of dairymen (Hathaway 1982; Wilson & Wetson, 1981). A vaccine for use in cattle has recently been introduced in this country.

Listeriosis
Listeria monocytogenes infection is widespread in domestic and wild animals and is also an important cause of meningitis and septicaemia in human neonates and the elderly. Infection of pregnant women and transplacental spread may lead to premature labour, stillbirth and early neonatal death.

The routes of transmission of listeriosis are not yet established but two recent outbreaks suggest that food may be an important vehicle of infection. In Canada an outbreak involving 7 adult cases and 34 perinatal cases was traced, by a case control study of possible exposure, to coleslaw salad which had been prepared from locally grown cabbage cultivated using infected sheep manure (Schleck et al, 1983). In N.W. England in 1981 a cluster of 11 cases was possibly associated with fresh cream (Hall, personal communication). It has been suggested that prolonged cold storage of raw foods may encourage the growth of *L. monocytogenes* so increasing the likelihood of infection.

Psittacosis/Ornithosis

Infection with *Chlamydia psittaci* is a well recognised hazard of pigeon fanciers and those dealing with exotic birds. Outbreaks of ornithosis in poultry industry workers, particularly those handling ducks in Eastern Europe and turkeys in USA, have been well documented (Schacter & Dawson, 1978). In the UK however no incidents were associated with commercially reared birds until 1980 when investigation of a small cluster of cases in East Anglia led to the identification of a problem in the duck industry (Andrews et al, 1981). It was estimated that 10% of the duck workers in the UK had been clinically ill with ornithosis in the winter of 1979/80 and that the greatest risk of infection was associated with handling viscera and feathers. A second outbreak amongst veterinary surgeons attending a course at one duck processing plant confirmed the association and feather processing workers were also established to be at risk (Palmer et al, 1981). The risk to the general public from ducks or feathers was considered to be negligible but employers, employees and general practitioners were alerted to the hazard.

Q Fever

Infection with *Coxiella burnetii* first described by Derrick in Australia in 1937 has since been found in all continents (Derrick, 1937). The reservoir of infection in Britain is probably sheep and cattle (Marmion & Stoker, 1958), where infection is usually asymptomatic but may cause abortion. *Coxiella burnetii* is shed in vast numbers in infected products of conception and can survive in dust and litter for several weeks. Human infection is acquired by inhaling dust, by direct contact with infected animals and possibly by drinking inadequately pasteurised milk. Acute symptoms include meningism, pneumonitis and occasionally hepatitis. The sinister feature of Q fever is chronic infection of the liver and heart valves. Q fever endocarditis has been considered a rare event but a recent review of laboratory-confirmed cases reported to CDSC suggested that up to 11% of hospital diagnosed cases fall into this category, that 3% of all reported endocarditides are due to Q fever and that a young population is affected (Palmer & Young, 1982). Recent reports have stressed the need for increasing awareness of Q fever endocarditis and the need to elucidate the epidemiology of Q fever in the UK (Tobin et al, 1982).

In 1982 two large outbreaks occurred in England and Wales. One involved scientific staff exposed to infected sheep (Hall et al, 1982), but the other involved 29 people living in an urban area with no direct contact with farm animals (Salmon et al, 1982). In the latter outbreak one patient subsequently died of Q fever endocarditis.

The cases were associated with one area of the town but no adequate explanation for contamination of this area was found.

DEVELOPMENTS IN MEDICO-VETERINARY LIAISON

Collaboration between doctors and veterinarians is crucial to the successful control of zoonoses and this applies both at the level of the individual patient and at the population level. Difficulties have been encountered in the past but joint investigations have proved possible and successful (Payne & Scudamore, 1977). An example is the identification of ornithosis in workers in the duck rearing and processing industry which was the result of a collaborative investigation. The epidemiological investigation of duck workers would not have been possible without the liaison with employers and employees provided by MAFF and private veterinarians. Furthermore, the initial suggestion that a problem might exist was raised when two geographically separate human cases of ornithosis were identified and proved to be associated as a result of discussion made possible by long-standing local veterinary and medical liaison (Palmer, 1982).

Local liaison groups
Since 1975, when the Zoonoses Order was introduced, informal local liaison groups have been created in England and Wales following the Scottish example (Sharp, 1977). These groups comprise community physicians, public health laboratory microbiologists, veterinarians and environmental health officers with the aim of building up a collaborative approach to zoonotic incidents. There are at least 14 groups in England and Wales to date, most of which were started by Nominated Officers.

Central Zoonoses group
In 1975 a central zoonoses group was created; members comprised the Chief Veterinary Officer, of the Ministry of Agriculture, Fisheries and Food the Chief Medical Officer of the Department of Health and Social Security, and representatives of the Public Health Laboratory Service, Department of Health and Social Security, and the State Veterinary Service. Its functions are to provide a forum for discussion on interprofessional problems and to brief heads of services (Payne & Lowes, 1976).

NATIONAL SURVEILLANCE

The Communicable Diseases (Scotland) Unit was established in Glasgow in 1967 to carry out surveillance of communicable disease in Scotland. The unit has an attached Veterinary Officer of the Department of Agriculture and Fisheries for Scotland. The role of this officer is to coordinate veterinary and medical information and to provide advice and training in the management of zoonoses.

In England and Wales, the Communicable Disease Surveillance Centre was created in 1977 by the Public Health Laboratory Service on behalf of the Department of Health and Social Security and the Welsh Office (Galbraith, 1982). In 1979 a Divisional Veterinary Officer from the State Veterinary Service was seconded to the CDSC. This posting has facilitated the collation of data from and the exchange of information between the State Veterinary Service and the Public Health Laboratory Service, encouraged the joint investigation of zoonotic incidents in the community and has made expertise available for advice on the control of zoonoses.

FUTURE NEEDS

There is little doubt that the zoonoses will continue to create important public health problems. New zoonoses will be discovered and changes in the incidence of established zoonoses will continue to occur. For example, surveillance data in the UK show that reported salmonella infection continues to increase and campylobacter infection may be even more common. If these problems are to be successfully investigated and controlled it is important that the present frameworks of medico-veterinary cooperation are maintained and strengthened. One development which has been suggested is the designation of a national team of doctors for liaison with the veterinary nominated officers (Bell & Palmer, 1983).

In the past, zoonoses which caused serious human illness in Britain such as bovine tuberculosis and brucellosis also caused serious loss of animal production and the financial loss resulting to farmers was the most important factor in introducing successful control measures. Today however, the zoonoses important in human illness cause little or no animal disease and therefore the identification of public health problems and the pressure for control will depend increasingly on the medical profession.

REFERENCES

Abbott J D, Jones D M, Painter M J, Sutcliffe E M, Barrell R A E 1983 Serotypes and biotypes of Campylobacter jejuni/coli isolated from (a) clinical infections in North-West England during 1982 — a collaborative study by 20 laboratories and (b) non-human sources in North-West England 1982–83. In: Campylobacter II: (Eds) by Pearson A D, Skirrow M B, Rowe B, Davies J R, Jones D M, PHLS, London: 90–92
Akiba T, Koyama K, Ishiki Y, Kimura S, Fukushima T 1960 On the mechanism of the development of multiple-drug resistant clones of Shigella. Japanese Journal of Microbiology 4: 219–227
Andrews B E, Major R, Palmer S R 1981 Ornithosis in poultry workers. Lancet i: 632–634
Bell J C, Jacob M, Palmer S R 1981 Legal and ethical aspects of salmonellosis. The Veterinary Record 109: 301–304
Bell J C, Palmer S R 1983 Control of zoonoses in Britain: past, present, and future. British Medical Journal 287: 591–593
Casals J, Buckley S M 1981 Lassa Fever. In: Viral Zoonoses Volume 2 (Ed) Beran G W CRC Handbook Series in Zoonoses Section B: Editor-in-Chief Steele J H CRC Press Inc.
Chattopadhyay B 1979 Group R Streptococcal infection amongst pig meat handlers — a review. Public Health London 93: 140–142
Cohen D R, Porter I A, Reid T M S, Sharp J C M, Forbes G I, Paterson G M 1983 A cost-benefit study of milk-borne salmonellosis. Journal of Hygiene Cambridge 91: 17–23
Communicable Disease Surveillance Centre 1980 Brucellosis: England and Wales. British Medical Journal 283: 1477
Communicable Disease Surveillance Centre 1982a Anthrax Surveillance 1961–80. British Medical Journal 284: 204
Communicable Disease Surveillance Centre 1982b Food poisoning and Salmonellosis Surveillance in England and Wales 1981. British Medical Journal 285: 1127–1128
Craun G F 1979 Waterborne giardiasis in the United States: A review. American Journal of Public Health 69: 817–819
Department of Health and Social Security and the Welsh office 1977: Memorandum on Rabies. HMSO, London

Derrick E H 1937 Q fever, a new entity: clinical features, diagnosis and laboratory investigation. Medical Journal of Australia 2: 281–299

Galbraith N S, Forbes P, Mayon-White R T 1980 Changing patterns of communicable disease in England and Wales. British Medical Journal 281: 427–430, 489–492, 546–549

Galbraith N S 1982 Communicable Disease Surveillance. In: Recent Advances in Community Medicine (Ed Alwyn Smith) Churchill Livingstone, London: p 127–141

Galbraith N S, Forbes P, Clifford C 1982 Communicable disease associated with milk and dairy products in England and Wales 1951–80. British Medical Journal 284: 17–21

Gardner S D 1983 Prevention of Rabies in Man in England and Wales. In: Rabies a Growing Threat (Ed) J R Pattison. Van Nostrand Reinhold Co Ltd. Wokingham: 39–49

George J T A, Wallace J G, Morrison H R, Harbourne J F 1972 Paratyphoid in man and cattle. British Medical Journal 3: 208

Gill O P N 1983 Serological survey of leptospirosis in fish farm workers. Part 2 Thesis for Membership of Faculty of Community Medicine London

Hall C J, Richmond S J, Caul E O, Pearce N H, Silver I A 1982 Laboratory outbreak of Q fever acquired from sheep. Lancet i: 1004–1006

Hall S M 1983 Congenital Toxoplasmosis in England, Wales and Northern Ireland: Some epidemiological problems. British Medical Journal 287: 453–455

Hathaway S C, Little T W A, Stevens A E 1982 Isolation of *Leptospira interogans* serovar *hardjo* from aborted bovine fetuses in England. The Veterinary Record 111: 58

Hendrickson R V, Osborn K G, Madden D L, Anderson J H, Maul D H, Sever J L et al 1983 Epidemic of acquired immunodeficiency in rhesus monkeys. Lancet i: 388–390

Jones P H, Willis A T, Robinson D A, Skirrow M B, Joseph D S 1981 Campylobacter enteritis associated with the consumption of free school milk. Journal of Hygiene 87: 155–162

Leech F B, Vessey M P, MacRae W D, Lawson J R, MacKinnon D J, Morgan W J B 1964 Brucellosis in the British dairy herd 1960–61 MAFF Animal Disease Surveys Report No 4. HMSO, London

Langmuir A D 1979 Guillain-Barré syndrome: the swine influenza virus vaccine incident in the United States of America 1976–1977, preliminary communication. Journal of the Royal Society of Medicine 72: 660–669

London W T, Madden D L, Gravell M, Dalakas M C, Hauff S A, Sever J L et al 1983 Experimental transmission of Simian acquired immunodeficiency syndrome (SAIDS) and Kaposi-like skin lesions. Lancet ii: 869–873

Lowes E 1975 The Zoonoses Order. Veterinary Record 97: 32–33

McCoy J H 1975 Trends in Salmonella food poisoning in England and Wales 1941–72. Journal of Hygiene (London) 74: 271–282

Marmion B P, Stoker M G P 1958 The epidemiology of Q fever in Great Britain. An analysis of the findings and some conclusions. British Medical Journal 2: 809–816

Ministry of Agriculture Fisheries and Food 1975 Zoonoses Order (SI No 1030). HMSO, London

Ministry of Agriculture Fisheries and Food 1981 Diseases of Animals (Protein Processing) Order (SI No 676). HMSO, London

Ministry of Agriculture Fisheries and Food 1981 Importation of Processed Animal Protein Order (SI No 677). HMSO, London

Ministry of Agriculture Fisheries and Food 1983 Milk (Special Designations) (Scotland) Order 1980 (SI No 1866). HMSO, London

Morbidity and Mortality Weekly Report 1982a Cryptosporidiosis: assessment of chemotherapy of males with acquired immune deficiency syndrome (AIDS) 31: 589–592

Morbidity and Mortality Weekly Report 1982b Outbreak of *Yersinia enterocolitica* — Washington State 31: 562–564

Newell D G (ed) 1982 Campylobacter; epidemiology, pathogenesis and biochemistry. MTP Press, Lancaster

Office of Population Censuses and Surveys 1977–1982 Mortality Statistics Cause Series DH2 Nos 2–7. HMSO, London

Palmer S R 1982 Psittacosis in man — recent developments in the UK: a review. Journal of the Royal Society Medicine 75: 262–267

Palmer S R, Andrews B E, Major R 1981 A common source of outbreak of ornithosis in veterinary surgeons. Lancet ii: 798–799

Palmer S R, Young S E J 1982 Q fever endocarditis in England and Wales 1975–81. Lancet ii: 1448–1449

Palmer S R, Gully P R, White J M, Pearson A D, Suckling W G, Jones D M et al 1983 Waterborne outbreak of campylobacter gastro-enteritis. Lancet i: 287–290

Payne D J H, Lowes E 1976 Preventing animal disease. British Medical Journal i: 521

Payne D J H, Scudamore J M 1977 Outbreak of salmonella food poisoning over a period of eight years from a common source. Lancet i: 1249–1251

Reilly W J, Sharp J C M, Forbes G I, Paterson G M 1983 Milk-borne salmonellosis in Scotland 1980 to 1982. The Veterinary Record 112: 578–580

Report 1969 Joint Committee on the use of antibiotics in animal husbandry and veterinary medicine Cmnd 4190. HMSO, London

Report 1970 Report on the Animal Health Services in Great Britain 1969. HMSO, London

Report 1971 Report on the Animal Health Services in Great Britain 1970. HMSO, London

Report 1983 Animal Health 1982 Report of the Chief Veterinary Officer. HMSO, London

Riley L W, Remis R S, Helgerson S D, McGee H B, Wells J G, Davis B R, Hebert R J, Okott E S, Johnson L M, Hargrett N T, Blake P A, Cohen M L 1983 Haemorrhagic colitis associated with a rare *Escherichia coli* serotype. New England Journal of Medicine 308: 681–685

Robertson M H, Clarke R I, Coghlan J, Gill O N 1981 Leptospirosis in trout farmers Lancet ii, 626–627

Robinson D A 1981 Infective dose of *campylobacter jejuni* in milk. British Medical Journal 282: 1584

Robinson D A, Jones D M 1981 Milk-borne campylobacter infection. British Medical Journal 282: 1374–1376

Rowe B, Hall M L M, Ward L R, De Sa J D H Epidemic Spread of *Salmonella hadar* in England & Wales. British Medical Journal 280: 1065–1066

Rowe B, Threlfall E J 1981 Multiple antimicrobial drug resistance in enteric pathogens. Journal of Antimicrobial Chemotherapy 7: 1–3

Salmon M M, Howells B, Glencross E J G, Evans A D, Palmer S R 1982 Q fever in an urban area. Lancet i: 1002–1004

Schachter J, Dawson C R 1978 Psittacosis in Human Chlamydial Infections PSG, Littleton Massachusetts 9–43

Schleck 111 W F, Lavigne P M, Bortolussi R A, Allen A C, Haldane E V, Wort A J et al 1983 Epidemic Listeriosis — evidence for transmission by food. New England Journal of Medicine 308: 203–206

Sharp J C M, 1977 Medical — Veterinary Liaison in Scotland. Veterinary Record 101: 200–201

Sharp J C M, Paterson G M, Forbes G I 1980 Milk-borne salmonellosis in Scotland. Journal of Infection 2: 333–340

Skirrow M B 1982 Campylobacter enteritis in the first five years. Journal of Hygiene 89: 175–184

Stableforth A W 1954 Brucellosis in animals and man: its cause, nature and prevention. Royal Sanitary Institute Journal 74: 686–699

Steele J H 1979 Editor-in-Chief CRC Handbook Series in Zoonoses. Section A, Bacterial, Rickettsial and Mycotic Diseases, Volume 1, Section Editors, Stoenner H, Kaplan W and Torton M, CRC Press, Inc.

Steele J H, 1980 Editor-in-Chief CRC Handbook Series in Zoonoses, Section A, Bacterial, Rickettsial and Mycotic Diseases, Volume 11, Section Editors, Stoenner H, Kaplan W and Torton M, CRC Press, Inc.

Steele J H, 1981 (a) Editor-in-Chief CRC Handbook Series in Zoonoses, Section B, Viral Zoonoses, Volume 1, Section Editor, Beran G W, CRC Press, Inc.

Steele J H, 1981 (b) Editor-in-Chief CRC Handbook Series in Zoonoses. Section B, Viral Zoonoses, Volume 2, Section Editor, Beran G W, CRC Press, Inc.

Teas J 1983 Could AIDS Agent be a new variant of African Swine Fever virus? (correspondence) Lancet i: 923

Tobin M J, Cahill N, Gearty G, Maurer B, Blake S, Daly K et al 1982 Q fever endocarditis. The American Journal of Medicine 72: 396–400

Walters T M H 1978 Hydatid disease in Wales i Epidemiology. The Veterinary Record 102: 257–259

Wilson D, Wetson R 1981 Leptospirosis — a diagnostic problem and an industrial hazard. Journal of the Royal College of General Practitioners 31: 165–167

World Health Organization 1959 Zoonoses: second report of the Joint WHO/FAO Expert Committee Technical Report Series, No 169. WHO Geneva

World Health Organization 1979 Human Monkeypox in West Africa Weekly Epidemiological Record 54: 12

World Health Organization 1982 Bacterial and Viral Zoonoses. World Health Organization Technical Report Series 682: WHO Geneva

12. Do locally based enquiries into perinatal mortality reduce the risk of perinatal death?

Diana Elbourne   Lesley Mutch

Public concern about perinatal mortality rates has focussed interest on methods by which the perinatal health services can be evaluated. The aim of this chapter is to go one step further and to evaluate the role of locally-based enquiries into perinatal death.

BACKGROUND

Although infant mortality rates have been used as an index of the health of a community for many years, public awareness of perinatal mortality as an issue was fired only in the last decade. The publication of two reports (Committee on Child Health Services, 1976; Department of Health and Social Security, 1976) focussed attention on both international and intranational differences in perinatal mortality rates, with the implication that these reflected a variable quality of care.

Politicians and the press responded to these issues, fuelled by the Spastic Society's 'Save A Baby' campaign and prompted the House of Commons Social Services Committee to investigate perinatal and neonatal mortality in 1979 (House of Commons Social Services Committee: Second Report, 1980).

Early in 1980 a study group of the Royal College of Obstetricians and Gynaecologists on Perinatal Audit and Surveillance recommended that confidential enquiries into perinatal death should be established with independent assessors reviewing the conduct of care along the lines of the established confidential enquiry into maternal deaths (Chalmers & McIlwaine, 1980) and the ongoing enquiry into perinatal deaths in Leicester (MacVicar, 1980). These recommendations were reiterated in the publication of the Report of the House of Commons Committee in 1980. Hence from 1976 on, Districts, Areas and Regions were increasingly bombarded with publicity on the need for such enquiries—and they responded (Enkin & Chalmers, 1980). This was particularly so in some areas which had been pilloried in the press as having relatively high perinatal mortality rates.

In this chapter we detail the type and extent of locally-based perinatal mortality enquiries between 1974–1981; relate the setting up of such surveys to the previous perinatal mortality rates in that area; and finally, by analysing rates for 1974–1981 look for evidence that surveys had any effect on the subsequent risk of perinatal death.

Materials

The National Perinatal Epidemiology Unit has obtained information about locally based perinatal surveys from specialists in Community Medicine, Regional Nursing Officers and personal contacts. Since 1981, this information has been assembled in an Archive of Locally Based Perinatal Surveys and this is updated periodically (Mutch &

Elbourne, 1983). In addition to data from this Archive, all the analyses will employ official statistics for the years 1974 to 1981.

Extent and type of perinatal surveys

There have been many different types of locally-based perinatal mortality enquiries. We have classified them according to their complexity and depth. Some consisted of a statistical review of routinely collected data, but most supplemented this using clinical case records. In some cases, further information has been obtained from the parents of the dead baby (Garcia, 1982). In addition, some surveys have also collected information about control babies, selected either from the relevant population or as part of case control studies (Paediatric Research Unit, Exeter, 1982). We classified the surveys as follows:

(a) statistical review of routinely collected data
(b) case note review of deaths
(c) case note review of deaths and interviews with parents
(d) case note review of deaths and population controls
(e) case control studies using case notes
(f) case control studies using case notes and interviews with parents.

The enquiries have been classified hierarchically so that if there was more than one study in any area at any time, the more 'complex' study has been given precedence.
    As Figure 12.1 shows, the earliest of these enquiries began in 1976, although we

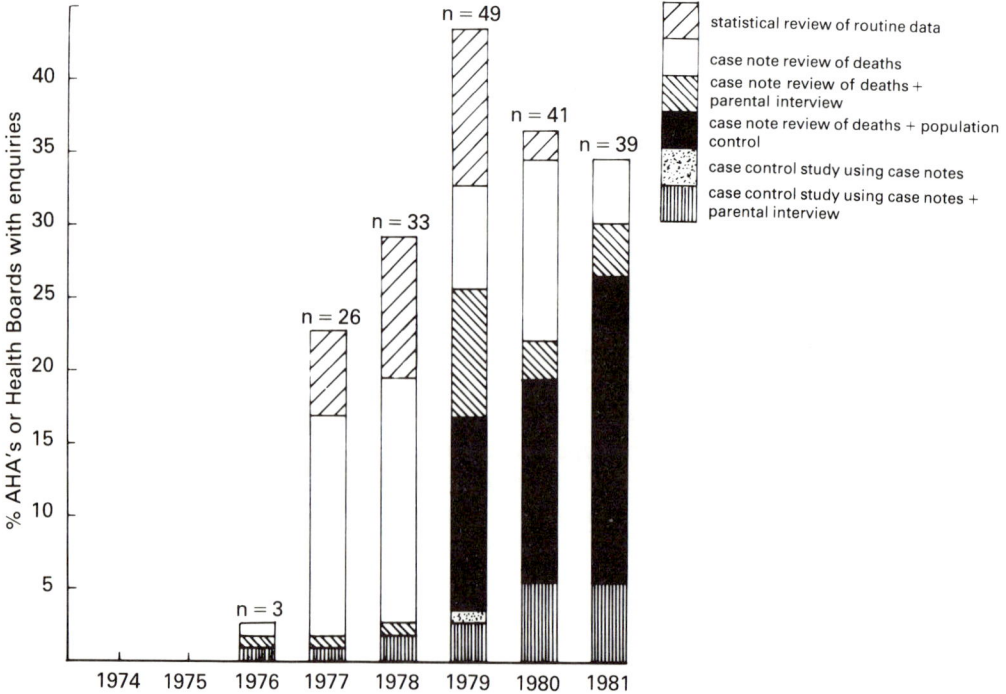

Fig. 12.1 Number (%) of AHAs (England and Wales) and Health Boards (Scotland) with different types of perinatal mortality enquiry, 1974–1981.

recognise that preparation for and discussion about them may well have begun much earlier. Between 1976 and 1981 some sort of locally based enquiry covered between 3% and 43% of the 98 Area Health Authorities (AHAs) in England and Wales and 15 Health Boards in Scotland. During this period six Regional studies in England and Wales as well as one covering the whole of Scotland were carried out. About a sixth of the enquiries were statistical reviews of routinely collected data; for nearly 40% of enquiries, some sort of control data was available. Interviews with parents were a feature of 20% of these enquiries.

Such studies can also be classified in another way. In some cases, a study is planned to examine deaths which have occurred in previous years, and in others a decision is taken to study deaths prospectively as they occur. These two broad types of enquiry we shall term 'retrospective' and 'prospective'. Two thirds of the studies were prospective by this definition.

Why do some areas undertake perinatal mortality enquiries?

It would seem very possible that those areas in which enquiries into perinatal deaths had been established were prompted to mount them because of a relatively high perinatal mortality rate. To examine this, we took as the index rate the perinatal mortality rate two years before either a prospective study was mounted, or the report of a retrospective study was published. However, we found that in only half of the areas in which studies had been undertaken was the perinatal mortality rate higher than that for England, Wales and Scotland combined in the index year (Table 12.1).

Table 12.1   Relationship between undertaking a perinatal mortality study and previous perinatal mortality rates

Year*	Number of studies	Study areas with PNMR in index year higher than that for England, Scotland and Wales combined	
		Number	Percentage
1976	2	2	100
1977	2	1	50
1978	5	3	60
1979	9	5	55
1980	5	3	60
1981	14	6	43
1976–1981	37	20	54

*Year of either a 'prospective' study being mounted or the publication of the report of a 'retrospective' study (see text).

Do locally based perinatal mortality enquiries have any effect on the subsequent risk of perinatal death?

The explicit aim of most enquiries into perinatal deaths is to reduce the perinatal mortality rate. By what pathways might we expect any effects be mediated, and how can these effects be determined?

The presumed route by which enquiries might be expected to have an effect is usually by identifying problem areas in the services and by making recommendations intended to lead to an improvement in outcome. However, there may be unintended consequences simply by virtue of examining the problem, regardless of the results of the survey—the Hawthorne effect (Roethlisberger & Dickson, 1939). For example, in a 'retrospective' study a decision taken in 1977 to study perinatal deaths for 1974–1976 is unlikely to have any effect on perinatal mortality rates until a report is published in, say, 1978. On the other hand, in a 'prospective' study a decision taken in 1977 to study future deaths as they occur in 1978 may have 'Hawthorne' effects while the study is in progress, long before any report is available.

METHODOLOGY

A possible framework for considering the effect of perinatal mortality enquiries on perinatal mortality rates is to examine ways in which the influence of maternal mortality enquiries on the rate of maternal mortality has been evaluated.

Although the present system of confidential enquiries into maternal deaths was not formally instituted in England and Wales until 1952, similar forms of investigation existed much earlier following a rise in the maternal mortality rate in the 1920s. Following several ad hoc enquiries in the early 1920s, Medical Officers of Health, in 1928, were invited to obtain information about every maternal death in their area and to send confidential reports to the Ministry of Health. Summary statements were included in the Chief Medical Officer's reports every year from 1932 to 1953. The present system was introduced in 1952 both in order to obtain completeness and also to ensure that it would be practising consultant obstetricians who would judge whether 'avoidable factors' were associated with the maternal death. Since then reports have been issued triennially. The most recent covered 227 of the 228 known maternal deaths in England and Wales between 1976 and 1978 (Department of Health and Social Security, 1982).

A priori, from Figure 12.2, there is no evidence of any increasing rate of fall in

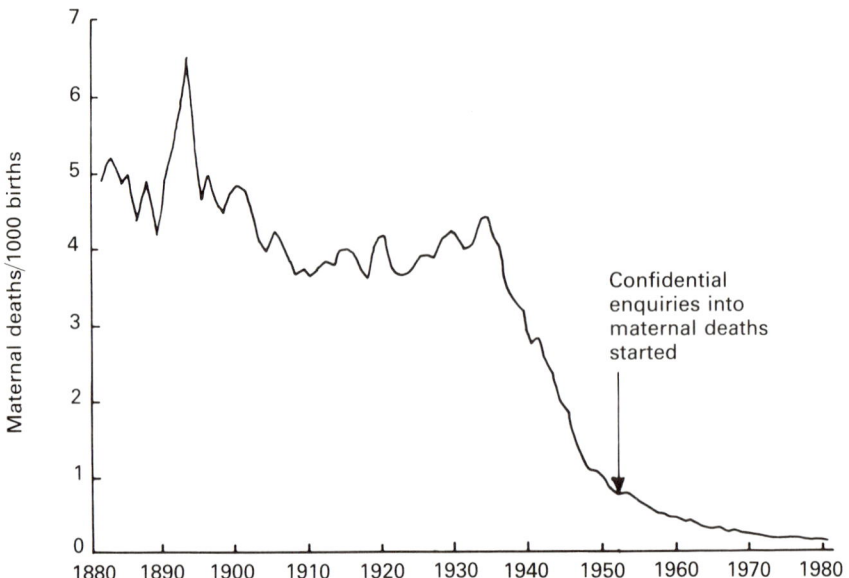

Fig. 12.2   Maternal mortality rates, England and Wales, 1881–1981.

maternal mortality in the 1950s. It might be tempting to suggest that the enquiries which began in the late 1920s and early 1930s were responsible for the fall in the maternal mortality rates from the mid 1930s. However, we do not know whether, rather than causing the fall, enquiries merely contributed to a fall which had begun for other reasons, such as the introduction of preventive and then curative measures against puerperal sepsis, or recovery from the worst aspects of the depression. There is also a statistical problem involved in interpreting whether the initial declines in mortality were consistent with random variation or were of a magnitude unlikely to occur by chance (Taylor & Dauncey, 1954). The basic problem is the comparison group. In the situation in England and Wales where coverage, if patchy between 1928 and 1952, was national, the only feasible controls are historical, with all the attendant problems of such controls (Doll & Peto, 1980).

Applying this method to perinatal mortality studies we cannot see (Fig. 12.3) any

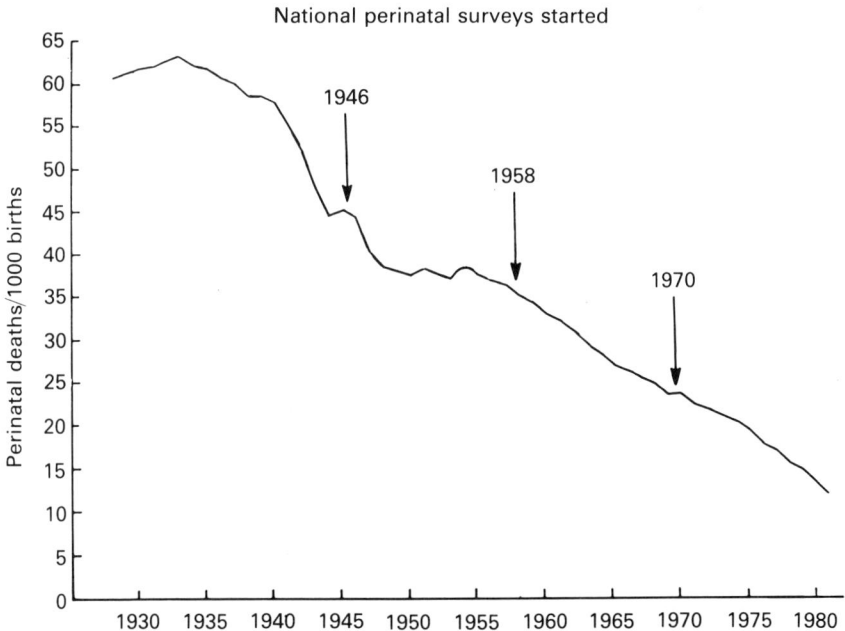

Fig. 12.3   Perinatal mortality rates, England and Wales, 1928–1981.

obvious influences of the three ad hoc national perinatal surveys (Joint Committee of the Royal College of Obstetricians and Gynaecologists and the Population Investigation Committee, 1948; Butler & Bonham, 1963; Chamberlain et al, 1975).

An alternative approach, and one more relevant to recent enquiries in England, Wales, and Scotland is that suggested by Grimes & Cates (1977). In the United States of America, state maternal mortality study committees closely approximate to the confidential enquiry into maternal mortality for England and Wales. Grimes & Cates compared the rates of decline in maternal mortality ratios by decades from 1938–1940 to 1968–1970 for states with such committees to those without. They found that although the two groups of states had nearly equal rates of decline during the first decade, states with committees had, however, smaller rates of decline during the two latter decades. An editorial (Pearse, 1977) accompanying the Grimes & Cates paper questioned the usefulness of continuing maternal mortality enquiries and concluded that the committees should concentrate their efforts on the larger problem of perinatal deaths.

Because perinatal mortality enquiries have not been in existence for anything like as long a period in England and Wales as maternal mortality committees have been in the USA, we cannot use exactly the same methodology as Grimes & Cates. But we have adopted a similar approach.

RESULTS

In Figure 12.4 we show the perinatal mortality rates for 1974 to 1981 for two groups of areas in England, Wales and Scotland—those which had, and those which did not have, any type of locally-based audit of their perinatal deaths at any time between 1974 and 1981. This demonstrates that the average perinatal mortality of those areas which undertook surveys was consistently higher than for those which did not undertake studies. If enquiries were to have an effect on these rates one would expect the distance between the two lines to narrow. But there seems no evidence of this from Figure 12.4.

An obvious solution to the question 'Why do we not see an effect of these studies?' is that there is none. This is certainly not an answer we can dismiss out of hand, particularly in the light of the Grimes & Cates paper.

Another possibility is that, although there has been an effect, it is masked by an artefact of the data. Studying a subject often leads to more complete reporting. This may have the effect of artificially increasing the number of perinatal deaths in those areas under investigation (Clarke & Clayton, 1980). If this were so, we might expect that, as the collection of statistics settles at some new plateau of efficiency, an effect of the enquiries may be seen at a later date.

There may be other explanations in terms of a delayed effect. It is possible that any effect on perinatal mortality rates will not occur, or be seen to occur, so soon after an enquiry has been instigated. This argues for a longer time scale. Unfortunately, the 1982 reorganisation of the National Health Service has rendered it impossible to look over a longer time period at official statistics for the geographical areas covered by the AHAs which existed between 1974 and 1981.

It might be that some types of surveys are more effective than others in reducing perinatal mortality. For example, it might be expected that the most complex kind of survey, which is a case control study involving parental interviews, would have a greater effect than that of a purely statistical review. In Figure 12.4 we are not able to demonstrate such an effect. However, it must be stressed that breaking down the analyses into these smaller categories means that the random variations associated with small numbers may confuse the issue.

Finally, we must address the problem raised by not comparing like populations. It may be that areas which do undertake enquiries differ in some ways from areas which do not. Grimes & Cates refined their analysis of the effects of enquiries on maternal mortality by taking into account the maternal age distribution of the populations under study. In the case of perinatal mortality it would be an appropriate refinement to consider the effect of differing proportions of deaths associated with congenital

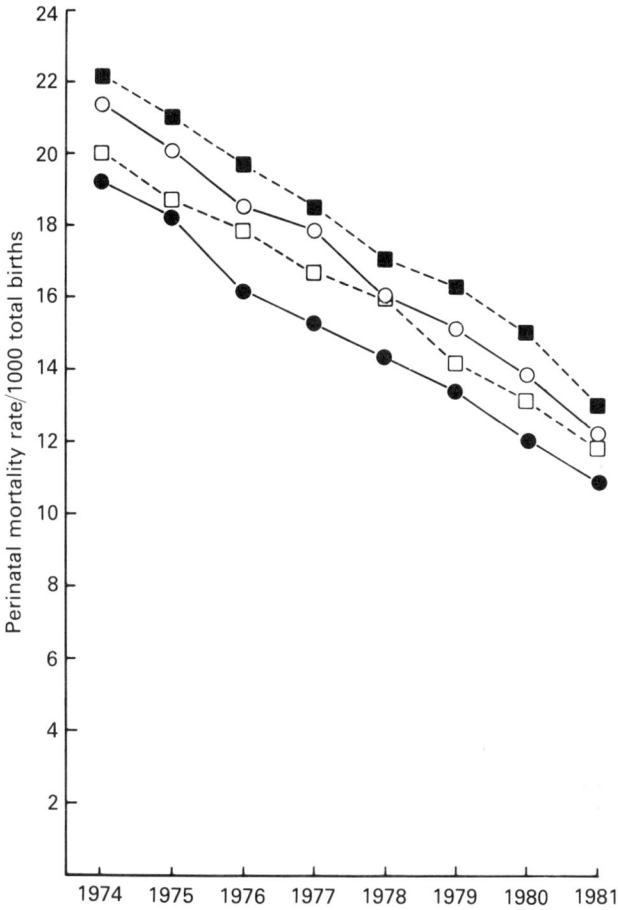

Fig. 12.4 Perinatal mortality rates in areas which did not undertake locally based perinatal mortality enquiries, and by selected types of enquiry England, Scotland and Wales, 1974–1981. ●—● Areas having no locally based enquiry into perinatal deaths at any time between 1974 and 1981; ○—○ areas having a locally based enquiry into perinatal deaths at sometime between 1974 and 1981; ■—■ areas having a statistical review of routinely collected information only, at some time between 1974 and 1981; □—□ areas having a locally based case control study of perinatal deaths involving parental interviews at some time between 1974 and 1981.

malformations in the two types of population. However the rates of decline in perinatal mortality excluding deaths due to malformations do not differ significantly between areas which have or have not undertaken locally based perinatal mortality enquiries between 1974 and 1981 (Fig. 12.5).

CONCLUSIONS

In our study, we have been unable to show any effect of population based perinatal mortality enquiries on perinatal mortality rates. However, there may be other advantages derived from undertaking such studies.

Commentators have suggested that parental interviews have therapeutic benefits for

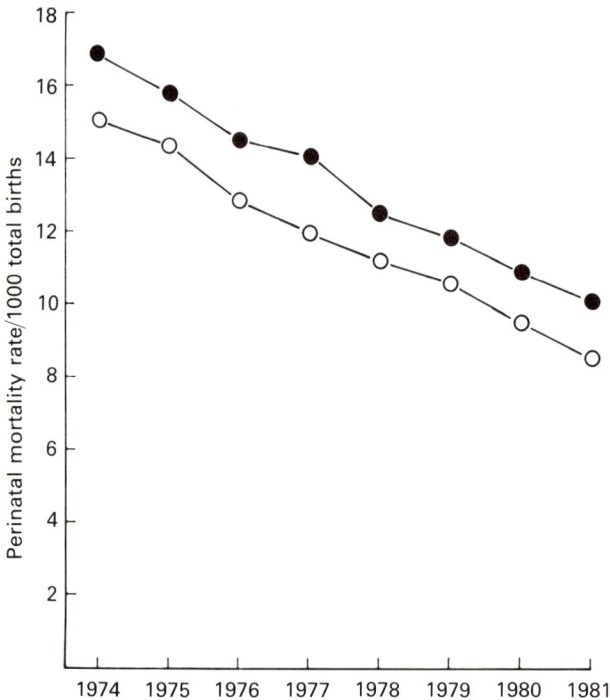

Fig. 12.5 Perinatal mortality rates, excluding deaths due to congenital malformation, in areas which did and did not undertake locally based perinatal mortality enquiries, in England, Scotland and Wales 1974–1981 (1981 figures provisional). ●—● Perinatal mortality rates in areas which had locally based enquiries at some time between 1974 and 1981; ○—○ perinatal mortality rates in areas which did not have locally based enquiries at any time between 1974 and 1981.

the parents (Cartwright, 1979; Gilligan, 1980; Garcia, 1982). They may also have an educative effect for both parents and those working in the services.

Enquiries may, by identifying deficiencies in the system, lead to changes in the organisation of care and the allocation of resources.

These perhaps less tangible benefits have to be weighed against the cost of administering such surveys on an ad hoc basis. Perhaps the way forward lies in an ongoing study of perinatal outcomes using routinely collected data such as that recommended by the working group on the Standard Maternity Information System (Thomson & Barron, 1980) and the Steering Group on Health Services Information (1982) for all births.

ACKNOWLEDGEMENTS

We should like to thank Iain Chalmers, Alison Macfarlane and Malinee Somwichong for their help and encouragement; and Dr Susan Cole for providing data for Scotland; and Jini Hetherington and Lesley Mierh for typing. Diana Elbourne and Lesley Mutch are supported by a project grant from the DHSS. Figures 12.2 and 12.3 are derived from OPCS mortality and fertility statistics with the permission of the Controller of Her Majesty's Stationery Office: Crown Copyright reserved.

REFERENCES

Butler N R, Bonham D G (eds) 1963 Perinatal Mortality: the first report of the 1958 British perinatal mortality survey. Churchill Livingstone, Edinburgh

Cartwright A 1979 The Dignity of Labour? Tavistock, London

Chalmers I, McIlwaine G (eds) 1980 Perinatal Audit and Surveillance. Proceedings of the Eighth Study Group of the Royal College of Obstetricians and Gynaecologists, London

Chamberlain R, Chamberlain G, Howlett B, Claireaux A 1975 British Births 1970, Vol I, the first week of life. William Heinemann Medical Books, London

Clarke M, Clayton D 1980 Interpreting case control studies. In: Chalmers I, McIlwaine G, (eds) op cit, 263–273

Committee on Child Health Services 1976 Fit for the future. Cmnd 6684, HMSO, London

Department of Health and Social Security 1976 Priorities for health and personal social services in England. HMSO, London

Department of Health and Social Security 1982 Report on confidential enquiries into maternal deaths in England and Wales 1976–1978. Report on public health and social subjects No. 26. HMSO, London

Doll R, Peto R 1980 Randomised controlled trials and retrospective controls. British Medical Journal 1: 44

Enkin M, Chalmers I 1980 A service note: inquiries into perinatal deaths at area health authority level (a status report winter 1979/80). Community Medicine 2: 219–224

Garcia J 1982 Women's views of antenatal care. In: Enkin M, Chalmers I (eds) Effectiveness and Satisfaction in Antenatal Care. Spastics International Medical Publications. William Heinemann Medical Books, London: 81–91

Gilligan M 1980 Perinatal mortality enquiries at district level. In: Chalmers I, McIlwaine G (eds). op cit, 148–158

Grimes D A, Cates W 1977 The impact of state maternal mortality study committees on maternal deaths in the United States. American Journal of Public Health 67,9: 830–833

House of Commons Social Services Committee (Chairman R Short) Second Report 1980 Perinatal and Neonatal Mortality. HMSO, London

Joint Committee of the Royal College of Obstetricians and Gynaecologists and the Population Investigation Committee 1948 Maternity in Great Britain: a survey of social and economic aspects of pregnancy and childbirth. Oxford University Press, London

MacVicar J 1980 Perinatal mortality — an area survey. In: Chalmers I, McIlwaine G, eds. op cit, 133–147

Mutch L M M, Elbourne D R 1983 Archive of locally-based perinatal surveys (unpublished paper)

Paediatric Research Unit, Exeter 1982 A suggested model for inquiries into perinatal and early childhood deaths in a health care district (unpublished)

Pearse W H 1977 Maternal mortality studies — time to stop? American Journal of Public Health 67,9: 813–816

Roethlisberger F J, Dickson W J 1939 Management and the Worker. Harvard University Press, Cambridge, Mass

Steering Group on Health Services Information 1982 Review of information about hospital clinical activities, maternity statistics and the report of the joint group A (Maternity)

Taylor W, Dauncey M 1954 Changing patterns of mortality in England and Wales II. Maternal Mortality. British Journal of Preventive and Social Medicine 8: 172–175

Thomson A M, Barron S L 1980 A Standard Maternity Information System. In: Chalmers I, McIlwaine G, (eds), op cit, 79–92

13. Collection, analysis and dissemination of vital and health statistics

M. J. Goldacre

Vital and health statistics are numerical records of births, marriages, sickness and deaths by which the growth and health of a community may be studied (Benjamin, 1968). The features of some of the main routine medical information systems have been described in earlier volumes of this series (Campbell, 1978; Anderson, 1978; Donnan, 1982; Galbraith, 1982) and elsewhere (Benjamin, 1968; Ashley, 1972; Alderson, 1974; Weatherall, 1978). The first part of this chapter describes briefly the main systems in England which include medical data, concentrating on the data collected in them, and comments on their uses. The description of the data collected is not exhaustive and, in particular, the details of such systems as Hospital Activity Analysis (HAA), cancer registries and the child health systems vary a little from region to region. The interested reader is recommended to obtain copies of local documents used for data collection. The second part of the chapter reviews the work of the Steering Group on Health Services Information and the development of Performance Indicators for the National Health Service (NHS). The third part discusses some organisational aspects of the collection, analysis and distribution of routine statistics.

COLLECTION OF DATA

Birth and death registration: general
The Office of Population Censuses and Surveys (OPCS) is responsible, through the Registrars of Births and Deaths, for recording every birth and death which occurs in England and Wales. A draft entry for each birth or death is completed by the registrar. Most of the particulars are then transferred to the register. Certain confidential particulars are entered on the draft, and forwarded to the OPCS for statistical purposes with a copy of the full entry, but are not entered on the public register.

Birth registration
A qualified informant (usually the mother or father) is statutorily required to provide registration details to the registrar within 42 days of the birth. The data recorded for a live birth include the surname and forenames of the child, father and mother; the child's sex, date and place of birth, birthweight and NHS number; the father's occupation, date and place of birth; the mother's maiden surname and usual address; whether the child was one of a multiple birth; legitimacy, the date of marriage if the child was of legitimate birth, whether the mother has been married more than once, and the number of children previously born alive and still born to the mother. Birthweight has only recently been recorded on birth registrations and is obtained by

linkage from birth notification records (Lewis, 1981). The details completed for a still birth are similar but they also include the duration of the pregnancy in weeks, the cause or causes of death, and whether or not a post-mortem was held.

Birth notification
In addition to the requirements of civil registration, the attendant at birth (usually the midwife) must notify the local health authority of each birth within the authority's boundaries. Many authorities now participate in the standard Child Health Computer System (see below) and use its recommended notification form.

Death registration
The OPCS is responsible, through the local registrars, for the collection of registration data from the informant and from the medical certificate of death. The data recorded include the surname and forenames of the deceased (and the maiden surname in the case of a married woman), date and place of death, date and place of birth, sex, usual address, occupation of the deceased (and of the husband of a married woman, or the parent of a child), civil state, NHS number, whether or not a post-mortem was held, the coroner's verdict in the event of a coroner's inquest, type of accident when relevant, and the cause or causes of death. A copy of each form is sent by the registrars to the OPCS. The OPCS is responsible for the analysis of mortality statistics and it also forwards a copy of each death certificate to the district medical officer of the district in which the deceased was resident.

Hospital inpatients
HAA covers all discharges from general hospitals and is processed by regions. The Hospital In-patient Enquiry (HIPE) is a one-in-ten sample of discharges from general hospitals, processed by OPCS, and its data are now usually obtained by sampling from HAA. Data about all patients discharged from psychiatric hospitals are collected through the Mental Health Enquiry (MHE) which is currently processed by the Department of Health and Social Security (DHSS). Data about maternity patients are collected through maternity HIPE as a national one-in-ten sample; and in some regions maternity HAA is collected on a 100% basis. Much of the data collected in HAA, the MHE and maternity HAA are common to all three systems and include the hospital and district of treatment, the patient's unit number, date of birth, sex, address, place of birth, marital status, category (e.g. NHS, private), source of admission, date on the waiting list (if relevant), dates of admission and discharge, consultant and department on admission and discharge, hospital ward, general practitioner, disposal, type of accident (if relevant), number of visits to theatre and days from admission to first operation (if relevant), main and other diagnoses, and main and other operations. Most regions do not collect the patient's occupation or social class and do not computerise patients' names.

Additional data collected in the MHE include the patient's name, NHS number, occupation, religion, mental category, legal status, and whether or not the patient has received previous psychiatric care.

Additional data collected in maternity HAA include the date of delivery and date of the mother's last menstrual period; number of previous live births, still births and abortions; antenatal diagnoses, and complications during delivery or the puerperium;

method of onset of labour and mode of delivery; information about analgesia, anaesthesia, episiotomy and sterilisation; the infant's presentation, sex, birthweight and disposal from hospital care; the presence of congenital abnormality or other disease; and whether or not the infant was transferred to a special care baby unit.

Outpatients
Counts of attendances are recorded by hospital, department, and according to whether the attendance is a new or repeat visit. No demographic or diagnostic information is routinely collected.

General practice
There is no comprehensive statistical coverage of patients seen in general practice. Some self-selected practices participate in a national morbidity study from which statistical tables are published periodically which give, for example, consultation rates by diagnosis and age-group (Royal College of General Practitioners, 1979).

Cancer registration
Cancers are registered at regional registries and registrations are forwarded to the OPCS. The data include the patient's surname (and maiden name of a married woman), forenames, NHS number, date of birth, sex, address, place of birth, hospital, unit number, the occupation and industry of the patient (and of the husband of a married woman, or the father of a child), the site of the primary growth, type of growth, whether microscopically confirmed, the anniversary date of registration, and the date of death.

Congenital malformation registration
Registrations are collected by district health authorities and forwarded to the OPCS. The data include the child's district of birth, date of birth, sex, birthweight, whether live or still born, whether single or multiple birth, mother's and father's occupation, mother's address and date of birth, number of previous live and still births, date of the mother's last menstrual period, and details of each congenital malformation. The form includes a form number, allocated locally, but no other personal identifiers.

Infectious diseases
Statutorily notifiable diseases are notified to the medical officer for environmental health. The data include the patient's name, address, age, sex, the disease and its date of onset, and further particulars required in cases of certain diseases. In addition, the Public Health Laboratory Service maintains a system of microbiological surveillance based on laboratory data from which weekly and quarterly reports are published.

Child health computer systems
These systems, now implemented to varying extents by many health authorities, contain a personal, cumulative record on each child. The Child Register includes details about births obtained from birth notifications. The modules on vaccination and immunisation, pre-school and school health include details of immunisation history, the results of certain screening procedures, of whether developmental checks have been undertaken, the results of hearing tests, and of other findings from school health examinations.

Handicap registers

Local authorities maintain registers of blind and partially sighted people and of people with certain other categories of handicap. The availability and type of handicap registers varies from place to place (e.g. Balarajan et al, 1982).

Sickness absence statistics

These are compiled nationally on the basis of claims by insured people for either sickness or injury benefit. The data include the diagnosis of illness as written on the medical certificate, date of birth, sex, marital status and the duration of the spell. Regulations on the certification of sickness absence have recently changed and statistics before and after the change will not be comparable.

General Household Survey

This is a national sample survey of the population, organised by the OPCS, which includes questions on a wide variety of subjects including health. Questions put to individuals cover, in very general terms, the prevalence of chronic sickness and, in defined periods preceding the interview, the occurrence of acute sickness, any consultations with general practitioners and any hospital outpatient attendances.

Other health service statistics

Other systems which contain information of clinical relevance include data on prescriptions processed by the Prescription Pricing Authority, data about dental treatment processed by the Dental Estimates Board, and statutory notifications of termination of pregnancy which are sent to the Chief Medical Officer at the DHSS. A wide range of other statistical returns are made to the DHSS on activity, manpower and costs in the health and personal social services. These have been listed in a recent publication by the DHSS (1983a).

USES OF HEALTH AND VITAL STATISTICS: A SUMMARY

The population base

Population statistics are derived from the decennial census. In intercensal years population estimates are calculated using data from the census adjusted for natural changes in the population (obtained from birth and death statistics), migration (obtained from the NHS Central Registry), and, in the case of estimates by age-group, adjusted for 'transfers' of people moving up to the next age-group (Benjamin, 1968). Population projections — projections into the future of the continuation of effects of existing trends in fertility, mortality and migration — are made in similar ways. Statistics on the size and composition of the population provide the population base-line for planning health services and for the calculation of population-based rates in epidemiology and in the study of health services' utilisation.

Community diagnosis

Information about the occurrence and distribution of disease is essential to measure the impact of disease on the population and to assess requirements for health care and the scope for prevention. Analysis of variation in disease frequency over time, in different places, and in different subgroups of the population provides guidelines for planning the direction of health services and contributes to the study of factors which may explain the distribution of disease.

Causes and risks

The use of routine health and vital statistics in the study of causes and risks of disease is, of course, well established. Some classic studies — such as those of daily numbers of deaths in relation to daily levels of atmospheric pollution, and the geographical mapping of cases of cholera in relation to water supplies — are discussed by McMahon & Pugh (1970), Lilienfeld & Lilienfeld (1980) and Alderson (1980). More recent studies, using routine statistics, of variation of disease frequency over time include those of trends in mortality from asthma (Inman & Adelstein, 1969) and heart disease (Marmot et al, 1981), registration of congenital malformations (Weatherall, 1982), seasonal variation in hospital admissions for asthma (Khot et al, 1983) and variation in coronary deaths by day of the week (Macfarlane & White, 1977). Geographical studies include those of coronary mortality rates and characteristics of water supplies (Crawford et al, 1971); and of cancer registration and mortality data in relation to environmental and dietary factors (Armstrong & Doll, 1975). Studies of disease in relation to personal characteristics, using routine data, customarily consider such factors as patients' age, sex, occupation, social class and marital status but, of course, any of the other variables collected routinely can be analysed. For example, MHE data have been used to study schizophrenics' season of birth (Hare et al, 1979) and HAA data have been used to study hospitalisation rates according to patients' place of birth (Cruickshank et al, 1980).

In addition to statistical analysis of the data base itself, routine medical information systems can be used (with appropriate consents) as diagnostic indexes to identify patients for person-based epidemiological studies in which further data are obtained from patients, their medical records, general practitioners or relatives; and for the follow-up of cohorts of patients. For example, in studies of contraceptive safety, mortality records, hospital diagnostic indexes, congenital malformation registrations and cancer registrations have all been used to initiate case-control studies (Inman & Vessey, 1968; Mann et al, 1975; Janerich et al, 1974; Adam et al, 1981); mortality records have been used to aid the follow-up of cohorts of women (Vessey et al, 1977); and the linkage of routine records has been used for record-based case-control and cohort studies (Goldacre et al, 1983). In epidemiological studies of leukaemia, mortality statistics have been analysed to study secular trends (Hewitt, 1955), mortality records have been used to identify individual cases of leukaemia for detailed study (Stewart et al, 1958), and data on cohorts of irradiated patients have been linked to cancer registration and mortality records (Modan et al, 1974).

Resource allocation, monitoring and planning

The formula for financial resource allocation in the NHS (DHSS, 1976) requires the use of population statistics, mortality statistics, HAA statistics on national utilisation rates and local cross-boundary flows (for inpatients in general hospitals) and MHE statistics (for psychiatric services).

In addition to the use of routine statistics in the RAWP formula, statistics on the local utilisation of services can be used for local negotiation about the distribution of resources and the provision of services. Consider, as an example, the data in Table

Table 13.1 Hip arthroplasty rates per 100 000 population, 1979–1982: (a) all operations undertaken in each district, and (b) operations on all residents of each district

	District					
	1	2	3	4	5	6
(a) Operations in district	63	38	31	4	57	135
(b) Operations on residents of district	48	59	49	29	54	58

Fom HAA in the Oxford Region.

13.1. The first line shows operation rates based on the number of patients treated in each district, irrespective of their place of residence. The second line shows operation rates based on the number of operations undertaken on residents of each district, irrespective of their district of treatment. The data raise a number of questions for local management. District 6, and to a lesser extent District 1, is a net importer of patients who undergo hip arthroplasty: are the orthopaedic services in these districts adequately provided with resources to undertake the imported workload? Relatively few such operations are undertaken in District 4: is access to hip replacement surgery adequate for its residents? Do the observed patterns of utilisation and cross-boundary care correspond with the policies established for the service and, if not, what remedial action might be taken?

Customary indicators to monitor the use of hospital services include admission rates, patients' duration of stay, throughput per bed and turnover intervals (Ashley, 1972; Heasman, 1964; Heasman & Carstairs, 1971; Yates, 1982). Other measures of medical care which have been studied using routine statistics include waiting times for hospital care (Buttery & Snaith, 1979; Duthie, 1981), duration of time spent in hospital prior to elective surgery (Heasman & Carstairs, 1971), variation in hospital admissions on different days of the week (Williams, 1979), trends in the use of obstetric procedures (Chalmers et al, 1976), and consultation rates according to patients' socioeconomic status (Collins & Klein, 1980). The use of routine statistics to monitor variation in the outcome of care is less often undertaken but examples include studies of hospital fatality rates (Ashley & Morris, 1967; Ashley et al, 1971) and of population-based variation in avoidable deaths (Charlton et al, 1983).

Planning decisions can be regarded as the resultant of historical precedent, the current distribution and use of services, negotiation between competing demands, and the assessment of need for services and of their effectiveness. Routine health and vital statistics can often contribute, in varying degrees, to these considerations. Nonetheless, the view is commonly expressed that data from routine information systems are used less for management purposes than one might expect. This criticism formed part of the background to the establishment of the joint NHS/DHSS Steering Group on Health Services Information.

THE STEERING GROUP ON HEALTH SERVICES INFORMATION

In 1979 the DHSS, responding to discontent expressed about information activities within the NHS, issued a consultative document on the Information Requirements of the Health Service (DHSS, 1979). Consultation was followed by the establishment of the Steering Group on Health Services Information chaired by Mrs E. Körner. The Steering Group's terms of reference included the tasks of reviewing existing health services information systems and agreeing principles and procedures to guide their future development. The Steering Group has made recommendations about information systems on hospital clinical activity, community health services, finance, manpower, paramedical services and transport services. At the time of writing, the extent to which the Steering Group's recommendations will be implemented is still under consideration. It seems unlikely, however, that the substantial task undertaken by the Group will be repeated in the near future and so its work on hospital clinical activity (DHSS, 1982a) and community health services (DHSS, 1983b) will be briefly reviewed.

The Steering Group's general approach was to make recommendations about 'minimum data sets' which should be collected throughout the NHS. It stressed that the recommended data sets represent only a minimum; and that many districts would require additional data to provide information relevant to local needs and circumstances. It stressed the importance of, and made recommendations about, the definition and classification of data items to ensure comparability of data between districts. Its working approach was that data should be relevant and timely; that the minimum data sets would represent a compromise between what was desirable, feasible and affordable to collect; and that, by identifying and recommending a minimum set of data, 'we imply that a district health authority and its officers who are not using such data are handicapped by being inadequately informed when fulfilling their responsibilities' (DHSS, 1982a).

Inpatients: the patient information system

The Steering Group's First Report (DHSS, 1982a) recommended that there should be a single integrated information system covering all hospital inpatients and, in particular, that the historical separation of systems covering the general specialties, psychiatry and maternity should not be continued. The data items recorded for all inpatients should include an 'identifier' (usually a district record number), the patient's date of birth, sex, marital status, address code, general practitioner code, category, date of admission, method of admission, source of admission, date of decision to admit (for elective admissions), management intention (day case or inpatient), consultant codes, ward codes, date of discharge, method of discharge, destination on discharge, diagnoses and operative procedures. One notable change to the present systems is the recommendation that, when patients are transferred between consultants or wards during a continuous inpatient spell, each episode of consultant care and each ward stay should be separately identified. Another major change is the recommendation to calculate district spells, i.e. the total continuous stay of a patient within a hospital or hospitals within a district, to reduce the problems associated with multiple counting of episodes when patients are transferred between hospitals within a district during the course of a single spell of care. Transfers of patients between districts during a continuous course of inpatient care will still be counted as two (or more) spells of care.

The report discussed a number of data items which were considered but not eventually recommended for the minimum data set: these included the patient's name, NHS number, occupation, social class, ethnic group, country of birth and religion.

Inpatients: mental illness and mental handicap

An internal DHSS review of mental health statistics has recommended that the DHSS should no longer maintain the MHE and suggested that the responsibility for collecting mental health statistics should be transferred to the NHS. The Steering Group's Report recommended that the NHS should collect information in the psychiatric specialties, in the same way as for other specialties, as part of the integrated patient information system. It commented on the use of statistics about 'first ever' admissions to psychiatric hospitals for epidemiological purposes and as indicators of workload in the psychiatric services. It recommended that information should continue to be collected on whether or not each psychiatric admission is a first ever admission for the patient in the care of the mental health specialties.

The report also recommended that an annual census should be carried out on all patients who have been in mental illness or mental handicap hospitals for a year or more. The census would include basic demographic, administrative and diagnostic information about each patient. It was also suggested that local health authorities should consider the use of measures of patients' social functioning as items in the minimum data set for the census.

Maternity

The report recommended that a minimum data set should be collected for all registrable births whether they take place in hospital or at home. The data items for the mother, and for each baby, should be the same as those for other patients in the patient information system (above) with a few items recorded as not applicable in the case of home deliveries. In addition, the birth notification would be used to obtain data items about the delivery. The data from the mother's record, the baby's record and the delivery/birth notification record would be brought together so that the whole would give information about the mother, delivery and offspring. Recommendations for data items collected by notification of each birth included the parity of the mother; the number of babies delivered and the baby's birth order at delivery; whether the baby was live- or still-born; birthweight; the use of resuscitation; the place of delivery, original intention for place of delivery and (when different from actual place of delivery) reasons for change, length of gestation, method of onset of labour, and method of delivery. In addition, it was recommended that parental occupation and the baby's NHS number should be obtained from the registration of each birth. The report also recommended a number of data items about the mother, the delivery and each baby as additional, local clinical options.

Outpatients, day care, and accident and emergency departments

The recommendations about these groups of patients were confined to the provision of counts of attendances in various categories (e.g. by department; first attenders and re-attendances). The minimum data set does not include data about the characteristics of patients (such as their age, sex, place of residence or diagnosis).

Community health services

The report on Community Health Services (DHSS, 1983b) distinguished between information about services to the community and information about patient care in the community. Recommendations on the former include the collection of statistics on the percentage of target populations covered by vaccination and immunisation programmes and reasons for non-completion of courses; the percentage of target populations covered by child health surveillance programmes and the number of children requiring follow-up action; the percentage of the target population covered by screening programmes, the percentage of test results which were positive on screening, and the percentage of positive results subsequently confirmed by diagnosis; and statistics about contact tracing, community antenatal and postnatal services, family planning services, school health services, and health education activities.

Recommendations about the care of patients in the community centred on statistics about the work of the community nursing services. The report noted that 'a review of general medical practice does not fall within our remit' (DHSS, 1983b).

Epidemiological data

The Steering Group also stated that 'in our work we have not directly considered information about the occurrence of disease or about the health needs of populations except in so far as these can be inferred from data about hospital episodes and certain community health programmes; nor have we made recommendations about data describing health status or the clinical and social outcomes of the use of health services' (DHSS, 1982a). The remit set for the Steering Group, with its orientation towards management information, has been criticised for being too narrow (McCarthy, 1983; Catford, 1983). The Faculty of Community Medicine (1983) has published a statement on strategic health information; and recently a joint working group of the Steering Group and the Faculty has been convened to report on the needs of community physicians for routine information. This group is expected to report later in 1984.

PERFORMANCE INDICATORS

In 1982 the Secretary of State for Social Services announced that the DHSS, in collaboration with the NHS, would develop Performance Indicators (PIs) to assess the delivery of health services (Hansard, 1982). The list of PIs (DHSS, 1982b; DHSS, 1983c) was compiled using currently available data from the NHS and, perhaps not surprisingly, the measures chosen are familiar ones. The activity indicators are aggregate measures of workload undertaken by acute specialties in each health authority. They include, for each specialty, the gross hospital admission rate per 1000 population served, average length of stay, throughput per bed, turnover interval, day cases expressed as a percentage of all hospital admissions, outpatient referral rates per 1000 population, and numbers of people on the waiting list per 1000 population. Districts are ranked on the basis of each indicator (DHSS, 1983c). The indicators do not take account of either demographic factors or diagnostic case-mix within specialties. The rates used in PIs are 'management rates' in that the numerators refer to all patients treated in each district, irrespective of where they live, and the denominators relate to residents of the district. Because patients may cross administrative boundaries for treatment, the rates do not necessarily accurately describe the uptake of services by residents of the district.

The finance indicators, which are used to rank individual hospitals within general categories, include average costs per case and costs per inpatient day, component costs per inpatient case and day, domestic and cleaning costs per unit of floor area, and laundry costs per 100 articles laundered. Manpower indicators include average staff costs per whole-time equivalent in the major staff groups, ratios of nursing staff per 1000 inpatient cases and per 1000 inpatient days, overtime as a percentage of total staff costs, part-time staff as a percentage of all staff, and various other ratios of one staff group to another. The list also includes PIs for ambulance services, such as costs per 1000 patients carried, and for estate management, such as maintenance expenditure and energy use per unit volume of building.

The current PIs are open to the criticisms that they lack an explicit conceptual framework of health care evaluation, it is generally uncertain whether high or low values are 'good' or 'bad', the PIs seem to be more concerned with measures of economy than of effectiveness or efficiency, and, in particular, they indicate little or nothing about the output and outcome of health services. These points have been discussed in detail by Klein (1982) who stressed that the NHS is distinguished by the complexity and heterogeneity of its activities; and by uncertainties about the relationships between its inputs and outputs. He suggested that 'performance evaluation can most usefully be seen as a process of argument' in which appropriately chosen indicators may contribute to the debate.

The progress report on PIs (DHSS, 1982b) recognised that 'no single indicator or combination of indicators could lead to a firm conclusion on whether the use of existing resources was efficient or inefficient, good or bad'. The aim was therefore to construct a 'sieve' which would focus attention on situations where detailed study of local circumstances would be worthwhile. It is interesting that similar points, about a similar range of indicators, were made many years ago by the Guillebaud Committee (1956).

Ease of interpretation of PIs is likely to depend considerably on the capability to analyse and present data at appropriate levels of detail. Lewis & Modle (1982) have written that the 'creation of indicators should start with extensive disaggregation by diagnostic condition and age-group, so that poorly correlated factors are not merged in to broad summarising statistics'. However, the provision of detail will itself present problems. The publication of even the current simple set of PIs illustrates a common dilemma in the presentation of statistics. The document (DHSS, 1983d) is simultaneously overwhelming in its sheer volume of data and yet, on any single topic, it often lacks sufficient detail to be illuminating. Nonetheless, if first-line PIs are to be used as 'sieves' to raise questions, second-line indicators must also be available to help answer the questions. Three main approaches are possible. The first is to take account of detail (e.g. case-mix) by using standardisation or other summarising methods in the calculation of aggregated PIs. The second would be to take a selective approach to the presentation of PIs by abstracting the most striking aspects of the data and relegating the detail to reference tables. The third approach would be to provide details of comparisons of second-line indicators (e.g. admission rates and lengths of stay by diagnosis and age-group) on suitable computer media which could be interrogated locally, selectively as required, to answer specific questions.

The development of appropriate indicators of health service performance, including indicators of outcome, remains an important challenge for community physicians.

SOME ORGANISATIONAL PRINCIPLES IN THE MANAGEMENT OF INFORMATION SERVICES

Information systems in the NHS have been criticised for being inaccurate and untimely (DHSS, 1979) and for a paucity of information amongst an abundance of data (Barr, 1977). Similar criticisms have been made of medical information systems abroad (Loup & Thompson, 1982) and of administrative information systems in business (McCosh, Rahman & Earl, 1981). This suggests, rather generally, that the attention given to data collection is not necessarily accompanied by close attention to organisational aspects of information systems. Probably the greatest single failing of information systems in the NHS at the local level is that inadequate consideration is given to the resources required to exploit their data. The functions which need resources are set out as the paragraph headings, below, and managers of information systems need to review periodically whether each function is adequately supported.

Setting objectives and planning programmes of work

Whether data are collected and processed locally, or obtained from elsewhere (e.g. the OPCS) for local use, it goes almost without saying that clear and realistic objectives should be set for the provision of local information from each data system. This implies that individuals are identified in the management of the information service who have the responsibility, resources and expertise to develop objectives and to plan programmes of work.

Statements of general intent — to monitor the efficiency of the health service, to aid planning, to aid research — are insufficient. They should be supported by detailed considerations of how the data will be used to meet these ends, by whom, which specific areas of knowledge might be advanced by the use of each system, and which kinds of decisions might be influenced by the information from the system. Consideration of who will use the system, with attention given to whether they have the resources to do so, may avert the introduction of 'orphan systems' in search of customers.

There are problems in setting objectives for information systems which need to be acknowledged. Firstly, one of the purposes of a routine monitoring system may be to alert the organisation to unusual or unexpected events and thus, virtually by definition, it is impossible to specify precisely in advance what these may be. Secondly, medical interests, management interests, patterns of illness and of service use change such that it is difficult to predict which problems may arise in the future for which the availability of past data might be valuable. Nonetheless, the *approach* to meeting objectives can be specified. For example, if an objective of an information system is to monitor geographical variation in the use of medical services, one can specify how the data will be analysed and by whom, how it will be presented and to whom, what problems of interpretation might be encountered and how these might be resolved, and what action might be indicated if variation is found. As a general principle, information systems should be supported by a planned programme of analysis to exploit their data within foreseeable time-scales, coupled with an element of foresight, and the extent to which objectives have been met should be periodically assessed.

Collection, preparation and input of data

Closest attention tends generally to be given to the resources required for the collection, preparation and computer input of data. It is usually readily apparent if resources are inadequate for these purposes. An important consideration, which may not be so apparent, is that staff time is required to maintain liaison with data collectors and with professionals, such as clinicians, on whose records the data are based in order to sustain awareness of the systems and motivation for providing accurate, timely information.

Monitoring standards of data collection

Attention is less commonly given to monitoring the collection of data in terms of their completeness, accuracy and timeliness. For the purpose of this discussion, HAA is used as an example; completeness is defined as the extent to which all eligible records, and all data items on each record, are captured by the system; accuracy is the extent to which data have been correctly recorded in the system; and timeliness is the extent to which data are available from the system on the time-scales required. There is often a trade-off between completeness and timeliness. For example, Table 13.2 shows that,

Table 13.2   Availability of HAA data for 1982 by dates of file status monitor in 1983: (a) completeness of records containing administrative data (by comparison with the SH3 returns), and (b) completeness of clinical details on received HAA records

Date of file status report	(a) HAA as % of SH3 District		(b) % of HAA with clinical details District	
	1	2	1	2
1.2.83	99.1	93.6	93.1	86.7
21.3.83	99.6	96.0	98.3	87.7
20.5.83	99.9	96.7	98.4	94.8

From HAA file status monitor, Oxford Region.

in the first part of 1983, the user wanting data from HAA for 1982 would have to choose between using data in the early months which were incomplete (to a variable extent, depending on the district) or waiting until later in the year for more complete data. There is a trade-off between completeness, accuracy and timeliness, on the one hand, and costs on the other. Most issues in the quality control of data are not conceptually problematic: the provision, training and supervision of staff can be increased, the abstraction and coding of records can be checked, key-punching can be verified, and edit checks and corrections can be made, if resources are available for these purposes. There are also important relationships between completeness, accuracy and timeliness, on the one hand, and the use of data on the other. The less complete, accurate and timely that data are, the less they will be used; the less they are used, the lower the priority is likely to be that data will be submitted completely, accurately and promptly in the future.

A finite level of omission and error is inevitable in the collection of large volumes of data. The important issue is therefore not whether data are wholly accurate but whether they are sufficiently accurate for their purposes. The level of acceptable accuracy will vary according to particular purposes. Consider, as an example, an HAA system which consistently allocates patients' addresses to the wrong town but right district, patients' diagnoses to the wrong diagnostic code of the International Classification of Diseases (ICD) but right ICD chapter, and patients' care to the wrong consultant but right specialty. None of these errors would have any practical effect on the way that the data are currently used in the RAWP formula. Some or all of the errors may matter in local planning. The data would be valueless to the individual clinician or the epidemiologist.

Albeit that standards for data are somewhat arbitrary, consideration should be given to setting them. They will represent a compromise between what is desirable and what is achievable. For example, current standards for HAA in Oxford are that (i) HAA records should be available for 99.5% of all discharges, (ii) all HAA records should include the patient's date of birth, sex, place of residence and a range of other specified items, and (iii) a diagnosis should be available on 98%, and the patient's occupation on 90%, of all records. The completeness of data on files from each district are monitored by regular file-status reports. When standards are met they can, of course, be raised for the future.

Key-punch verification by duplicate punching may be done and edit checks may be used whereby computer programs identify format, range and logical errors in the data. The accuracy of data in a system can, of course, also be quantified by sampling its records and checking back to source documents. Such sampling may be done either as a continuous monitor or as periodic surveys. The obvious benefit of checking records is that it enables the level of error in the system to be quantified. Limitations are that it adds to the cost of a system; and that unless each error is investigated individually, or unless the sample size is very large, it may not be possible to distinguish between systematic errors (e.g. the hospital which consistently codes one diagnosis wrongly) and random errors. With few exceptions (Goldacre, 1981), a low level of random error does not usually matter much in the analysis of statistics. Systematic errors may matter and there is no alternative but to attempt to identify and reduce them. One way of reducing errors is to ensure that data collection and coding staff are adequately trained for their tasks; another is to encourage the analysis and use of data, and to request feedback on suspected errors identified by use of the system.

Random checks are not commonly made as a routine. For example, in mid-1982 I sought information from all English regions on whether HAA records were sampled and assessed for accuracy by checking back to source documents. One region did this routinely for all HAA records which included a diagnosis of cancer. Otherwise, no region did routine sample checks.

A number of ad hoc studies have been published on the accuracy of medical information systems (e.g. Heasman & Lipworth, 1966; Martini et al, 1976; West, 1976).

Analysis and distribution of statistics
General strategies which may be considered for analysis are as follows and, if adopted, the resources required for each type of output must be assessed.

i. Routine tables
It is usual to produce certain suites of tables, considered to be required by a wide range of customers on a regular basis, as a routine. For example, central government departments publish routine tables from most of the main national systems on an

annual basis (e.g. OPCS, 1982, 1983a–e) or at other regular intervals (OPCS, 1978). Local managers of information services need to decide, both for locally managed systems and for locally relevant data from national systems, whether to produce and distribute routine tables of statistics. Decisions are needed on the content of such tables, the customers to whom they will be distributed, and whether they will be produced with or without textual commentary. It is usual in the production of routine tables to maintain similar content over a number of years so that series of comparable data can be built up over a period of time.

ii. Reference tables
Suites of reference tables may be produced, containing more detailed analyses than routine tables, for in-house use. The distinction between routine and reference tables is obviously arbitrary but, as an example, we produce a number of routine tables from HAA for grouped diagnoses on such measures as admission rates, lengths of stay and cross-boundary care. We also produce, for reference, much more detailed tables which give similar statistics for each diagnosis separately at the three-digit level of the ICD. The first purpose of reference tables is to provide ready access to information to answer questions on points of detail without burdening potential users by routine distribution of volumes of additional data which may be of no interest to them. (The need for reference tables for this purpose depends to some extent on the ease with which ad hoc analyses can be obtained, see below.) The second purpose of reference tables is to allow the information service itself to scan data across a wide range of topics, as a monitoring exercise, and to alert others to findings which may be worth pursuing. For example, such scanning alerted us to the fact that hospital admissions for whooping cough had risen in the late 1970s (Goldacre & Harris, 1981a) in close parallel with the debated rise in infectious-disease notifications for the condition.

iii. Ad hoc analysis
High priority should be given to the capability to respond to individual requests for data. The number, range and complexity of ad hoc requests is, of course, unpredictable but speed of response is one of the criteria by which information services can be judged. Types of request tend to show some consistency (e.g. numbers of cases, age distribution, geographical variation, seasonal variation) and it is often worth considering the production of generalised parameter-driven software or other 'user-friendly' packages which can readily be used to produce similar analyses on different topics as needs arise.

iv. In-house research
When an objective of an information system is to aid research, decisions must be made about whether there will be an in-house research programme or whether it will be wholly left to others to use the data to meet this objective.

v. Peripheral access
Consideration should be given to the provision of local access to data, either by terminal access or by physical transfer of data on magnetic media, for frequent users. For example, it may be appropriate for districts or hospitals which make frequent use of data to be able to analyse regional files directly. In these circumstances, procedures

have to be developed to protect data security and confidentiality (e.g. by the production of anonymised statistical subfiles) and to agree on transfers of responsibilities for the custodianship of data.

vi. Contribution to national and other data banks
A number of locally organised systems, such as HAA and cancer registries, contribute data to national data bases. Some cancer registries pool data for international comparisons (Waterhouse et al, 1982). Allowances need to be made for the resources required to contribute data in these ways.

Analysis by use of subfiles
The analysis of large sets of data can present practical difficulties. One expedient which we have increasingly used is to analyse data in two main steps by the construction of files of aggregated statistics (Goldacre & Harris, 1981b). The first step entails the extraction, sorting and totalling of data from the large data base into much smaller subfiles of aggregated statistics which are held on computer in the format of a 'raw data' file for further analysis. The statistics on this file can then be manipulated without the need either to return repeatedly to the main file or to invest clerical effort in further analyses. The data can be combined in different ways for different purposes; mathematical calculations can be undertaken on them; the data can be presented as tables in different formats, as required for particular purposes; and statistical subfiles of data in the same format for each new year can be added to produce tables over a period of years without needing to re-analyse the historical data on the main data files. Statistical subfiles on magnetic media can also be provided to local users for local analysis.

Interpretation and presentation
Resources may be required to advise users on the interpretation of data. The advantage of using routine information systems is that investigators do not need to invest time in collecting their own data; but they may need to be advised about the ground rules of the system, the way that variables are classified and coded, and other aspects of interpretation which may not be readily apparent to the occasional user (Goldacre, 1981).

Resources will be required to ensure that data are adequately presented. Busy potential users may have neither the time nor the inclination to work through large quantities of poorly presented data.

Evaluation
It is easier to suggest that health information systems should be evaluated than to suggest how this can best be done. One problem is that the contribution of routine systems to knowledge may not be easily quantified. For example, facts about international variation in the incidence of individual types of cancers, or about smoking-related diseases in Doll's cohort of doctors, pass into general medical knowledge without there necessarily being a general appreciation of the contribution of pooled data from cancer registries to the former and the flagging of death records through the NHS Central Registry in the latter (Waterhouse et al, 1982; Doll & Peto, 1976). Information from local statistical systems may pass second- and third-hand into

papers for management meetings, may contribute to 'an informal climate of opinion' (Williams, 1983) and may influence local decision-making, without general knowledge of its sources. Even when sources are well understood, the difficulty remains of quantifying the role of routine statistical data, considered alongside a variety of other factors, in contributing to decisions and policies. Despite these difficulties, managers of information systems should, at the least, maintain an inventory of the readily identifiable uses of the systems and a bibliography of any publications resulting from use of the systems.

Other considerations

Two other points deserve brief consideration. Firstly, enthusiasts for information systems may overestimate the extent to which customer departments have the resources to assimilate and use statistical information. The collection, analysis and distribution of routine health statistics should be tailored to customers' capacities to use them. Secondly, the role of each system should be considered alongside the overall intelligence activities of the organisation. Organisations require information for both operational and strategic purposes: no amount of operational information (e.g. on the costs or use of a service) will compensate for inadequate information about strategy (e.g. on the effectiveness of the service). Health authorities' requirements for intelligence include the use of information from routine statistics, from the published literature, and from ad hoc surveys. An important role for community physicians, as the principal advisors on medical information services, is to ensure that an appropriate blend of resources is available to meet the information requirements of the NHS.

REFERENCES

Adam S A, Sheaves J K, Wright N H, Mosser G, Harris R W, Vessey M P 1981 A case-control study of the possible association between oral contraceptives and malignant melanoma. British Journal of Cancer 44: 45–50
Alderson M 1974 Central Government Routine Health Statistics. In: Maunder W F (ed) Reviews of United Kingdom Statistical Sources, Volume II. Heinemann Educational Books, London
Alderson M 1980 An Introduction to Epidemiology. The Macmillan Press, London, chs 2, 3
Anderson H R 1978 The epidemiological value of hospital diagnostic data. In: Bennett A E (ed) Recent Advances in Community Medicine, Number One. Churchill Livingstone, Edinburgh
Armstrong B K, Doll R 1975 Environmental factors and cancer incidence and mortality in different countries, with special reference to dietary practice. International Journal of Cancer 15: 617–631
Ashley J S A 1972 Present state of statistics from hospital inpatient data and their uses. British Journal of Preventive and Social Medicine 26: 135–147
Ashley J S A, Morris J N 1967 Deaths from appendicitis and appendicectomy. Lancet i: 217
Ashley J S A, Howlett A, Morris J N 1971 Case-fatality of hyperplasia of the prostate in two teaching and three regional-board hospitals. Lancet ii: 1308–1311
Balarajan R, Weatherall J A C, Ashley J S A, Bewley B R 1982 A survey of handicap registers for pre-school children in England and Wales. Community Medicine 4: 315–324
Barr A 1977 Information for management and planning in the NHS. The Hospital and Health Services Review 73: 387–390
Benjamin B 1968 Health and Vital Statistics. George Allen and Unwin Ltd, London
Buttery R B, Snaith A H 1979 Waiting for surgery. British Medical Journal 2: 403–404
Campbell H 1978 Appendix on mortality. In: Bennett A E (ed) Recent Advances in Community Medicine, Number One. Op cit
Catford J C 1983 Positive health indicators — towards a new information base for health promotion. Community Medicine 5: 125–132
Chalmers I, Zlosnik J E, Johns K A, Campbell H 1976 Obstetric practice and outcome of pregnancy in Cardiff residents 1965–1973. British Medical Journal 1: 735–738

Charlton J R H, Hartley R M, Silver R, Holland W W 1983 Geographical variation in mortality from conditions amenable to medical intervention in England and Wales. Lancet i: 691–696

Collins E, Klein R 1980 Equity and the NHS: self-reported morbidity, access, and primary care. British Medical Journal 2: 1111–1115

Crawford M D, Gardner M J, Morris J N 1971 Cardiovascular disease and the mineral content of drinking water. British Medical Bulletin 27: 21–24

Cruickshank J K et al 1980 Heart attack, stroke, diabetes and hypertension in West Indians, Asians and whites in Birmingham, England. British Medical Journal 2: 1108

DHSS 1976 Sharing resources for health in England: report of the Resource Allocation Working Party. HMSO, London

DHSS 1979 Information Requirements of the Health Services. HN 79(21). DHSS, London

DHSS 1982a Steering Group on Health Services Information. First Report to the Secretary of State. HMSO, London

DHSS 1982b Performance Indicators in the NHS. RA (82)34. DHSS, London

DHSS 1983a A guide to health and social services statistics. DHSS, London

DHSS 1983b Steering Group on Health Services Information. A Report from Working Group D: Community Health Services. DHSS, London

DHSS 1983c Health Services Management: Performance Indicators. HN(83)25. DHSS, London

DHSS 1983d Performance Indicators. National Summary for 1981. DHSS, London

Doll R, Peto R 1976 Mortality in relation to smoking: 20 years' observations on male British doctors. British Medical Journal 2: 1525–1536

Donnan S 1982 Cancer registration — advance or retreat? In: Smith A (ed) Recent Advances in Community Medicine, Number Two. Churchill Livingstone, Edinburgh

Duthie R B (chairman) 1981 Orthopaedic Services: waiting time for outpatient appointments and inpatient treatment. HMSO, London, ch 5

Faculty of Community Medicine 1983 Strategic Information Systems. Faculty of Community Medicine, London

Galbraith N S Communicable disease surveillance. In: Smith A (ed) Recent Advances in Community Medicine, Number Two. Op cit

Goldacre M J 1981 Hospital inpatient statistics: some aspects of interpretation. Community Medicine 3: 60–68

Goldacre M J, Harris R I 1981a Hospital admissions for whooping cough in the Oxford Region, 1974–1979. British Medical Journal 1: 106–107

Goldacre M J, Harris R I 1981b Use of 'interim results' files to facilitate analysis of large data sets: with reference to Hospital Activity Analysis. Community Medicine 3: 140–143

Goldacre M J, Holford T R, Vessey M P 1983 Cardiovascular disease and vasectomy: findings from two epidemiologic studies. New England Journal of Medicine 308: 805–808

Guillebaud C W (chairman) 1956 Report of the committee of enquiry into the cost of the National Health Service. Cmnd 9663. HMSO, London

Hare E H, Bulusu L, Adelstein A 1979 Schizophrenia and season of birth. Population Trends 17: 9–11

Hansard 1982 Volume 16, January 22, cols 211–212

Heasman M A 1964 How long in hospital? Lancet ii: 539–541

Heasman M A, Carstairs V 1971 Inpatient management: variations in some aspects of practice in Scotland. British Medical Journal 1: 495–498

Heasman M A, Lipworth L 1966 Accuracy of certification of cause of death. Studies on Medical and Population Subjects No 20. HMSO, London

Hewitt D 1955 Some features of leukaemia mortality. British Journal of Preventive and Social Medicine 9: 81–88

Inman W H W, Adelstein A M 1969 Rise and fall of asthma mortality in England and Wales in relation to use of pressurised aerosols. Lancet ii: 279–285

Inman W H W, Vessey M P 1968 Investigation of deaths from pulmonary, coronary and cerebral thrombosis and embolism in women of child-bearing age. British Medical Journal 2: 193–199

Janerich D T, Piper J M, Glebatis D M 1974 Oral contraceptives and congenital limb-reduction defects. New England Journal of Medicine 291: 697–700

Khot A, Evans N, Lenney W 1983 Seasonal trends in childhood asthma in south east England. British Medical Journal 2: 1257–1258

Klein R 1982 Performance, evaluation and the NHS: a case study in conceptual perplexity and organisational complexity. Public Administration 60: 385–407

Lewis A F 1981 Linking birthweight and birth registration data: a postscript. Community Medicine 3: 38–39

Lewis A F, Modle W J 1982 Health indicators: what are they? An approach to efficacy in health care. Health Trends 14: 3–8

Lilienfeld A M, Lilienfeld D E 1980 Foundations of Epidemiology, 2nd edn. Oxford University Press, New York, chs 5–7

Loup R J, Thompson B J 1982 Control of quality in a medical record information system. WHO/HS/Nat.Com/82.374. World Health Organisation, Geneva

McCarthy M 1983 Epidemiology: a losing cause? British Medical Journal 1: 1682–1683

McCosh A M, Rahman M, Earl M J 1981 Developing Managerial Information Systems. The Macmillan Press, London, chs 1–3

Macfarlane A, White G 1977 Heart attack deaths: the weekly cycle. Population Trends 7: 7–8

MacMahon B, Pugh T F 1970 Epidemiology: Principles and Methods. Little, Brown and Company, Boston

Mann J I, Vessey M P, Thorogood M, Doll R 1975 Myocardial infarction in young women with special reference to oral contraceptive practice. British Medical Journal 2: 241–245

Marmot M G, Booth M, Beral V 1981 Changes in heart disease mortality in England and Wales and other countries. Health Trends 13: 33–38

Martini C J M, Hughes A O, Patton V A 1976 A study of the validity of the Hospital Activity Analysis information. British Journal of Preventive and Social Medicine 30: 180–186

Modan B, Baidatz D, Mart H, Steinitz R, Levin S G 1974 Radiation-induced head and neck tumours. Lancet i: 277–279

Office of Population Censuses and Surveys 1978 Occupational mortality: decennial supplement 1970–1972. HMSO, London

Office of Population Censuses and Surveys 1982 General Household Survey 1980. HMSO, London

Office of Population Censuses and Surveys 1983a Mortality Statistics 1982. HMSO, London

Office of Population Censuses and Surveys 1983b Hospital In-patient Enquiry: main tables 1980. HMSO, London

Office of Population Censuses and Surveys 1983c Communicable disease statistics 1982. HMSO, London

Office of Population Censuses and Surveys 1983d Cancer statistics 1980. HMSO, London

Office of Population Censuses and Surveys 1983e Congenital malformation statistics 1971– 1980. HMSO, London

Royal College of General Practitioners and Office of Population Censuses and Surveys 1979 Morbidity statistics from general practice 1971–1972. Second national study. HMSO, London

Stewart A, Webb J, Hewitt D 1958 A survey of childhood malignancies. British Medical Journal 1: 1495–1508

Vessey M P, McPherson K, Johnson B 1977 Mortality among women participating in the Oxford/Family Planning Association Contraceptive Study. Lancet ii: 731–733

Waterhouse J, Muir C, Shanmugaratnam K, Powell J (eds) 1982 Cancer Incidence in Five Continents, Volume IV. IARC Scientific Publications No. 42. International Agency for Research on Cancer, Lyon

Weatherall J A C 1978 Congenital malformations: surveillance and reporting. Population Trends 11: 27–29

Weatherall J A C 1982 A review of some effects of recent medical practices in reducing the number of children born with congenital abnormalities. Health Trends 14: 85–88

West R R 1976 Accuracy of cancer registration. British Journal of Preventive and Social Medicine 30: 187–192

Williams A 1983 The practice of health services research. Community Medicine 4: 317–320

Williams B T 1979 Admission to hospital and the day of the week. Public Health, London 93: 173–176

Yates J 1982 Hospital Beds. A problem for diagnosis and management? William Heinemann Medical Books, London

14. Screening for cervical cancer: an opportunity for change

Patricia Hobbs   Andrea Knopf Elkind   Dave Haran
Anne Eardley   Brenda Spencer   Laura L. Pendleton
Diana K. Chisholm

The effects of cytological screening in the United Kingdom have so far been disappointing. The opportunity has now arisen to reconsider the basis of the provision of screening services and to examine ways in which it might be improved. The closing of the NHS Central Registry at Southport and the transfer of responsibility for recall for screening to the District Health Authorities has coincided with the DHSS proposals for the computerisation of Family Practitioner Committee records. This combination of circumstances allows for the development of a system of call as well as recall for screening. However, before launching new schemes an examination of the reasons for the failure of the existing system is necessary if past mistakes are not to be perpetuated.

The experience of several countries (Hakama, 1982) suggests that very substantial reductions in both incidence and mortality are possible following well-organised programmes of screening. This has not been the case in the United Kingdom, despite a similar investment per unit population [2.9 million cervical smears per annum (Roberts, 1982)] during the two decades in which it has been available.

In this chapter we examine the reasons underlying this failure, put forward some principles for the development of a more effective screening service, and describe a system incorporating such principles.

PART 1: THE PROBLEM

A mismatch between policy and practice

The incidence of cervical cancer increases with age and reaches a peak among women aged 55–64 (Office of Population Censuses and Surveys, 1983a). Although considerable attention has been paid recently to the growing incidence of both positive smears and mortality amongst younger women (Draper & Cook, 1983; Wolfendale et al, 1983), it remains the case that, in terms of numbers, it is older women who are most vulnerable to developing the disease (Burslem, 1983). Women from social classes IV and V are at greater risk than those in other groups (Hakama et al, 1982; Wakefield et al, 1973; Grünfeld et al, 1975; Robinson, 1982). Other high-risk groups include women with an early age of first sexual intercourse and first parity, and women with a history of multiple sexual partners (Hulka, 1982), divorced women, and those who were widowed when young (Leck et al, 1978; Sibary et al, 1978). Underlying these factors is the undisputed link between cervical cancer and sexual behaviour. However, the causes of the disease are far from being fully understood (see, for example, Robinson, 1982 for a comprehensive discussion of the evidence about possible carcinogens).

The official screening policy of the last few years (Draper, 1982) corresponds closely with the epidemiological evidence, in that it seeks to include all sexually active women, with particular emphasis on those aged 35 or more. However, it is clear that the service as actually operated in the UK has failed to achieve the results which the number of tests undertaken might lead us to expect. Every year, in England and Wales, approximately 4000 new cases of cervical cancer are diagnosed and over 2000 women die of this disease (Office of Population Censuses and Surveys, 1983b). Further, there has been no marked decline in the mortality from cervical cancer and, in fact, recent authors have documented a marked increase in mortality among younger women (Draper & Cook, 1983; Wolfendale et al, 1983). These authors have raised the possibility that the screening programme has been successful in that it may have prevented an actual increase in mortality, and contained an even greater rise among younger women. Nevertheless, the fact remains that a majority of women with invasive carcinoma of the cervix had not previously been screened (Spriggs & Boddington, 1976). Knox (1976) has shown by computer modelling that the number of examinations presently carried out, if deployed as prescribed by official policy, would be expected to reduce mortality from cervical cancer to something like a quarter of its present level.

An examination of the characteristics of women who have undergone screening points to the simple conclusion that the wrong women have been screened. British studies indicate that the at-risk groups have been inadequately represented in the population of screened women. Studies carried out in the decade or so following the inception of screening noted a marked under-representation of women from social classes IV and V (Wakefield & Sansom, 1966; Sansom et al, 1970; Sansom et al, 1971a). More recent studies, however, suggest that this trend may have become less marked (Andrews & Davies, 1980; Parkin et al, 1981). Under-representation of widows and divorcees has been noted (Sansom et al, 1971a; Sibary et al, 1977; Parkin et al, 1981), but perhaps the most frequently reported factor associated with low response is age. A majority of smears are taken from younger women (under 35 years of age) (Wakefield & Sansom, 1966; Sansom et al, 1970; Brindle & Wakefield, 1976; Brindle et al, 1976; Parkin et al, 1981), whereas those most at risk of developing cervical cancer are women aged over 35 (Office of Population Censuses and Surveys, 1983b).

Pathways to screening
Having indicated the existence of a mis-match between those at risk of cervical cancer and those covered by the existing screening programme, we now seek explanations for this state of affairs. We begin with an examination of the means by which women currently enter the screening programme.

The first and most important aspect of cervical screening in the United Kingdom is that there is no system for routinely inviting women to have a test. Responsibility for the organisation of screening programmes lies at the local level, and the way provision has been organised has varied widely. Given these local variations, however, several general points can be made. There are three possible pathways by which a woman may enter the screening system: having the test as part of another procedure, by the woman herself requesting a test, or as a result of an invitation.

Many women have a cervical smear test as a routine part of another procedure (i.e., essentially by chance), for example, ante-natally, post-natally or when seeking family planning advice. Because of the likely age of such women, it is not surprising that younger women tend to predominate in the screened population. Wakefield (1976) found that only 28% of women under 35 had had a test by choice (i.e., as a screening procedure for reasons unconnected with pregnancy or contraception), compared with 49% of older women. Conversely, Sansom et al (1971b) found that most of the women who had themselves requested a test were aged 35 and above. Clearly, then, the older the woman the more likely it is that she will have to take the initiative herself to obtain a screening test, either from her own family doctor or at a District Health Authority clinic.

Family doctors may themselves offer screening to their patients, either on an individual basis, by offering special sessions, or by sending out invitations. However, the likelihood of a woman receiving an invitation to be screened will depend on factors outside her control, namely, on the willingness of her family doctor to offer such a service. That there is marked variation between practices in the amount of cervical screening undertaken has been well documented (Wakefield, 1972; Evans & Semmence, 1975). Of particular interest is the fact that this variation does not appear to be random, but related to the perceived social characteristics of patients. Wakefield (1972) found that family doctors who judged their practices to be serving mainly the lower socio-economic groups or mixed working class and middle-class patients were less likely to be taking smears than those with an exclusively middle-class clientele.

Women may also be invited to attend screening organised either at their place of work—the so-called industrial clinic—or at a mobile unit visiting their locality. Again, factors outside the control of the woman herself will determine whether or not such a service is available to her.

Explaining the mis-match: two hypotheses

The problem of under-representation of at-risk women in the screening programme has frequently been defined in terms of the failure of women 'to avail themselves of this facility' (Adelstein et al, 1981). In other words, the blame has been placed squarely on the women who do not attend rather than on any attributes of the screening system itself. Thus an editorial in the *British Medical Journal* (1980) states that 'unfortunately the value of screening programmes is limited by the fact that those women most at risk of developing cervical cancer are the *least likely to come forward*';* and in a discussion of cervical screening in general practice, Jackson (1979) writes 'it is particularly unfortunate that older, poorer women are often the ones that are *least likely to come forward** for cytological tests'. Chamberlain (1983) asserts that 'it has repeatedly been shown that older women are *less interested in preventive medicine*'* and that 'there is a pronounced social class trend (in incidence) with cervical cancer being commoner in unskilled, less educated classes who are also *less easy to convince of the value of preventive measures.*'* The definition of the problems of the cervical screening programme in these terms has now been taken up and further distorted by the mass media; thus a journalist writing in *The Guardian* newspaper (Veitch, 1983) states that 'women most at risk of the disease . . . *simply did not turn up for their appointments.*'*

It may be suggested that the underlying assumption of this 'failure to attend'

---

* Our italics.

hypothesis is that it is the attributes of the woman herself that determine whether or not she attends for screening. Such a view, however, is too narrow and fails to take into account the attributes of the service that is being offered. We will suggest as an alternative hypothesis that the screening system has not only failed to take the initiative in routinely inviting women to be screened, but that it has also failed to meet the needs of the very women it must attract in order to have a substantial impact on mortality. The underlying assumption of a provider-initiated, user-oriented system that such a hypothesis suggests is that the attributes of the service as well as the women must be taken into account. Let us examine the available evidence for these competing hypotheses.

Evidence about response from records
One source is demographic data from records of women who have attended for screening. As we have already noted, such records suggest that older, working-class women and those with broken marriages are the least likely to attend for screening, but such differences do not, in themselves, explain a great deal. This has not prevented frequent speculations, of the type described above, as to the attitudes and values of the broad groupings revealed in analyses of this type, but as MacIntyre (1979) has pointed out, 'the problem with theories attributing social action to sub-culturally held values is that they often provide no evidence for the hypothesised values other than the observed behaviour they seek to explain.' Moreover, it has already been shown that older, working-class women are the least well-served by the system as it is presently organised, since they are most likely to be the women who must themselves take the initiative if they are to have a test.

The second important drawback to using attendance records to consider why women have not had a test is that they fail to distinguish between those women who have refused a specific invitation to be tested (hereafter termed 'refusers') and those who have not had a test simply by default, i.e. they have never made a conscious decision *not* to have a test because the question has never been posed to them (hereafter termed 'non-attenders'). In other words, given the current organisation of screening facilities in the UK, with no system for routinely inviting women for a smear, it is unjustifiable to make the assumption that women who have not had a smear would not be willing to have one, given the right circumstances.

Evidence about response from invitation studies
Several studies have considered what occurs when women are specifically invited for a test, and provide the opportunity to examine the real differences between acceptors and refusers of such invitations. They give us a better indication of the willingness of women to take part in screening than data derived from records. In Table 14.1 they are divided into two categories: studies of women who have been invited to have a test who have never had a test before or whose screening history is unknown (initial invitation studies) and studies of women recalled for a repeat test some years after a previous test (recall studies).

What do the response rates obtained by such studies tell us? First, they show that in the right circumstances a high proportion of women are willing to have a smear test when invited, i.e. when the system is provider-initiated in character. As long ago as 1969, Saunders & Snaith concluded that 'about seven women out of ten under the

Table 14.1 Response to an invitation to attend for cervical screening

Type of study	Author	Year	Venue	Response (%)
Initial invitation	Houghton	1968	GP	70
	Saunders & Snaith	1969	Choice: clinic or GP	72.5
	Thompson	1969	Industrial clinic	70–89; higher rate where supervisors involved in campaign
	Miller	1969	Industrial clinic	77
	Scaife	1972	GP	23–36 initially; 88 after visiting
	Semmence & Mellors	1975	GP	51
	Carruthers et al	1975	Choice: clinic or GP: Cytopipette for use at home	41 / 53
	Cardiff Cervical Cytology Study	1980	Local Authority Clinic	65
	Standen & Rivalland	1982	Industrial clinic	31–39
Recall	Allman et al	1974	Left to women to choose	41 crude response; 64 of those eligible initially; 85 of those eligible after contact by nurse
	Sansom et al	1975(b)	Left to woman to choose	48 crude response 72 of those eligible

age of 70 years can be persuaded to be examined if they are told individually and in simple language just what is being offered and are accorded an appointment at a service source of their own choice'. Although it is clear that some studies have achieved or bettered the response rates predicted by Saunders & Snaith, others have patently failed to reach anything approaching this level. What accounts for this wide variation in response?

There are three factors to be borne in mind when interpreting this evidence. Looking first at initial invitation studies, the responses are based on populations of varying size, ranging from women at particular places of work (Thompson, 1969; Miller, 1969; Standen & Rivalland, 1982), through family doctor practice lists (Houghton, 1968; Scaife, 1972; Semmence & Mellors, 1975), to the population of particular geographical areas (Evans et al, 1980; Saunders & Snaith, 1969; Carruthers et al, 1975).

A second factor to be considered is that the methods of invitation and the amount of effort made to persuade women who did not respond initially varied from one study to another. In fact, it is not possible to make a true comparison between studies, since none of the authors reproduce the material supplied to the invited women. The reader is not therefore able to assess the nature of the message conveyed or the quality of the information supplied about the test. However, enough detail about the method of invitation and amount of follow-up is given for it to be clear that there were marked differences. Thus, some studies report that one or more letters of invitation were sent (Houghton, 1968; Carruthers et al, 1975), others that 'non-responders' received a home visit (Scaife, 1972). In the study by Evans et al (1980) on the other hand, personal contact only was used, and the invitation offered by a field worker visiting every house in the area.

A further reason why response rates reported by both initial invitation studies and response to recall studies should be interpreted with caution, is that a number of factors may contribute to their appearing misleadingly low. Close scrutiny of the evidence reveals that not all those who failed to respond to their invitation ('non-responders') were necessarily 'refusers'. These studies suggest that invitations do not always reach their intended recipients because they had moved house (Houghton, 1968; Allman et al, 1974; Sansom et al, 1975a). Interestingly, Sansom et al (1975a) suggest that women from the lower social classes are likely to be over-represented amongst those who did not receive an invitation for recall, since a common reason for change of address was re-housing as a result of slum clearance. Furthermore, there may be medical grounds for non-response; for example, some women may have had a hysterectomy; others may have already had a smear test in the interim period (Houghton, 1968; Allman et al, 1974; Sansom et al, 1975a; Sansom et al, 1975b). Some non-responders may even have died (Sansom et al, 1975a).

The experience of recall studies is of interest in this regard. Although these studies (Allman et al, 1974; Sansom et al, 1975a, b) suggest on first sight that response to recall is poor, when women ineligible through removal out of the area or on medical grounds are excluded from the study population, it becomes clear that a high response to recall is actually obtained. Furthermore, these studies suggest that once women are in the screening system in the sense that they have already had a smear, the differential effects of age and social class are much less marked or do not operate at all.

As far as true refusers are concerned, the evidence suggests that for a proportion a variety of social factors may be operating, for example, working women may find it more difficult to attend (Sansom et al, 1975b), as may women with heavy family commitments (Houghton, 1968; Allman et al, 1974). Transport and accessibility may also pose problems (Houghton, 1968; Carruthers et al, 1975). Such refusers are not necessarily unwilling to have a test but may be unable to do so, given their circumstances.

Taken singly such 'excuses' as family commitments, lack of time, problems with transport and so on seem trivial in the extreme. Cumulatively their impact may be considerable, in that those women who have been identified as 'poor' responders— the elderly, the divorced and widowed, and those from lower socio-economic groups—are probably more likely than others to face such practical obstacles. Any method of organising a screening service which seeks to attract such women must take their needs for accessibility and convenience into account. Thus, not only must a service be provider-initiated, it must also be user-oriented.

Evidence about the needs of women
The concept of provider-initiation, user-orientation may be developed further by considering the knowledge and attitudes of women towards the smear test. The available evidence comes both from invitation studies and public opinion surveys. Such data have, in the past, been interpreted in relation to the 'failure to attend' hypothesis as providing the basis for an understanding of the attributes of women who do not 'avail themselves' of the service that is provided. However, we argue that such data may also be interpreted in relation to the 'failure of the screening system' hypothesis, namely, that such attributes inform us of the needs of women that must be met if the screening programme is to succeed.

What then, do we know about these needs? It is our contention that the 'failure to attend' hypothesis has seriously under-estimated the pre-requisites of regular screening behaviour. Not only must a woman know of the test's existence, she must also have some positive concept of its function and a belief both in its efficacy and its relevance to her. She must find the prospect of both the experience of the test itself and its implications acceptable. Finally, she must know where to obtain a test, and the venue and its system of organisation must be acceptable to her. The absence of any of these pre-requisites will constitute a deterrent to participation. Our analysis bears certain similarities to the Health Belief Model (1974). However, by taking the implications of this evidence a stage further than is usually the case, it is possible to recognise that the onus for change lies with the system rather than the user.

What barriers exist to participation in screening? With regard to knowledge of the test, public opinion surveys in the early 1970s suggested that about one in five women had never heard of the cervical smear test (Williams et al, 1972; Davison & Clements, 1971), although the position may have improved somewhat since then (Bluck, 1975). Women in social classes IV and V are the least likely to have heard of the test (Williams et al, 1972), and older women in an inner city area were less likely than their younger counterparts to have adequate information (Davison & Clements, 1971).

Turning to knowledge of the test's function, several studies suggest that some women either do not know what the test is for or, more frequently, believe its function is the detection of cancer rather than its prevention (Davison & Clements, 1971; Bluck, 1975; Knopf, 1976). Bluck (1975) suggests that this distinction—essentially one that reflects a difference between the lay and medical conceptions of the test—is not important, provided women know of its existence. However, the belief that the intention is to detect an existing cancer rather than prevent its development may be detrimental. For example, Davison & Clements (1971) point out that 'an emphasis on this as a test for cancer in national propaganda may have been self-defeating in view of the strongly expressed reluctance of many women to face the prospect of discovering in themselves a disease which large sections of the population still regard with revulsion and dread'. Thus it must always be borne in mind that women are being expected to participate in what is for them an anxiety-provoking exercise. There is some suggestion also that the common practice of not routinely informing women of the outcome of a test when the result is negative militates against their willingness to respond to invitations for recall (Wakefield, 1972).

Women will respond favourably to an invitation only if they believe the test to be effective as a means of preventing cancer, and furthermore that they are themselves susceptible to the disease. Houghton (1968) found refusers were less likely to be in favour of regular check-ups, were less likely to think that cervical cancer can usually be cured and tended to rate cervical cancer as more serious than did the tested group. Similarly, Carruthers et al (1975) found that a smaller proportion of untested than tested women would want to know if they had a disease before they experienced any symptoms and were also less likely to think that cancer could be cured. King (1983) noted a belief among women who had experienced the menopause that they were no longer at risk of any disease of the reproductive organs. Misconceptions about the meaning of the menopause and symptoms connected with it are also reported in other studies (Clements & Wakefield, 1971; Knopf, 1974).

Inherent in the test itself are features that may deter women from undergoing the procedure. It is seen as embarrassing, unpleasant or painful (Davison & Clements, 1971; Knopf, 1974; King, 1982). Moreover, these beliefs are often based on experience. Sansom et al (1975b) found that women who failed to respond to recall were more likely to have found the original test unpleasant or embarrassing, suggesting that women contemplating a test are influenced by their own or by other people's previous experiences of it or of gynaecological examinations in general (see, for example, *SHE* magazine (1983) for one woman's account of her experiences).

Publicity surrounding the test frequently emphasises the role of sexual behaviour, and particularly promiscuity, in the aetiology of the disease. For example, an article appeared in the *Sunday People* (1983) which reported the findings of Wolfendale et al (1983) regarding the increased incidence in abnormal cervical smears among younger women in Milton Keynes. Although the article correctly reported that the increase was in cell abnormalities rather than in cancer, the headline reads 'Cancer Shock for the New Town Lovers', and opened with the statement that 'A new town's free-loving young women have been given a shock cancer warning'. The relative incidence of the disease in nuns and prostitutes is reported with tedious repetition in both the general and academic press. The damaging effects of such publicity are hard to estimate, but the linking of cancer and promiscuity is likely both to reiterate in the public's mind the image of cancer as retribution, and to associate the stigma of sexually transmitted disease with a positive finding from the test (King, 1982; Charlton, 1983).

If a woman is not offered a smear routinely the onus is on her to find out where she can obtain the test, and many women do not possess this knowledge. This appears to be especially true of older women (Davison & Clements, 1971). For those with some knowledge an obvious first port of call is the family doctor, but not all family doctors do cervical screening. Furthermore, there is some indication that not all women are happy to have the test carried out by their doctor. Saunders & Snaith (1969) found that a majority of women preferred to have the test done at a local authority clinic by a woman doctor. Sansom et al (1971a) noted that local authority clinics were more successful than family doctors in attracting older women; and in a later study found these clinics were favoured over other agencies by women who had asked for the test themselves (Sansom et al, 1975b). Most recently, in a study of women's preferences in cervical screening, Cullum & Savory (1983) found that a substantial minority of women said they would prefer a midwife to do the test rather than their family doctor. These findings suggest that some refusers of family doctor invitations to attend for screening might more properly be described as women who would prefer to have the test carried out by someone other than their own doctor. It may be speculated that this is related to embarrassment about having a male doctor perform the test. If women are unaware of other venues, do not know where to find them, or do not know that health authority clinics are frequently staffed by women doctors, these can pose important barriers to obtaining a cervical screening test.

Even when the woman has accurate knowledge about the purpose of the test and is convinced of its worth and knows where to obtain it, she must have the time and the means to get to the surgery or clinic and she must make arrangements for an appointment. A long delay between the woman taking the initiative and making an appointment and the appointment itself leads to considerable dropout (Wakefield, 1972). We have already noted that women with practical difficulties to overcome, such as illness in the family (Houghton, 1968), going out to work (Sansom et al, 1975b) or living in a rural area (Carruthers et al, 1975), are less likely to accept an invitation to be tested.

Meeting the needs of women

These then are the barriers to participation. What evidence is there to suggest that the system itself may be instrumental in removing these barriers by acting positively to meet women's needs? If we accept that many of those most in need of cervical cytology are currently having to surmount more barriers than those in less need of the service, the way forward would appear to lie in the direction of considerably greater initiatives on the part of the service provider.

It is clear that the single most important initiative that can be taken is that women aged 20 and over should be personally invited to attend for screening. Since it is estimated that nearly 80% of women under that age are currently being screened (Adelstein et al, 1981), it is essential that efforts are now concentrated on older women, whose risk of contracting cervical cancer is considerably greater. The evidence of the invitation studies summarised in Table 14.1 is that it is possible to attract a high percentage of previously unscreened women. There is other evidence, both from the field of cytological and breast screening, that a proportion of women who accepted an invitation had not previously engaged in other forms of preventive behaviour or would not have known about the test had they not been invited. Twenty-eight per cent of women who had had the test done as part of another examination, and at the doctor's suggestion, had known nothing about the test beforehand (Sansom et al, 1971b). Hobbs (1981) found that more than half of the women who accepted an invitation for breast screening had not previously had a smear test. She also found that the effect of a personal invitation from the woman's family doctor neutralised the effect of social class on response, and weakened the effect of age. This suggests that women who have not hitherto engaged in preventive health behaviour should not be branded as 'apathetic' or uninterested in their own health. Given the right approach, there is scope for attendance rates to be considerably boosted.

Turning to the way in which women perceive the test, in terms of its purpose, efficacy, acceptability and relevance, it should not be assumed that attitudes detrimental to participation are fixed and unchangeable. Women's knowledge and views about cancer can be changed in a positive direction (Aitken-Swan & Paterson, 1959; Knopf, 1976). Little attempt has been made hitherto to judge the efficacy of different types of invitation and any accompanying health education material. Spenser's (1972) plea that invitation letters 'should be quoted verbatim in any future reports' has unfortunately been ignored, with the result that it is impossible to come to any conclusions about the reasons for the size of a particular response. Yet failure to pay attention to the ways in which women interpret what they hear about the test leads to a perpetuation of the erroneous ideas reported by King (1983). At the most basic level, it is essential that any health education material be assessed for its readability (Flesch, 1948)—an important consideration in a country with an estimated two million adults who are functionally illiterate (Simonite, 1983).

Where the service provider takes the initiative in inviting a woman to be screened, the barrier of not knowing where to go to be tested is automatically removed, provided that a specific venue is designated and that the woman is not merely invited to attend her 'nearest clinic'. The clear implication to be drawn from the literature on women's preferences for particular venues is that choice is essential. Although many women may be happy to have their doctor do the test [and Sansom et al (1971b) found the family doctor an effective persuader of women to have the test], others may not see their GP as the obvious person to carry it out. Women who have always received their family planning advice and pregnancy care from agencies other than their family doctor may regard the surgery as an inappropriate venue for obtaining their smear test. In addition, with the broadening of the base of health care for women that has come about through the expansion of well-women clinics and other self-help initiatives, many women may find these venues to be the natural choice for obtaining a preventive health check. A recent analysis of attenders at a well-women clinic showed that it attracted older working-class women — precisely the group known in the literature as hard to reach (Spencer et al, 1982).

Attendance for screening is essentially voluntary. This being so, it is important that women's views should be ascertained if a comprehensive service which meets the needs of a variety of women is to be established. However, when considering the type of choices that women are offered, it needs to be borne in mind that the different venues are not equally successful in obtaining a response for repeat smears. Both Allman et al (1974) and Sansom et al (1975b) found that much smaller percentages of women who had had their first test at an industrial clinic responded to requests for recall, compared with women who had the test at the doctor's surgery or in a local authority clinic. Furthermore, when interviewing women about their intentions regarding future tests, the latter study found that the majority who had not responded to a recall invitation, and who said they would prefer to go somewhere different for further tests, had had their initial test at an industrial clinic.

With regard to the practical obstacles faced by some women, including many in high-risk groupings, in making and keeping an appointment for a smear test, any initiative that a service provider can take to remove these obstacles can only improve the effectiveness of the screening service. In Hobbs' (1981) study, reply-paid cards were employed, giving provisional appointments, together with the option of choosing a more convenient time. This type of flexibility in organising screening sessions is essential if the needs of women with family, work and other commitments are to be adequately catered for.

Figure 14.1 represents a model of how we believe the population of women eligible for cervical cytology is best viewed. At one end of the continuum are women who will take the initiative themselves to have a test and be prepared to overcome any obstacles in their way. At the other extreme is a small group of women who will be refusers, no matter how propitious the circumstances. In the middle are the large majority of women who are potential users of the system. Their participation will depend on the type of system that they are offered. When a programme of screening fails to take account of women's needs, expects women to take the initiative in making an appointment, and is organised in a way to suit the convenience of the provider rather than the user, then it is less likely that women will make use of the service. Conversely, in a provider-initiated, user-oriented system, we hypothesise that a much greater proportion of women will attend. Corroboration of our model is found in Hobbs' (1981) study of breast screening, where a similar continuum of willingness to participate was noted.

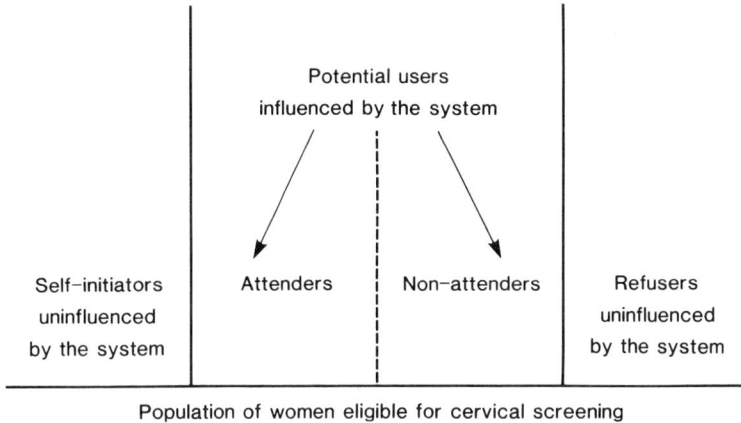

Population of women eligible for cervical screening

84.02.03.04.

Fig. 14.1   Model of utilisation of cervical screening. The broken line indicates that the proportion of screened women will increase in size in relation to the extent that the system offered incorporates the principles of provider-initiation and user-orientation.

To summarise, a provider-initiated, user-oriented system would take account of the following principles. First, it would aim to ensure complete coverage of the target population by inviting all eligible women to attend for screening, and by making provision to ensure that these women are subsequently recalled for repeat tests at appropriate intervals. Second, the invitation would be accompanied by careful health education which takes account of issues relating to efficacy, function, relevance and acceptability of the test. Such education would seek to deal in advance with women's fears and anxieties. Finally, the invitation would offer women a choice both of appointment and venue to ensure convenience and flexibility.

PART 2: THE PROPOSALS

Planning a provider-initiated, user-oriented system
In this section we describe the planning of a system to implement these principles. Its essence is to create a link between the user and the provider which takes into account a number of characteristics, not only those of the user. It consists of the creation, monitoring and maintenance of a communication channel between the provider and the user which is user-oriented rather than provider-oriented.

Creating the communication channel
The *providers* of a screening programme are the District Health Authority (DHA) and the general practitioner for clinical services, the DHA or Region for laboratory services. The traditionally recognised venues for screening are the GPs' surgeries, health centres, group practices, DHA health and clinic centres. Alternative venues are mobile clinics or the woman's own home. The *venues* require medical, nursing, clerical and other support staff. Some general practitioners prefer not to carry out the tests themselves. For their patients it seems logical for the DHA clinics to be

responsible for providing a cytology service. The *users* are women identified as eligible to have the test.

The *communication channel* to link these three elements needs to identify and invite eligible women, to offer a choice of appointment and venue, to arrange the provision of test results and to ensure that all elements in the system are provided with the information they need to maintain an efficient and effective service. To facilitate and coordinate these various responsibilities and activities a *management system* is necessary. This system works for and on behalf of the general practitioners, health authority and laboratory services and, ultimately, the users. This system requires a *database*. Such a database, that will cover all screening, whether by the GP or the DHA, is provided by the Family Practitioner Committee (FPC) registers. The recent DHSS proposal for the computerisation of such registers and the development of suitable computer programs by the Family Practitioner Services Unit in Exeter makes this an attractive option. The use of the FPC records as the database provides an economy of scale without becoming too unwieldy to be responsive to local needs. Our proposals therefore are based on the use of the FPC computerised registers as the database.

The initial data are the family practitioner records, data from the Central Register concerning women due for recall and from any regional cervical cytology scheme. These enable women to be identified for both call and recall.

A prime requirement is to identify general practitioners or group practices as 'participating', i.e., undertaking the screening themselves on their own premises, hereafter described as P-GPs, or 'non-participating', hereafter described as NP-GPs, whose patients should be invited to attend DHA screening clinics.

The management system

The management system is designed and located in conjunction with the database and is primarily a facilitator of provider functions. It facilitates the achievement of their various aims by standardising procedures while retaining flexibility. The initial reaction of the reader might be to suppose that this will create a whole series of problems but we will show that a provider-initiated, user-oriented approach lends itself to the design of an efficient management and support system.

The management system has three functions: to initiate the invitation, to monitor whether or not a smear test has been carried out and, when it has not, to initiate a follow-up procedure. These three functions can be carried out automatically by a computer system providing the computer is supplied with up-to-date information. By this means the burden of arranging an appointment for screening has been taken away from the woman, but the bulk of the administrative load does not fall on the provider, being instead taken up by the computerisation of these functions. This creates the channel of communication between provider and user but it is still necessary to ensure that the character of the communications is user-oriented.

System of invitation

In order to initiate the invitation the computer first identifies women due for screening or rescreening and generates the letter of invitation. Prior to despatching the invitations NP-GPs are given the opportunity to check the eligibility of their patients. P-GPs can check this eligibility on receiving the monthly batches of invitations. Letters relating to those considered ineligible are returned to the FPC, giving reasons

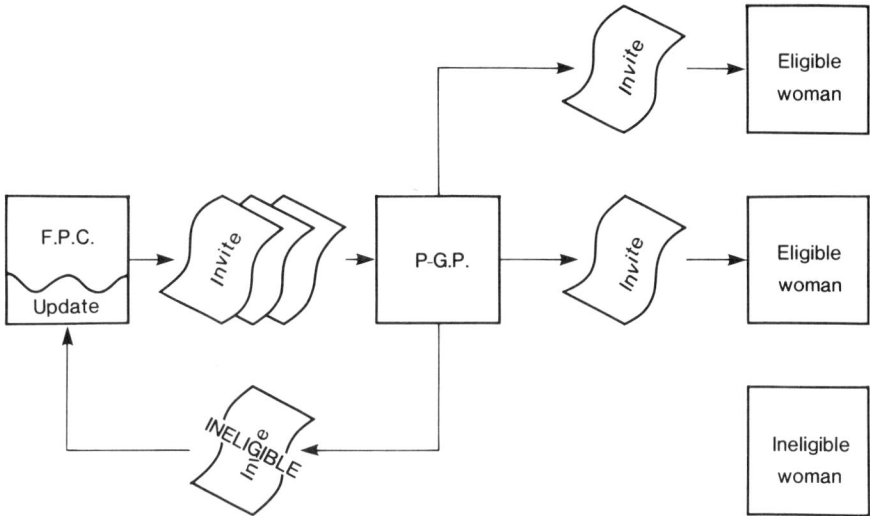

84.02.03.04.

Fig. 14.2 System for invitation. Batches of invitations go to P-G.P. who forwards them to eligible women. Invitations for ineligible women are returned to the F.P.C. indicating an appropriate recall date.

for their exclusion and suggesting an appropriate repeat invitation date. The NP-GP lists request similar responses (Fig. 14.2).

At the surgery, invitation letters are completed by inserting a choice of two appointment dates and times. In using these choices of appointments to create screening session lists some initial overbooking may be advisable until the average level of response becomes clear.

The letters of invitation

In the case of *P-GP patients*, the invitation is styled as if coming from the family doctor, recommending the advisability of being screened and providing an invitation which seeks to maximise the likelihood of a woman accepting a smear test. To this end it offers a choice of appointments, the option to choose to have the test at a DHA clinic and an opportunity to decline the test either for the time being or completely. Because of this element of choice a reply is required from the woman and this she indicates on an easily completed reply form which she returns in the envelope provided.

The reply goes to the P-GP so that provisional appointments can be confirmed or cancelled and the choice of clinic or refusal forms sent on to the FPC. Clinic choices are forwarded with the next clinic list (Fig. 14.3). Refusals pro tem are entered on the computer for recall in one year, total refusals for recall at the standard interval (five years).

In the case of *NP-GP patients*, the letter is styled as from a DHA clinic over the name of the District Medical Officer. Again the letter offers a choice of appointments, an opportunity to decline the test and, in this case, an option to choose a different clinic. The reply goes to the clinic to allow confirmation or cancellation of provisional appointments. Other clinic choices and refusals are sent to the FPC for processing as above.

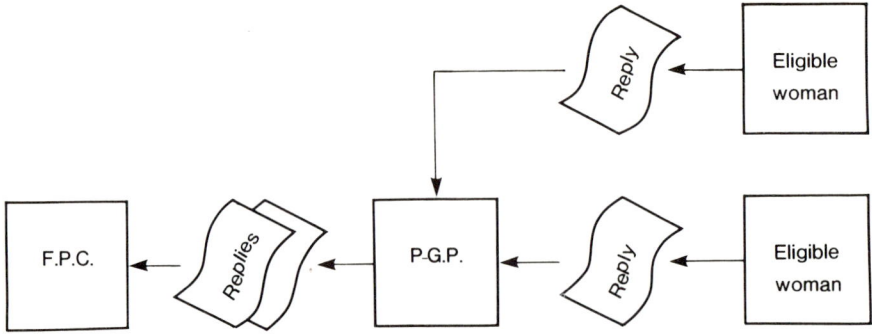

84.02.03.04.

Fig. 14.3   The system for reply. Women reply to the P-G.P. who notes accepted appointments and forwards to the F.P.C. those requesting a clinic appointment or refusing.

In both types of invitation the tenor of the letter is to encourage women with doubts or questions about the test to discuss these with their family doctor. Enclosed with the letter are a list of the DHA clinics, with addresses, clinic days and times and telephone numbers, and health education material.

The coordination of the general practice and DHA clinic services, the issuing of findings and the monitoring of follow-up procedures are designed to ensure that no one slips through the net at any point. This is not to say that refusals to be screened are not honoured but that every care is taken to bring women into the screening system and to extend that care to the final outcome.

Health education material
The invitation is itself a health education message and its presentation and wording place value on the woman's participation in and self-determination concerning screening. In addition, factual information dealing simply with basic questions is provided in an enclosed leaflet which has a low reading-age score. Because some women will wish to have information in more depth, a more detailed leaflet is made available at screening venues and referred to in the simple leaflet.

The woman
The simplest outcome is when women accept one of the appointments offered and attend for the test. There will be some cases where a woman fails to reply or to keep an agreed appointment. In these cases a repeat invitation is sent as soon as this becomes obvious. Those who do not respond to the reminder are identified routinely by regular computer reviews of invitation responses. Some providers may wish to extend the system by arranging for a practice nurse or health visitor to call to check if there is a health or social problem preventing a woman from replying and to see that she still lives at that address.

Where a woman indicates that she does not want the test just now her computer record is updated for recall in one year. If, however, she refuses the test altogether the computer program gives her a test date five years hence. This provides the opportunity for a woman to change her mind without feeling she is being badgered.

The replies of women choosing to have the test at a DHA clinic in preference to their GP are forwarded to the FPC for inclusion in the next month's list for that clinic. The computer record is altered so that future invitations come from that clinic.

Taking the smear
GPs may wish to organise the taking of smears in their practices by arranging special screening sessions, as opposed to trying to fit occasional tests into surgery hours. The former has the greater potential for maximising response, particularly if sessions are not always held on the same day of the week. Screening evokes a different atmosphere in the doctor/patient relationship, involving a more active, interventionist role for the doctor yet not requiring the woman to adopt the sick role. For both doctors and patients it is easier to adopt this changed stance in the context of a special screening session. It is also more efficient to set up equipment and staffing requirements for a session than for individual tests.

The attitudes, often unconscious, of the doctors, nurses and clerical staff of the practices and clinics can convey powerful messages to women being screened and these should not be at variance with the invitation and support material approach. Thus, the more detailed leaflet should be readily available and personal details should be taken in privacy. Careful attention needs to be given to correct recording of social data such as husband's occupation, which is increasingly recognised as a potentially significant factor in the prevalence of cervical cancer. Accurate completion of these forms will undoubtedly add to our epidemiological knowledge of the aetiology and natural history of cervical cancer and its precursors.

Giving results
The anxiety women feel awaiting results of the test varies but if it is acute or prolonged it may militate against re-screening. Three weeks is the maximum anyone should have to wait. If pressure on the laboratory is so great that this cannot be achieved, screening sessions may have to be reduced until the load is more manageable. If a DHA or GPs cannot afford to send individual letters giving the result, a slip can be enclosed with the invitation to indicate how soon after the test the results may be expected and that the woman can obtain them by telephoning or calling at the surgery or clinic (Fig. 14.4). The enclosed slip also asks women who wish to receive results by post to bring in a stamped addressed envelope when they come for the test. There is no justification whatsoever for the provider to take the approach that 'if you don't hear within three weeks you can assume all is well'.

Each GP determines the administrative arrangements regarding non-normal findings since it is inappropriate for a clerk/receptionist to have this responsibility. Except for abnormal findings, the DHA clinics are responsible for sending results to the women they screen. For unsatisfactory smears the clinic arranges with the patient to take the repeat test; negative findings are given directly to the woman. Where it is necessary for a woman to see her own doctor because inflammation or infection has been found, the wording of a verbal message needs to be carefully determined. It is anticipated that the woman's doctor will react promptly to abnormal findings. Nursing and clerical staff need to be guided on how to ensure that the woman sees her doctor promptly without exacerbating her anxiety.

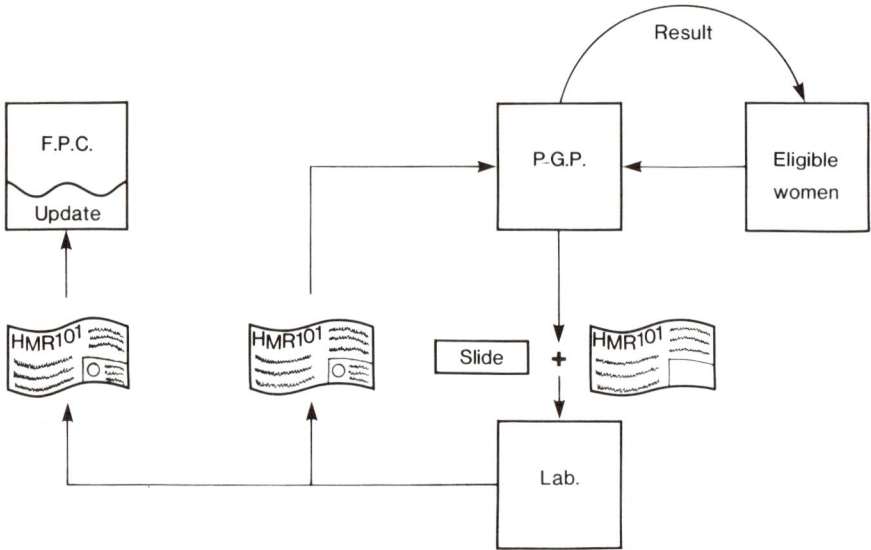

84.02.03.04.

Fig. 14.4 The system for processing the smear. The woman attends for the test; the slide and result form (HMR101) are sent to the laboratory; the laboratory sends completed forms to the F.P.C. to update the record and to the P-G.P. to inform the woman.

The cytology laboratory

Where the laboratory does not provide special kits for the transfer of slides and their identifying forms, the P-GPs and DHA clinic staff need to take special care to ensure that a slide and its accompanying form do not become separated (Fig. 14.4). The laboratory staff read the slide and send out the result in triplicate. One copy goes to the GP, one to the FPC to update the computer record, and one to the DHA clinic if the test was taken there.

It is possible that during the early years of this system there will be some increase in laboratory workload. It is a mistake to allow this pressure to build up into a backlog of work resulting in delay in making results available. The planning of the phasing-in of the new system together with the question of reducing the volume of frequent repeat smears from women at low risk are matters of concern to the laboratory service. The emphasis on providing results to women as soon as possible serves to support laboratories in asking for temporary reductions in workload when necessary.

The computer-managed support system

In addition to providing the functions of managing the screening invitation and its follow-up, the computer system facilitates the overall administration of the service for the providers and produces data for epidemiological studies. By keeping a record of smears taken, and by whom, the computer serves to facilitate FPC administrative and financial procedures and to reduce form-filling by individual doctors. The computer program allows for the assessment of the target population at any given time, the invitation response rates, and the levels of screening achieved. It also provides profiles of screening findings over different time periods. In the long term this information can be related to incidence and mortality data from cancer registries so that a more accurate picture of the effect of cervical cytology screening on the control of cancer of the cervix can be obtained.

With regard to these functions an important aspect of the computer software is its flexibility. Undoubtedly, the criteria for target populations will change over time and the computer program must be able to adjust to these easily. In the same way, administrative and epidemiological requirements may alter, so the software package must be amenable to adjustments to cope with these.

No innovation in the provision of health services can be expected to succeed without the cooperation of all personnel involved. Their ability to participate effectively is enhanced when they understand the total system rather than only being informed about their function within it. We therefore see that significant benefit will be obtained from the provision of in-service courses for staff at all levels, which provide a view of the service as a whole, in addition to detailed information on their particular tasks within it.

Practical implementation

A cervical cytology call and recall scheme such as we have described has been designed by the authors in conjunction with FPCs in the Manchester area. The problem of developing the necessary computer programs has been solved by opting to employ the software specially developed by the Family Practitioner Services Computer Unit in Exeter (Fisher & Head, 1983). A close evaluation by the authors indicated that this software adequately meets the requirements of the planned cytology system.

We feel that the system as described here offers the best means of producing the kind of response from the invited women that will in time reduce the incidence of and mortality from cervical cancer. Flexibility is built in so that changes can be made to the system in operation to maximise response rates. In order to know where and when such changes may be required it is necessary to monitor the functioning of the scheme. Much of the information required for this monitoring will be routinely provided by the computer system and the Department of Epidemiology and Social Research will be conducting an evaluation of the scheme in its early years. In many ways the operation of the scheme in Manchester will act as a pilot for other areas which may wish to develop similar systems.

In total, the effect of this shift from a user-initiated to a provider-initiated system is to produce a user-oriented screening service which we suggest will attract the vast majority of those potential attenders who have hitherto remained unscreened. On the basis of evidence from other countries, the implementation of a computer-managed call and recall scheme, which invites *all* women in the currently defined target population, should reduce the incidence and mortality from cancer of the cervix, providing that it achieves a sufficiently high response rate. Moreover, a high response rate must be achieved within those sections of the community considered to be at highest risk. The particular needs of older and lower social class women have been met in this system design. No special campaigns should therefore be necessary to encourage them to attend unless it is found that the level of response is lower than anticipated. Since the evaluation of the effect of screening on morbidity and mortality can only be achieved in the long term it is necessary to define the aims of the service in the shorter term by response rates.

As long ago as 1972, McKinlay pointed out that the trend of research into the use of health services was to move away from an emphasis on the 'personal pathologies of "under-utilisers" towards a concentration on various types of organisational impedimenta'. Our thesis is that this trend has not been reflected in the understanding of the uptake of cytological services. We have presented here a system which, we believe, overcomes many of the problems previously experienced. By implementing and evaluating the system the strengths and weaknesses of our thesis will be demonstrated.

ACKNOWLEDGEMENT

This work was financed by the Department of Health and Social Security.

REFERENCES

Adelstein A M, Husain O A N, Spriggs A I 1981 Cancer of the cervix and screening. [Letter]. British Medical Journal 282: 564
Aitken-Swan J, Paterson R 1959 Assessment of the results of five years cancer education. British Medical Journal i: 708–712
Allman S T, Chamberlain J, Harman P 1974 The National Cervical Cytology Recall System: report of a pilot study. Health Trends 6: 39–41
Andrews G S, Davies M 1980 Reflections on a cytology screening service. Tumori 66: 159–171
Becker M H (ed) 1974 The health belief model and personal health behaviour. Health Education Monographs 2: 4
Bluck M E 1975 Public and professional opinion on preventive medicine. Tenovus Cancer Information Centre, Cardiff
Brindle G, Wakefield J 1976 Screening by cervical cytology: its uses and abuses. Journal of Family Planning Doctors 2: 26–28
Brindle G, Wakefield J, Yule R 1976 Cervical smears: are the right women being examined? British Medical Journal 1: 1196–1197
British Medical Journal 1980 High-risk groups and cervical cancer [Editorial] 281: 629–630
Burslem R W 1983 Cervical cytological screening for users of oral contraceptives [Letter]. The Lancet ii: 968
Carruthers J, Wilson J M G, Chamberlain J et al 1975 Acceptability of the cytopipette in screening for cervical cancer. British Journal of Preventive and Social Medicine 29: 239–248
Chamberlain J 1982 Screening for early detection of cancer: general principles. In: Alderson M (ed) The Prevention of Cancer, Edward Arnold Ltd. ch 8, p 227–258
Chamberlain J 1983 Cancer Education Coordinating Group: Report of Working Party on Screening for Cervical Cancer, Belfast, 10 June 1983
Charlton A 1983 Young people's knowledge of the cervical smear test. Social Science and Medicine 17: 235–239
Clements J E, Wakefield J 1972 Symptoms and uncertainty. International Journal of Health Education 15: 113–122
Cullum D E, Savory J N 1983 Patient preference for cervical cytology. British Medical Journal 287: 329–332
Davison R L, Clements J 1971 Why don't they attend for a cytotest? Medical Officer 125: 329–331
Draper G J 1982 Screening for cervical cancer: revised policy. The recommendations of the DHSS Committee on gynaecological cytology. Health Trends 14: 37–40
Draper G J, Cook G A 1983 Changing pattern of cervical cancer rates. British Medical Journal 287: 510–512
Evans D, Hibbard, B, Jones J et al 1980 The Cardiff Cervical Cytology Study: enumeration and definition of population and initial acceptance rates. Journal of Epidemiology and Community Health 34: 9–13
Evans J H, Semmence A M 1975 The computer. In: Hart C R (ed) Screening in general practice, Churchill Livingstone, London, p 61
Fisher H, Head A 1983 Cervical cytology recall system: draft description. Report from Exeter FPS Computer Unit
Flesch R 1948 A new readability yardstick. Journal of Applied Psychology 32: 221–233
Grünfeld K, Horwitz O, Lysgaard-Hansen B 1975 Evaluation of mortality data for cervical cancer with special reference to mass screening programs, Denmark 1961–1971. American Journal of Epidemiology 101: 265–275

Hakama M 1982 Trends in the incidence of cervical cancer in the Nordic Countries. In: Magnus K (ed) Trends in Cancer Incidence, Hemisphere Publishing Company London, p 279–292

Hakama M, Hakulinen T, Pukkala E et al 1982 Risk indicators of breast and cervical cancer on ecologic and individual levels. American Journal of Epidemiology 116: 990–1000

Hobbs P 1981 Acceptors and rejectors of breast screening. In Tiffany R (ed) Cancer Nursing Update, Proceedings of the Second International Cancer Nursing Conference, Baillière Tindall, London, p 53–56

Houghton H 1968 Response to cervical screening. The Medical Officer 6 December, 334–338

Hulka B S 1982 Risk factors for cervical cancer. Journal of Chronic Diseases 35: 3–11

Jackson J 1979 Screening in general practice: cervical cytology for higher risk women. Public Health (London) 93: 300–305

King J 1982 Health beliefs, attributions and health behaviour. PhD Thesis, University of Oxford

King J 1983 'It's silly but I just don't want to know'. The Health Services, 11 May, p 13

Knopf A 1974 Cancer: changes in opinion after 7 years of public education. Manchester Regional Committee on Cancer, Manchester

Knopf A 1976 Changes in women's opinions about cancer. Social Science and Medicine 10: 105–109

Knox E G 1976 Ages and frequencies for cervical cancer screening. British Journal of Cancer 34: 444–452

Leck I, Sibary K, Wakefield J 1978 Incidence of cervical cancer by marital status. Journal of Epidemiology and Community Health 32: 108–110

MacIntyre S 1979 Some issues in the study of pregnancy careers. The Sociological Review 27: 755–771

McKinlay J 1972 Some approaches and problems in the study of the use of services — an overview. Journal of Health and Social Behaviour 13: 115–152

Miller D M 1969 Cervical cytology consent rate [Letter]. The Lancet ii: 491

Office of Population Censuses and Surveys 1983a Cancer Statistics: Registration Series MBI No 12. HMSO, London

Office of Population Censuses and Surveys 1983b Trends in Cancer Mortality 1951–1980. Series DHI No 11. HMSO, London

Parkin D M, Collins W, Clayden A D 1981 Cervical cytology screening in two Yorkshire areas: pattern of service. Public Health (Lond.) 95: 311–321

Registrar General 1980 Classification of Occupations 1980. OPCS London

Roberts A 1982 Cervical cytology in England and Wales 1965–1980. Health Trends 14: 41–43

Robinson J 1982 Cancer of the cervix: occupational risks of husbands and wives and possible preventive strategies. In: Jordan J A, Sharp F, Singer A (eds) Pre-Clinical Neoplasia of the Cervix. Proceedings of the Ninth Study Group of the Royal College of Obstetricians and Gynaecologists, October 1981. Royal College of Obstetricians and Gynaecologists, London p 11–27

Sansom C D, MacInerney J, Oliver V et al 1975a Recall of women in a cervical cytology screening programme: an estimate of the true rate of response. British Journal of Preventive and Social Medicine 29: 131–134

Sansom C D, MacInerney J, Oliver V et al 1975b Differential response to recall in a cervical screening programme. British Journal of Preventive and Social Medicine 29: 40–47

Sansom C D, Wakefield J, Yule R 1971a Trends in cytological screening in the Manchester Area 1965–1971. Community Medicine 126: 253–257

Sansom C D, Wakefield J, Pinnock K M 1971b Choice or chance? How women come to have a cytotest done by their family doctor. International Journal of Health Education 14: 127–138

Sansom C D, Wakefield J, Yule R 1970 Cervical cytology in the Manchester region: changing patterns of response. The Medical Officer 123: 357–359

Saunders J, Snaith A H 1969 Cervical cytology consent rate. The Lancet ii: 207

Scaife B 1972 Survey of cervical cytology in general practice. British Medical Journal 3: 200–202

Semmence A M, Mellors B E 1975 A cervical cytology recall system based on general practice and assisted by computer. Symposium on Information Systems in the Health and Social Services, Oxford. Organised by the Oxford Community Health Project, June 27.

SHE magazine 1983 Give us gynae with dignity. November, p 161

Sibary K, Burslem R W, Wakefield J 1978 Cause of high risk of cervical cancer in socially unclassified women. British Journal of Cancer 38: 166–168

Sibary K, Davis F, Wakefield J et al 1977 Women with cervical cancer detected through population screening. International Journal of Health Education 20: 205–211

Simonite V 1983 Literacy and numeracy: evidence from the National Child Development Study. National Children's Bureau

Spencer B, Gray S, Dunham M et al 1982 An evaluation of the Manchester Well Women Clinics. Manchester Community Health Councils

Spenser J T 1972 A survey of cervical smear screening in general practice. In: Wakefield J (ed) Seek Wisely to Prevent. Ch 9, p 111. HMSO, London

Spriggs A I, Boddington M M 1976 Protection by cervical smears [Letter]. The Lancet i: 143

Standen P J, Rivalland P R 1982 Cervical screening: reaching the non-attenders. Journal of the Institute of Health Education 20: 19–26

Sunday People, 25 September 1983

Thompson C. 1969 Cervical cytology consent rate [Letter]. The Lancet ii: 385

Veitch A 1983 How the lives of 1000 women could be saved each year. The Guardian 31 August, p 11

Wakefield J (ed) 1972 Seek Wisely to Prevent. HMSO, London

Wakefield J 1976 Studies of response to cervical screening. Tumori 62: 315–318

Wakefield J, Sansom C D 1966 Profile of a population of women who have undergone a cervical smear examination. The Medical Officer 116: 145–146

Wakefield J, Yule R, Smith A et al 1973 Relation of abnormal cytological smears and carcinoma of cervix uteri to husband's occupation. British Medical Journal 2: 142–143

Williams E M, Cruikshank A, Walker W M 1972 Public Opinion on Cancer, a survey of knowledge and attitudes in SE Wales. Tenovus Cancer Information Centre, Cardiff

Wolfendale M R, King S, Usherwood M McD 1983 Abnormal cervical smears: are we in for an epidemic? British Medical Journal 287: 526–528

15. A strategy for health in old age

J. A. Muir Gray

The last 20 years have seen a significant advance in the care of old people but developments in geriatric medicine, impressive as they have been, have not resulted in the development of a strategy for the development of services to meet the challenge posed by the ageing of the population in an era in which resources devoted to health and social services are unlikely to increase. Geriatric medicine has played a very important part in the development of a more enlightened philosophy and has developed many effective means of treating and rehabilitating elderly patients who were formerly considered to be untreatable. However, such treatments, although often complicated to devise and deliver, are simply tactics. The definition of tactics given in the Shorter Oxford English Dictionary is that it is 'the art or science of deploying . . . forces in order of battle'. It is obviously important to deploy one's forces in proper order but tactics by themselves are of limited effectiveness unless they are part of a strategy, defined in the same dictionary as 'the art of projecting and directing the larger movements and operations of a campaign'. To cope with the challenge posed by population ageing requires more than the right philosophy and a collection of useful tactics. It requires a carefully planned campaign, a strategy based on that philosophy and embracing those tactics, to ensure that resources are deployed as effectively as possible. The contribution of community medicine to the care of older people is to facilitate the development of such a strategy.

The development of a strategy does not necessarily begin with a consideration of the present pattern of services. No matter how radically these services may be analysed and criticised it is inappropriate to focus on the pattern of services until other issues have been considered.

(1) The nature of the challenge.
(2) The objectives of health care in old age.
(3) The interventions that are effective in achieving those objectives.
(4) The indicators that can be used to evaluate progress.

Only after these issues have been clarified should the pattern of services be considered.

THE NATURE OF THE CHALLENGE

In the 1960s it was demonstrated in many centres that old people could benefit from an active approach to diagnosis and treatment. The arguments advanced by the pioneers of geriatric medicine have been accepted and the need for an active therapeutic approach to the problems of older people is generally recognised. In the

1970s three other aspects of the problems of older people became more clearly understood.

The impact of social problems

The first was the fact that many of the problems of old people were caused neither by disease nor by the ageing process but by social factors, and notably by poverty. The 'social problems' of older people were not only the social difficulties they experienced; these also included the way they were treated by younger members of society, including doctors and nurses. The term 'ageism' entered common currency, due in part to the activities of voluntary organisations like Age Concern and Help the Aged, in part to the committed campaigning of the Grey Panthers, and the National Institute of Aging. Professionals began to accept that the problems of older people were not all attributable to biological processes, associated with ageing or simply to the shortage of resources: some were due to the beliefs, attitudes and behaviour of the professionals themselves. This appreciation has obvious implications for professional training, because there is disturbing evidence that some of the prejudices which students have on entering training are actually reinforced, rather than diminished, by professional training.

The impact of disuse

The second important change was the growing appreciation of the importance of unfitness in old age. The term 'fitness' has had strong connotations of youth and sport for many years but the concept is equally important for people in their eighties as for people in their twenties. The reason for this is that part of the loss of functional ability that occurs with age is due to a loss of fitness. In part, of course, the loss of ability is due to the ageing process and the effect of the ageing process is to reduce the maximum capacity for work, due to changes in a number of different systems, for example due to a decline in the maximum attainable heart rate. For the majority of people, however, the rate of decline that occurs is faster than that which would take place if the ageing process were the only process operating and the reason for the increased rate of decline is a progressive loss of fitness. At any age there is a gap between the actual level of ability and the best possible level of ability. This gap may be called the fitness gap and it widens with age (Fig. 15.1).

Ageing *per se* does not result in a loss of fitness but the two processes are inter-related because the older people lose fitness more quickly if their level of physical activity decreases and regain it more slowly if the level of physical activity is increased. The main cause of the progressive loss of fitness is the decreasing level of physical activity that characterises the lives of people from an early age, usually from the age of leaving school or university, but sometimes before this, and sometimes after if the person has a job that is physically demanding or participates in active leisure pursuits (Shephard, 1978; Smith & Serfass, 1981).

Disease and loss of fitness are also inter-related and one of the achievements of geriatric medicine has been to demonstrate that the effects of immobilising diseases such as arthritis are due not only to the pathological process but also to the effects of immobility. The reason why disease accelerates the loss of fitness is in part biological, for some diseases make physical activity difficult or painful, but it is also social. Many elderly people and their relatives believe that rest is always indicated in disease with

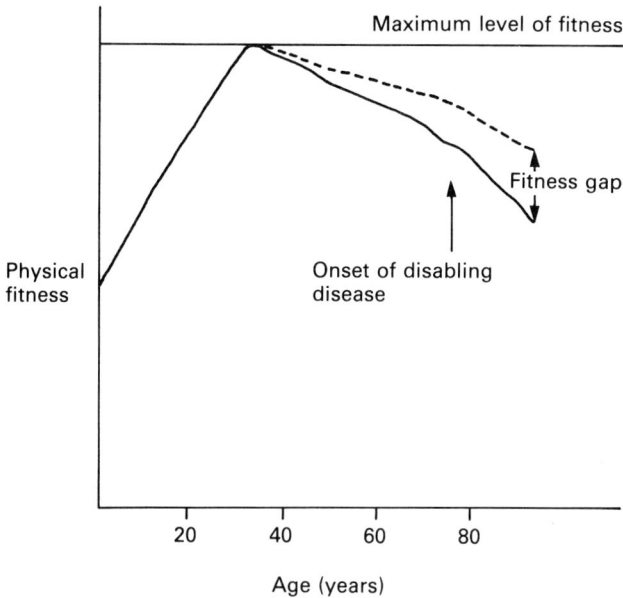

Fig. 15.1   Rate of change of physical fitness with age. Broken line = rate of decline due to ageing if fitness is not lost. Continuous line = actual rate of decline. Source: Gray 1983a.

the result that elderly people who are disabled either expect, or are expected to, sit still and have everything done for them with the result that the fitness gap widens after the onset of chronic disease

Disuse produces many of the changes that have hitherto been assumed to be due to the ageing process (Table 15.1) but it has been shown in well-designed research,

Table 15.1   Changes formerly considered to be the result of the ageing process but which have since been observed as a result of disuse due to bedrest or weightlessness

Decline in	Increase in
VO$_2$ max. (Maximum oxygen carrying capacity)	Systolic blood pressure
Cardiac output	Peripheral resistance
Stroke volume	Sensitivity of balance mechanism
Lean body mass	Thrombotic tendency in
Body water	blood
Concentration of red blood cells	Blood cholesterol
Total body calcium	Body fat
Muscle mass	Nitrogen excretion
Bone thickness	

Source: Bortz 1982.

principally in Sweden and North America, that many of the effects of disease can be reversed by increasing the individual's level of physical activity sufficiently to apply a load that requires the old person to work to overcome it irrespective of their age or the presence of a chronic disabling disease.

These findings have important implications not only for those involved in preventive medicine but also for all those providing services for elderly people. Many of the services for old people are prosthetic, they perform some task that the old person can no longer perform, for example by the provision of meals on wheels or a home help. The sequence of events which leads to the introduction of such a prosthesis is usually that the old person or a friend perceives some difficulty and requests help with the request for help being met by the provision of a prosthesis. Such a response is not perhaps surprising when the referral is made to a social services department but it is disappointing when a doctor's reaction to the report that an old person is having increasing difficulty in preparing meals is simply to suggest meals on wheels without asking whether the decline in function could be due to a treatable disease and without asking what effect the provision of meals on wheels on three days a week will have on fitness and ability. This level of service may remove three hours of purposeful activity from the life of the old person thus accelerating the rate of decline.

The importance of self-care and informal care
The third important fact to emerge from research in recent years is the major contribution to care made by old people themselves and by their families and voluntary helpers. The preoccupation with the organisation of professional services that characterises many of the papers written about old age has obscured the importance of self-care and informal care but it is increasingly appreciated that most old people are independent and active in looking after themselves and others. Only a minority are heavily dependent and even those who are make an important contribution to their own care. Furthermore, recent research, both epidemiological and historical, has demonstrated that families care for their elders as well as families ever did, provided they are given adequate support from the professional services and live near enough to do so (Moroney, 1976).

SETTING OBJECTIVES

There has been an increase in the expectation of life in old age in the last twenty years but this has not been the result of a conscious policy, and seems to have resulted from a number of factors such as the more effective treatment of disease in old age, advances in the use of treatments that were formerly not used in old age (for example the increasing ability of anaesthetists to prepare elderly people for surgery) and the increasingly good state of health of people reaching old age. The prolongation of life in old age is not the principal aim of the health services and most old people themselves would agree that the principal aim of health care in old age is 'not to add years to life but to add life to years;' to improve the quality of life rather than the quantity.

As a basis for service planning it is essential to define specific objectives. A set of objectives that most people would agree as being appropriate for service planning are:

(1) To prevent unnecessary loss of physical ability;
(2) To prevent a decline in the quality of life due to the development of preventable or treatable symptoms such as pain or depression, or due to the development of social problems such as poverty;
(3) To prevent family breakdown;

(4) To keep old people in their own homes;

(5) To provide good quality long-stay care for those who cannot be supported at home;

(6) To help old people have a good death as well as a good life.

Obviously such a set of objectives can be criticised. These objectives include normative terms such as 'good' and 'quality' and they may not always be endorsed by elderly people themselves but they are useful as a basis for discussion with elderly people themselves and with the general public.

Increasingly, objectives are being quantified to produce targets. For example, the United States Surgeon General in his report on *Healthy People* stated that his target was 'to reduce the average annual number of days of restricted activity due to acute and chronic conditions by 20%, to fewer than 30 days per year for persons aged 65 and older', and it is simple to devise targets for service development (Table 15.2).

Table 15.2   Examples of targets for service development

By 1985 the proportion of old people dying at home will be 5% greater than the present level

By 1985 no old person living alone will be admitted to long-stay care until she has been offered seven day domiciliary care with two visits a day on Saturdays and Sundays

By 1990 the proportion of elderly people who do not have a telephone will be reduced to half the present proportion

By 1990 the proportion of elderly people receiving artificial hips annually will be at least equal to the present national average in all Regions of the NHS

The setting of targets is not always popular with planners and politicians but it does provide a definite focus for professional and public effort and a yardstick by which progress, or the lack of it, can be measured.

IDENTIFYING EFFECTIVE INTERVENTIONS

Having agreed on a set of objectives it is essential to identify the specific interventions that will allow those objectives to be achieved. It is important not to identify the means of achieving the objective in terms of development of a certain service or certain profession, for example as being 'more domiciliary care', or 'more physio-therapy'. The present pattern of services and professions is the result of a series of disparate and unconnected developments and even though the interventions identified as being effective may eventually be delivered by these professions and services, it is important to think of the interventions independently from the systems which will deliver them. The reason for this is that there is greater scope for changing the service or the profession if the primary focus of attention is the intervention. For example, if the intervention that is desired is 'the education of people suffering from disabling disease about the benefits of physical exercise and about the type, duration, intensity and frequency of exercise', it is important to state this rather than that 'an increase in physiotherapy' is required. If the latter is the stated intervention then it is probable that the service will simply deliver more of the same, namely more physiotherapy treatments, to those elderly people who happen to be referred to a physiotherapist. If, on the other hand, attention is focussed on the educational intervention then physiotherapists will be encouraged to think of ways in which they can educate all elderly people with disabling disease and this may lead to links with adult education service, with leisure centres, and with the post-basic education of health and social service staff, thus having a much greater impact, albeit indirectly, than can be achieved by increasing the number of elderly people treated by physiotherapists directly.

INDICATORS OF HEALTH IN OLD AGE

The World Health Organisation has suggested four different types of health indicator:

Health policy indicators; for example, the proportion of resources devoted to services for elderly people.

Health status and quality of life indicators; for example, the prevalence of common diseases, disabilities and handicaps and measurements of people's satisfaction with life at home or in residential care.

Health service indicators; for example, the proportion of the population receiving specific services.

Social and economic indicators; for example, the mean income of elderly people and the proportions of elderly people in households with a car and a telephone.

Such indicators have to satisfy the criteria generally agreed for health indicators; that is they should be valid, reliable, sensitive and specific. It is, however, also essential to consider the feasibility and cost of collecting such indicators and to distinguish between those data that can only be reliably collected by research workers following a carefully designed protocol and using a validated assessment tool, and those that can be reliably collected by health service managers.

Health status and quality of life are extremely difficult to measure accurately because there are so many sources of bias (Kane & Kane, 1981) and it would not be feasible to collect such data routinely. An objective of research should therefore be to determine which health service and social indicators are the most valid proxies for health status and quality of life. It is important not only that each health authority should collect health service and social indicators but also that agreement be reached on the set of indicators that every health authority should use. At present it is impossible for a health authority to compare its own performance in the provision of series for the elderly with that of other authorities, and it would probably lead to an improvement in the effectiveness of health care if this type of competitive audit could be developed.

Health service indicators are obviously important and many health and local authorities would claim to be collecting such data at present. Often, however, the indicator is a simple financial indicator, for example the amount spent on geriatric or home help services per thousand population. This type of information, the cost of a single service or group of services, does not take into account the full range of costs. It is, for example, common to calculate the cost of 'community care' without including the discounted cost of the dwelling in which the old person lives and it is very uncommon to make any attempt to cost the burden borne by family and friends. It is, therefore, more appropriate for health service managers to concentrate on health service and social indicators until detailed studies have identified the financial data that might serve as valid indicators of the true cost of the services provided for an elderly population (Cullis & West, 1982).

Indicators of efficiency

These are indicators of health but it is also necessary to have indicators of health service efficiency. It is relatively easy to calculate the financial cost of an intervention and to express this as cost per treatment, or per patient treated, but great care has to be taken with such indicators. Costs calculated by dividing the total cost of a service by the number of units of service, do not give a valid indication of cost-effectiveness. The unit cost of a service can be used as a measure of efficiency but only when the costs of two comparable services are set against one another, for example when the average cost of a chiropody treatment in one authority is compared with the average cost of chiropody treatments in a similar authority, which again emphasises the need for a common set of performance indicators, as suggested by the Korner Committee (1982).

The patient's point of view

A major weakness of all these indicators is that they reveal neither the patients' views nor the views of their relatives. It is possible to prevent functional decline in ways that may result in dissatisfaction or disappointment or even in an increase in suffering, namely in a deterioration in the quality of life. For example, an increase in ability may result in an old person losing the services of her home help and district nurse: to the doctor the outcome is independence; to the patient the result is increased loneliness.

No suitable data are routinely collected. We have to depend on our 'sensitivity' or 'professional expertise' or the complaints made to the health authority or Community Health Council. The latter are more valid but still biased and only by soliciting the opinion of a sample of patients could suitable information be obtained. The introduction of such a data collection system need not be prohibitively expensive.

PLANNING FOR HEALTH CARE

These elements of the planning process can be brought together into a coherent plan not only by setting them in sequence but also by basing them on a set of principles such as those proposed by the World Health Organisation for primary health care planning. These are:

Services should be planned to meet the needs of the whole population;
There should be effective and efficient use of resources;
Health service planning should be incorporated with the planning of other services;
There should be participation of the community at all levels of planning and
  management (Gray, 1982; Gray, 1983b).

Using these principles and the objectives, interventions and indicators can be synthesised into a set of programmes designed to achieve the defined objectives (Tables 15.3–15.8).

The changing challenge

In looking to the future it seems likely that the nature of the challenge will change as new cohorts reach advanced old age. There are still too few longitudinal studies to

Table 15.3   Plan for prevention of functional decline

Objective	Interventions	Indicators

1. Prevention of loss of functional ability	Education of elderly people and their relatives
	Accurate diagnosis and effective treatment of acute and chronic diseases
		Proportion of elderly people attending adult education classes
		Proportion of elderly people using swimming baths
		Age specific rates of:
		   hip replacement
		   pacemaker insertion
		   cataract extraction
		Proportion of elderly people receiving treatment from:
		   day hospital
		   chiropodists
		   domiciliary occupational therapists
		Proportion of elderly population receiving regular prescriptions of:
		   no drugs
		   more than three drugs
		   major tranquillisers
		   minor tranquillisers
		   hypnotics

Table 15.4   Plan for maintenance of quality of life

Objective	Interventions	Indicators

2. To maintain the person's quality of life at the level it was when he retired	Effective control of distressing symptoms:
	   Anxiety
	   Depression
	
	   Pain
	   Incontinence
	
	Provision of adequate income
	Satisfactory housing
	
	Measures to reduce isolation
	
	Provision of opportunities for involvement in service planning and management
		
		Tranquilliser prescription rates
		Anti-depressant prescription rates
		Suicide rate
		Numbers of elderly people with depression seen by psychiatrists
		Analgesic prescribing rates
		Number of incontinence pads per thousand population
		Uptake of benefits
		Proportion of elderly people lacking inside toilet
		Proportion of elderly people attending day centres and day hospitals
		Proportion of community health council and health authority members over the age of 60 and over the age of 80

allow an accurate prediction of such changes but it is reasonable to assume that the people who are becoming old will be fitter than those who are very old today; that they will be better educated and more assertive; and that they will be wealthier as the proportion of people retiring with occupational pensions will increase. The prevalence of certain of the disabling diseases, notably dementia, cataract, macular degeneration and Parkinson's disease, shows no prospect of declining but the prevalence of chronic obstructive airways disease, rheumatic and ischaemic heart disease, and stroke may decline depending upon factors such as changes in the prevalence of smoking and in the effectiveness of the health services in preventing stroke by the detection and treatment of high blood pressure.

Table 15.5   Plan for family support

Objective	Interventions	Indicators
3. Prevention of breakdown of informal support offered by relatives and friends	Provision of financial help Introduction of housing policies that allow elderly people to move to live *near* their children Practical help in the home to relieve relatives Relief given by day care and by planned short stay admissions	Uptake of Invalid Care Allowance Numbers of elderly people rehoused by National Mobility Scheme Numbers from outside local authority area rehoused by housing associations Number of elderly people living with relatives who receive home help or home nursing Numbers of elders living with relatives given day care Numbers of elderly people living with relatives admitted for planned short stay care

Table 15.6   Plan for domiciliary care

Objective	Interventions	Indicators
4. To keep old people out of long stay care	Those summarised under 1, 2 and 3, together with: Seven day home care for old people living alone with two visits daily on Saturday and Sunday The provision of relief to families looking after elderly people which amounts to at least one third of the total time, for example two weeks' admission in every six weeks	 Number and proportion of elderly people admitted to long stay care who were not receiving this level of support at the time of admission Proportion of elderly population in long stay and mean duration of stay (not good indicators because they are mainly a function of number of long stay beds available)

Table 15.7   Plan for good quality long stay care

Objective	Interventions	Indicators
5. Provision of long stay care which is of good quality and enjoyable	Those summarised under 1, together with: Development of policies that will increase resident participation and community involvement Increased staffing levels Provision of physiotherapy and occupational therapy skills Staff training Modification of homes to increase proportion of residents in single rooms Publication of a *Bill of Rights* to set standards	 Staffing levels Number of hours spent by occupational and physiotherapists in homes Proportion of residents in single rooms Proportion of residents receiving hypnotics Proportion of residents receiving tranquillisers

Table 15.8 Plan for terminal care

Objective	Interventions	Indicators
6. To help old people have a good death	Development of evening nursing service and night sitting service	Percentage of old people dying at home
	Development of hospices for education and training of community health workers, in addition to the services	Numbers of old people receiving injections of analgesics at night
	Hospice day hospital services	Numbers of old people helped by night sitting service
	More widespread use of interventions shown to be effective in: pain control mouth care care of the skin	

The continual evolution of the challenge poses problems for the health planner but the strategist has to develop a strategy which can cope with a degree of uncertainty and which is based on an educated guess as to the way in which the campaign is likely to unfold.

REFERENCES

Bortz W M 1982 Journal of the American Medical Association 248: 1203–1208
Cullis J G, West P A 1979 The Economics of Health, p 167–194. Martin Robertson
Department of Health and Social Security 1982 Report of the Steering Group on Health Services Information (Korner) HMSO
Gray J A M 1982 Health for all elderly people by the year 2000. Lancet ii: 1036–1038
Gray J A M 1983a Prevention in old age. p 66–73 in Practising prevention, British Medical Association
Gray J A M 1983b Four box health care: health service development in a time of zero growth. Lancet: in press
Kane R A, Kane R L 1981 Assessing the elderly: a practical guide to measurement. Lexington Books
Moroney R M 1976 The family and the state: considerations for social policy. Longman
Shephard R J 1978 Physical activity and ageing. Croom Helm
Smith E L, Serfass R C eds 1981 Exercise and ageing: the scientific basis. Enslow

16. Current issues in handicap due to intellectual impairment

T. Fryers

INTRODUCTION

The field commonly called 'mental handicap' is in a most exciting state of ferment. Attitudes have been changing radically and rapidly; vague hopes of better services have given way to expectations and demands, fed by new ideas and new knowledge. A genuine commitment by governments has led to finances being made available even at a time of economic retrenchment.

Concepts of comprehensive, integrated, community-based services, inter-disciplinary team-work, inter-agency management, and the demand for monitoring and evaluation of programmes of prevention, habilitation and care, have located many developments within the domain of public health and the responsibility of the community physician. Increasing acceptance of the philosophy of 'normalisation' as a guide to the provision of care, will naturally be welcomed by community physicians who value their traditional role in promoting the health of the community, and whose professional roots lie in the ecology of health, sickness, disability and disorder in human communities.

The issues discussed in this chapter are related predominantly to the British scene, and fall generally into the two principal areas of Community Medicine practice. Sections I–IV are concerned with investigation of the size and nature of the 'problem', chiefly by epidemiological and related methods; sections V–IX are concerned with promotion of health, that is control of the problem, chiefly through involvement in management of health care and related systems. They tie up at each end, since concepts in epidemiology (I) are equally important for service development, and management information (IX) should be informed by epidemiological methods and support continuing investigation. As with any field of Community Medicine activity, they are bound together and form a satisfactory entity by a common overall objective; the improvement of health (in the widest sense) and the enhancement of life for this client group, their families and the wider community. It is this commitment which gives meaning to the practice, and legitimacy to the existence of Community Physicians.

Names inevitably keep changing to reflect current concepts, and acceptability with parents is as important as scientific precision. 'Mental' is seen to be offensive and promotes confusion with psychiatric illness. 'Handicap' in this use conflicts with current epidemiological terminology. Many terms are in use, world-wide; here I have tried to be consistent with the WHO (1980) terminology, by using 'intellectual impairment' usually, 'learning disabled' where appropriate and 'handicap (due to intellectual impairment)' for the field of professional interest.

CONCEPTS AND CLASSIFICATION: IMPAIRMENT, DISABILITY AND HANDICAP

Terminology relating to abnormality, disfunction and disadvantage has recently been codified by WHO (1980): Impairment is an abnormality of psychological, physiological or anatomical structure or function; disability is restriction of ability to perform activities in the manner or within the range considered normal; handicap is the resulting personal disadvantage which limits individual fulfilment of normal, expected social roles. This is peculiarly appropriate to the field under discussion here, clarifying the relationship between apparently disparate scientific and professional contributions.

Impairment of structure is the main focus of aetiological diagnosis, which is important for primary prevention and helping parents to come to terms with their child's problem. Impairment of function is the main focus of neurological diagnosis, which is important for secondary prevention, limitation of disability and control of common additional impairments such as epilepsy and cerebral palsy.

Disabilities experienced by intellectually impaired people are legion, but bear little relationship to aetiological diagnosis. Epidemiologically, measurement of disability is problematic, but the development of instruments for careful description and classification of specific abilities and disabilities is encouraging exploration of 'syndromes of disability', and offering a clearer focus on individual habilitation needs, based on precise formulations of disabilities of, for example, speech, hearing, vision, mobility and social inter-action.

Handicap is much more difficult to define because it is necessarily situation-specific and individual-specific. It can be classified or compared only in broad descriptive terms, but a clear analysis for each individual of the components of handicap, and the factors which contribute to it, facilitate intervention to diminish it in terms of the inter-personal, social and organisational environment, as well as reducing specific disabilities themselves, even where basic impairments are not susceptible to amelioration.

Handicap as experienced therefore is far more than that determined directly by impairments and disabilities. Family responses to an impaired child, their degree of understanding, how they were told, the child's particular characteristics, may all increase or decrease handicap, as do the responses of others in the community. Ageing is likely to modify these responses, and itself eventually to add other handicapping factors.

Societal response in the provision of services also has positive and negative effects on handicap. Unfortunately, we cannot claim that services have generally aimed to minimise handicap, when many have been deliberately restrictive or punitive in character, and starved of resources of imagination, skill and money. Generally, separation, institutionalisation and psychiatric medicalisation of services have added to the burden of stigma, and precluded stimulating, challenging and habilitating inter-actions in society by which global handicap might be minimised. The picture is more complex because intellectually impaired people often require assistance in developing normal functions and activities, and neglect of positive intervention by others will increase both disabilities and handicap. Epidemiologically we need to be able to relate specific disabilities to preventable factors to allow positive action at an early stage. Early stimulation programmes already demonstrate the possibilities (Cunningham & Sloper, 1984)

In spite of its collective ambiguity, 'handicap' due to intellectual impairment is virtually all we have to designate the group as a whole, to study changes in overall prevalence. A classification based upon intelligence quotients fits rather uneasily into the impairment, disability and handicap system, illustrating the ambiguities and confusions which have characterised their use. Since intellectual function controls the development and application of learning capacity, serious diminution could be considered as either impairment or disability, but the former is probably better. Reduced learning capacity, by limiting the opportunities and effects of inter-action with the outside world, has a global effect upon the individual, physically, mentally and socially. Though 'learning disabled' is a more precise term, it is thus not entirely unreasonable to use measures of intelligence as a proxy, albeit an insufficient one, in defining categories of 'overall handicap'. There are, of course, other reasons, including validity and reliability of measurements, why IQs have fallen into some disrepute among psychologists, but as one of several types of assessment they may yet regain a useful place (Warren, 1977).

There is a further complication. No individual exists alone, and intellectual impairment necessarily imposes special characteristics, problems, challenges and costs upon the family. A humane society will wish to minimise individual handicap and maximise satisfaction in life, but not at the cost of inordinate demands, restriction or damage to others. Accepting the challenge and commitment is not necessarily damaging of course, many have found it life-enhancing, but the community as a whole needs to share the burdens and minimise the restrictions.

To summarise, there may be unalterable impairments leading to unavoidable disabilities, producing inevitable elements of handicap for the individual, but this is overlain by avoidable disabilities and reducable handicaps which are not the necessary sequelae of the impairments, and may even be unrelated directly to them. The objectives of epidemiology and the aims of the service are:

To identify causes and causal processes; to prevent impairment wherever possible.

To study the distribution of specific disabilities in relation to causal factors and to identify disability syndromes: to maximise personal function and minimise disability.

To identify handicapping factors in family, community and services and methods of control: to counter them in order to maximise normal life opportunities and satisfactions, and thereby to minimise handicap; to provide appropriate and sufficient assistance to families of affected people, and to other carers, to minimise their handicaps.

To identify temporal, cultural and environmental variables affecting prevalence: to co-ordinate planning, implementation and evaluation of comprehensive community based care.

Increased clarity of concepts and categories, and better measures have provided community medicine with better tools to do the job.

IMPAIRMENT, AETIOLOGY, DIAGNOSIS

In the last decade, interest in intellectual impairment has increased dramatically among paediatricians. Multi-disciplinary assessment centres or child development centres have multiplied usually from a paediatric base (see Court Report: DHSS, 1976). Specialist paediatric neurologists are now contributing a new precision to diagnosis and assessment following developments in Sweden (Hagberg, 1978; 1980) . Comprehensive early assessment has long had its advocates (Mackay, 1976) but it has not always been accepted that seriously impaired children (or adults) have the same right to thorough investigation as others (Iivanainen, 1981). The relationship of neurological impairments related to learning disability and those related to cerebral palsy and epilepsy are of special current interest both clinically and in research. Approaches are wide ranging and include investigation by EEG (e.g. Gasser et al, 1981), CT Scan (Snyder et al, 1979) and Radiography (Iivanainen, 1981) as well as new methods of clinical examination. Such studies will bring new possibilities for primary and secondary prevention.

Already they have added a new dimension to our understanding of people with mild intellectual impairment. It has usually been considered that few members of this group have demonstrable pathologies seen almost universally in association with severe impairment, and the title 'subcultural' has added vague implications of 'social' causation. It is now clear that almost all such people reveal some degree of neurological impairment when precise techniques of paediatric neurology are applied (Cooper et al, 1979; Iivanainen, 1981). Such impairments are not limited to those with learning disability nor does such finding preclude limitations of genetic endowment and a collage of social disadvantage as contributory factors in poor educational achievement. But the more thorough our understanding of the relationship between genetic endowment, neurological disorder and social environment, the more likely we are to be able to provide helpful interventions, medical, educational or other.

Similarly, there have been widespread developments in medical genetics bringing increased understanding of the genetic contribution to intellectual impairment. With the success of preventive programmes for phenylketonuria and similar disorders, there has been increasing hope of the possibilities of primary prevention. Unfortunately, because almost all genetically determined syndromes are extremely rare, they pose serious difficulties in both measuring their incidence in specific populations, and evaluating screening programmes or other preventive measures. Genetic registers have developed in a number of communities to keep track of vulnerable families and major surveys have identified practical potential for counselling (Van Den Berghe et al, 1981; Linna et al, 1981; Evans, 1972). The one major contribution of chromosome disorders, Down's Syndrome continues to be the subject of much fundamental research, producing more understanding of the long and complicated causative processes involved, but ultimate causes still escape us.

In recent years there have been some claims that the 'fragile X' syndrome is almost as important a contributor to intellectual impairment as Down's. Research results have varied, but it will be interesting to see how many 'unknown' diagnoses this eventually explains (Crawfurd, 1982).

Two environmental factors have gained new prominence as possible causes of intellectual impairment in the last decade. Lead in water, food and air is well documented but its precise relationship to neurological disorder is not established. It may well contribute a little to mild impairment but is probably not important in severe intellectual impairment. More certain in its effects but similarly doubtful in its frequency, is fetal alcohol syndrome. There is no doubt that regular consumption of alcohol through early pregnancy can cause serious brain damage including intellectual impairment. Reports from North America have suggested large numbers of children affected, but others claim never to have seen it in their communities. Patterns of alcohol consumption vary, but other factors are presumably also at work. Even small amounts of alcohol may reduce birth weight and increase vulnerability, and the Royal College of Psychiatrists has recently advised that the only safe practice at present is no alcohol at all, even just before conception! (Anon, 1983).

Another current debate concerns the proportion of children with severe intellectual impairment who can be given a satisfactory diagnosis. Until recently it has generally been claimed that only 30–40% can be given a diagnosis, mostly Down's Syndrome. There is little dispute that this has increased with the number of syndromes identified now running into many hundreds, and with improvements in investigation and assessment. Some claim that the numbers added in any one population with a satisfactory diagnosis are very few because the new syndromes are all rare, and that as many as 50% of severely impaired children in community surveys can still be given no cause (Crawfurd, 1983). However, five total community surveys in Sweden, England and Denmark, one hospital contact survey of 1000 cases in Finland, and one institutional population survey in Belgium have recently identified aetiological diagnoses in 80–90% of children (Gustavson, 1981; Fryers & Mackay, 1979b; Bernsen, 1981; Corbett, 1981; Iivanainen, 1981; Van Den Berghe et al, 1981). Partly the dispute revolves around the use of the words aetiology and diagnosis; it is true that the whole process of causation is not fully understood, but this is particularly true of Down's Syndrome where the ultimate cause is quite unknown, yet all would include it in their list of 'known' causes. It seems likely that, where paediatric assessment facilities are of the highest quality and serve whole populations, over 80% of severely intellectually impaired children can be given a diagnosis with aetiological implications with reasonable confidence.

The dispute also arises from the intrinsic problems of studying such populations and identifying syndromes. Many studies produce only proportions rather than incidence or prevalence data for specific aetiological groups. Sometimes the base population is not known or the study is of an institutional group. There is no doubt wide variation in the balance of causes in different communities; it would be extraordinary if it were not so with such a diversity of processes and factors, all of them rare, and many subject to social, demographic and medical care determinants. Proportions cannot be compared since each is subject to variations in incidence in all other groups, and population frequencies are difficult to establish without very large study populations. Similar standards and criteria for diagnosis are not necessarily applied in different centres, and there remain problems of definition of the category 'severe intellectual impairment', which increase in practice as service provision becomes more flexible. Nevertheless the importance of a change in status for diagnosis in this field should not be minimised. It should give a boost to epidemiological work to establish much needed population frequencies, and even incomplete knowledge of aetiological processes may give genuine opportunities for preventive intervention.

Currently, prevention is having some success though the numbers are mostly very small. Screening for phenylketonuria and similar disorders is now effective nation-wide in Britain and screening for hypothyroidism should soon be equally available, mounted on the same programme. Genetic registers allowing counselling to 'at risk' families and improvements in obstetrical and neonatal care have almost certainly improved the chances, not only of survival, but of undamaged survival for even the smallest of babies. Modern management of Rhesus incompatibility has virtually eliminated kernicterus: hypoglycaemia in the new born should now be recognised and treated (Steiner & Neligan, 1983). Immunisation against measles and rubella generally needs to be tightened up; for pertussis, immunisation has been effectively cleared of causing encephalopathy, and will prevent similar risks from the wild virus (DHSS, 1981a). The prospects for prevention of impairment due to lead, accidents or alcohol are not so good; changing social behaviour on sufficient a scale to have measurable effects has proved difficult with more compelling objectives than these.

For Down's Syndrome, primary prevention becomes less and less tenable as knowledge increases, since it would need to span generations. Amniocentesis and abortion for women 35 years and over may have taken effect in some districts in reducing the numbers born but national notification rates are low and make trends in prevalence at birth difficult to interpret (Weatherall, 1982) Certainly some local data indicate that the dramatic reduction in birth rate in older women during the 1970s significantly reduced the potential of intervention in pregnancy (Fryers & Mackay, 1979a). Most Down's children are now born to younger mothers because there are few others! Ensuring that older women fully understand the risks and contraceptive options available may be a more effective as well as a more acceptable means of reducing numbers.

MEASUREMENT OF DISABILITY

For decades, intelligence tests have been used to classify those with intellectual impairment, direct their placement in services, especially educational services, and provide a ground for expectations of parents and professionals. None of these objectives is wholly fulfilled by conventional IQ scores, though repeated, detailed, professional, culturally appropriate tests may give valuable guidance to the potential and changing potential of an individual, and for simple classification we have had nothing much better. IQs have thus been used virtually to imply global handicap and this they cannot do. Devised to indicate intrinsic learning ability, they are not independent of achievement, determined also by experience, environment and intervention. Specific learning tests have been used less frequently and are less standardised. Test batteries provide a profile rather than a score, more useful for clinical or educational guidance, but less useful for simple classification. In Britain currently, few districts appear to have test results available and categories tend to be assumed from educational placement! IQs do have value if placed in a context of other assessments serving complementary needs (Clark, 1974; Warren, 1977; Gould, 1981).

Recently there have been very encouraging developments in the measurement and epidemiology of disabilities. Broad indication of learning disability by IQ score has never related closely enough to the daily experience of parents and professionals, which largely related to more specific disabilities particularly problems of communication and mobility. There have been many attempts to measure or record in standardised form aspects of behaviour, psychological function and social performance. The American Association on Mental Deficiency, Adaptive Behaviour Scales record coping behaviour in specific areas of development and mal-adaptation, and have been widely used in North America (Grossman, 1973). In Britain the Gunzburg Progress Assessment Charts have been used to identify self-help skills, and aspects of communication, socialisation and occupation (Gunzburg, 1974). The Vineland Social Maturity Scale provides a 'social age' score from a wide range of behaviours and skills and has been used on both sides of the Atlantic largely for research purposes (Doll, 1953). Gould (1981) has briefly reviewed the variety of tests available.

These are the background to recent developments in Britain pioneered by Kushlick with a very simple assessment of three problem areas; continence, ambulence and general behaviour. He derived two broad groups, with constituent sub-groups, of the 'CANs', who were continent, ambulent and exhibited no behaviour disorder, and the 'CAN'Ts' who were incontinent, non-ambulent and showed behaviour disorders (Kushlick et al, 1973). Devised for service planning rather than research, this had the great merit of simplicity and could be used in a standard way by care staff throughout the whole of a community service. This was adapted for use and publication by the National Development Group (DHSS, 1978a). It now includes aspects of communication and additional impairments, and from its use four 'NDG Categories' were derived. This has encouraged positive attitudes towards those with intellectual impairment and a focus on the practical issues of habilitation rather than global problems, by carers and planners. It has also emphasised the need for careful observations, accurate description and validated categories, and other projects have developed this further from a more thorough research base.

One of the most important is Wing's comprehensive Handicaps, Behaviour and Skills Schedule (HBS) which has been used in epidemiological studies of at least four very different communities to assess the total child population in terms of detailed scales of specific abilities and disabilities (Wing, 1981; Bernsen, 1981; Ort & Liepmann, 1981). Results from these surveys have raised important questions about ethnic differences in disability profiles, individual programme planning, defining new syndromes of disability and the possibilities of new parameters for classification. The HBS is essentially a research tool, but Wing has developed from it a small practical schedule for use in service contexts using what had emerged as the most important aspects of mobility, communication and social interaction. The resulting Disability Assessment Schedule (DAS) is being used in several communities as a source of high quality routine data for a total population. Given appropriate personnel with a brief but necessary training, the data are standardised and eminently suitable for micro-computer processing. There are several possible objectives.

(1) They promote clear thinking about specific abilities and disabilities and encourage a more professional approach to care and habilitation.

(2) They may facilitate individual programme planning and monitoring of progress on a standardised record.

(3) They can provide small-scale planning data suitable for initial identification of people with particular patterns of need who may then be personally selected for particular substitute homes, families or other services. They may also be an aid to monitoring the progress of a group and evaluating the provision of care. They may also be useful to guide and monitor re-location of people from the big hospitals in alternative forms of care (Wing, 1983).

(4) They can provide information on the distribution of disabilities in a whole population for more general planning use. It is hoped to monitor changes in the

patterns of need as improved services develop. The information should also be of value in guiding staffing and training.

(5) They may identify new syndromes of disability. Many 'syndromes' in medical use are mere collations of signs and symptoms occurring commonly in association. This could imply common aetiological factors or merely common needs. With disabilities, causal implications are perhaps unlikely, but focussing on common special needs can be invaluable. Autism is an example of a syndrome of disabilities, not implying common causality but allowing special help to be given to a group of children with special problems in common.

(6) Causal hypotheses may be generated. There is accumulating evidence of different patterns of disability, particularly relating to mobility and social interaction, in different ethnic groups in Britain (Wing, 1979b; Akinsola, 1983). Although not yet conclusive, the hypotheses generated deserve further research on bigger populations.

The classical epidemiological problems of definition, classification, standardised measures and reliable recording apply particularly to disability assessment. It is an important development in the epidemiology of intellectual impairment that these difficulties are being seriously tackled, and with some evidence of success. It is also a development which should have immediate practical effects upon the service.

HANDICAP DUE TO SEVERE INTELLECTUAL IMPAIRMENT: CHANGES IN PREVALENCE

The literature on prevalence in the last 20 years has been extensive but difficult to use. Until recently most authors have claimed remarkable consistency in the prevalence of severe intellectual impairment, independent of time and place. This would indeed be remarkable and extremely difficult to explain, in a group so difficult to define consistently, measure accurately and include comprehensively. In a group with such a diversity of specific pathologies and aetiological processes, subject to a multiplicity of genetic, demographic, environmental and medical care factors affecting both incidence and survival, widely divergent findings would be expected.

The concept of incidence is difficult to apply to this group as a whole. Some conditions leading to severe intellectual impairment are present at conception; others arise during fetal life; the hazards of the perinatal period add yet more and there are diminishing additions as childhood progresses. During the whole of this period, relatively high mortality takes its toll. Indeed, the periods of highest incidence tend also to be the periods of highest mortality; early fetal life, the perinatal period and early infancy. Factors affecting either will affect the prevalence of severe intellectual impairment at all subsequent ages. It is complicated further by inevitable delays in ascertainment and designation, so that identified prevalence ratios, particularly at the earliest ages, will be affected by variations in coverage, quality and style of child assessment services (Fryers, 1984a).

Comparison of published prevalence studies is made difficult by frequent absence of criteria for definition and inclusion, estimates of thoroughness of case finding or accuracy of base population figures, and the presentation of figures only for wide age groups (e.g. 0–19 or all ages) which mask cohort variations in incidence, mortality and ascertainment. Even without these difficulties, prevalence ratios in demographically, cultural and environmentally different communities, for different age groups representing different cohorts of conceptions or births, and studied at different times, cannot be compared as they stand.

Recent work has related prevalence ratios for small age groups of children to their years of birth, allowing the confounding variables of place and time to be disentangled (Fryers, 1981, 1984b). This has exploded the myth of consistency and particularly demonstrated significant time trends in prevalence ratios for severe intellectual impairment. The considerable geographical differences in studies related to children born in the same period are to be expected and elucidation of reasons would require large-scale co-operative studies. More importantly, consistent time trends over 20 years reveal a rise from $\simeq 1.5\text{--}4.0/1000$ related to years of birth in the early 1950s, to $\simeq 3.5\text{--}5.5/1000$ related to years of birth in the mid 1960s, with a subsequent fall to $\simeq 2.5\text{--}4.0/1000$ for the mid 1970s. This is shown in general by reliable published data from the developed world, and also specifically by a twenty year study of one community, Salford (Fryers, 1984b). The analysis originally performed in 1978 has been confirmed by subsequent reports of recent prevalence surveys from Bristol, Dumfries and Galloway, Eire and Sheffield (Russell & Hall, 1980; Cunningham, 1981; Mulcahy et al, 1983; Martindale, 1983) whose results have been consistent with the general trend predicted. The general pattern of change is true for Down's Syndrome alone, where general expectation of life from birth has radically changed (Fryers & Mackay, 1979a) and for all others, though not at quite the same times.

The explanation of the increase of prevalence at 'school' ages is almost certainly an increase in survival affecting all or most aetiological groups, due to advances in pre and neo-natal care from the early 1960s (Fryers & Mackay, 1979b). We would expect similar processes throughout the developed world, though not necessarily at exactly the same time.

The more recent decrease in prevalence at 'school' ages is not so easily explained except perhaps in Down's Syndrome. Prevalence at birth of Down's Syndrome has diminished considerably over the past ten years with lower birth rates especially at higher maternal ages (Fryers & Mackay, 1979a) and amniocentesis and abortion have probably added to this more recently. The demographic effect could be reversed in the future. The reduction in numbers of non-Down's children with severe intellectual impairment is probably the product of many factors, for example; specific preventive programmes, improved antenatal and perinatal care and fewer high risk pregnancies. A few severely impaired children, having received effective stimulation and habilitation may have moved from the severe category, but none of these can account for more than very small numbers in any one community. We must assume that mortality is continuing to fall so that decreasing prevalence at school ages must reflect real decreases in prevalence at birth and/or incidence of disorders leading to severe intellectual impairment. Perhaps only a prospective study in a very large population would produce the precise information we need.

Survival has also increased at all subsequent ages and this has a cumulative effect on prevalence ratios in older age groups. The age structure of the severely intellectually impaired population has been changing very significantly over the last 20 years. In most developed communities there are now likely to be three to four times as many severely impaired adults as children. The cohort which experienced the dramatic increase in survival (at the same time as high birth rates in general) is now a young adult group putting great pressure on the services for adults. Prevalence ratios for this cohort are not uncommonly $\simeq 5.0/1000$, and they will continue to benefit from increased life expectancy as they move through the age groups over the next 40 or 50 years. Already there have been significant increases in age groups over 45 years. Reliable data are scarce, but from recent studies we might currently expect $> 2.0/1000$ at 45–54 years, $\simeq 2/1000$ at 55–64 years and $> 1/1000$ at 65–74 years (Innes et al, 1978; Russell & Hall, 1980; Cunningham, 1981; Fryers, 1982, 1984a; Mulcahy et al, 1983). Problems of ageing added to those of severe intellectual impairment and a lifetime's experience of poor services are becoming ever more common. Only recently has this received much attention (Sweeney & Wilson, 1979; Anglin, 1981). Many are in long-stay hospitals, which also include many with milder degrees of intellectual impairment whose life expectancy will be essentially that of the general population.

The implications of this change in age structure are important for community medicine. The field is largely concerned with adults rather than children. The paediatric interest may need to be matched by the interest of the geriatrician and psychogeriatrician. The great advances in education for children with severe intellectual impairment in the last ten years will need continuing adaptation to the changing context. Preparing a severely impaired child and his family for a life expectancy of 50 years or more requires a different perspective, but neither should habilitation and learning stop at 19. The metamorphosis of 'adult training centres' to 'social education centres' is slow, but day provision, whether educational, social, occupational or other in objectives, is inadequate in serving both numbers and needs. Increased life expectancy also has profound implications for residential care, since most severely impaired people will now outlive their parents and will eventually require a substitute home. A large proportion of older severely impaired people are in the large hospitals and we cannot predict the particular characteristics and needs of their successors who do not experience prolonged institutional care, but the ageing of current residents adds to the difficulties of re-location in community based care. Community Medicine is necessarily involved with Social Service Departments in resolving these difficulties.

Another surprising aspect of received epidemiological wisdom is the apparent lack of social class gradient in severe intellectual impairment. Mild intellectual impairment has been predominantly located in 'lower' occupational social classes and associated with elements of deprivation. Most measures of morbidity and mortality in developed communities favour occupational classes one and two (Townsend & Davidson, 1982). The varied nature of severe intellectual impairment might well produce some gradient, as many environmental factors affect processes of aetiology and mortality, though causal implications would be very different from the mild group. Some recent work has challenged the conventional view. A major thorough survey of the Mannheim population revealed marked occupational class differences for severe intellectual impairment (Cooper et al, 1979). Approaching from a different angle, work in Sheffield, Cardiff and Bristol have related prevalence to characteristics of small urban communities (Martindale, 1980; Russell & Hall, 1980; Humphreys et al, 1981). These pose methodological problems of area definition, relationship to occupational classification, accurate denominators and variations with small numbers, but each case suggested that severe impairment is more common in the areas of 'low social class'. Twenty years data from the Salford Register confirm neither Cooper's findings nor the small area analyses. Distributions of disability assessment data revealed remarkably similar patterns in three small areas chosen for their social diversity.

The hypothesis is advanced that a social class distribution in incidence of aetiologies leading to severe intellectual impairment has usually been masked by a similar social class distribution of mortality in those conditions which feature severe intellectual impairment, thus producing even distribution of prevalence ratios after the first few years of life. As early mortality diminishes, the social class gradient of causes will be increasingly revealed. Current research findings are equivocal and further work is needed not merely to test hypotheses, but to clarify important implications regarding factors affecting aetiologies, determining disabilities and increasing total handicap (Cooper & Lackus, 1981).

In summary the knowledge that the prevalence of severe intellectual impairment varies from place to place and consistently with time has profound implications for planning. There is no single prevalence ratio to provide crude guidance for everybody, and this is now officially recognised (DHSS, 1980). On the other hand, the common experience of developed communities over the last 20 years may provide reasonable prediction of the likely age-specific or cohort prevalence ratios if the planning population is large enough (Fryers, 1984b). Even this is probably not as useful as it sounds; information needs to be far more subtle than this if planning is worth doing. Local variations in aetiologies, patterns of disability, birth cohort and small area prevalence, affect prevention and new patterns of care, and require relatively sophisticated information services, such as registers, discussed later (Körner, 1983). Like other epidemiological information, prevalence statistics only have meaning when related to specified small age groups, specified times and specified populations.

PHILOSOPHY OF CARE; NORMALISATION

Over the last decade there has been increasing acceptance amongst professionals of the philosophy of 'normalisation'. The ideas are not new but aggressive promotion of normalisation as an alternative to convention and orthodoxy, is now giving way to demands that 'abnormal' traditional patterns of care must justify any continued existence.

Several factors have encouraged this. Increased involvement of parents, parent associations and other voluntary bodies has challenged common assumptions and expectations, and the worst of professionalism. The 'campaign' element of public health tradition has been taken up by such bodies as MIND, and the Campaign for Mentally Handicapped People, backed by increasing numbers of professionals. The diversity of professional involvement has increased and the dominance of doctors reduced, as total subsumption under 'health care' has given way to genuine education and social services responsibility for non-medical needs (Mittler, 1979).

The advocacy and 'patients rights' movements have also played a part, particularly in North America (Wolfensberger & Zanha, 1973). Listening to parents has moved to working with parents and listening to intellectually impaired people themselves (Williams & Shoultz, 1982). A better understanding of the potential of even severely impaired people to develop, grow, mature and exercise choice, to enjoy a range of relationships and environments and to contribute something to others, should not raise unrealistic expectations, but should inform the objectives of education, support and care.

Comprehensive community based habilitation and care is a worldwide movement promoted by WHO, UNICEF, and Rehabilitation International. 'Community' is conceived in human rather than administrative terms, and there are problems in applying such ideas to major urban centres, though British health districts and social service divisions usually represent reasonable communities. Comprehensive community based care proposes that services should generally be local and accessible to all, co-ordinated, meeting special needs within generic services and primary care based, supported by specialists. As an organisational concept this has provided a fertile context for the philosophy of normalisation to develop.

Normalisation was succinctly summarised by Wolfensberger (1972) as 'The utilisation of culturally valued means in order to establish and/or maintain personal behaviours, experiences and characteristics that are culturally normative or valued'. It firstly accords to intellectually impaired people, the same human value and rights as others. They are developing people with a wide range of abilities, preferences and needs, and should be involved in decisions affecting their lives wherever possible. They should be helped to participate in those activities and experiences which give value in our society. Within the variety of normal life, they should be encouraged to enjoy as wide a range as possible of experiences, opportunities, relationships and choices. They should not usually be segregated from the rest of the community, and should wherever possible be supported in their own homes, whatever form these take. Financial support should ideally be individual and allowing choice. Special needs should usually be met by the generic education, employment, housing, social and health services. Where specialist care is required, it should be the least restrictive form possible, and objectives should always include maximising independence, adoption of normally valued lifestyles, and participation in normal social networks (Nirje, 1970).

It must be emphasised that 'normalisation' is a philosophy of care, has a humanitarian ideological basis, and can provide principles and a framework within which services may be developed, but is not a plan, a system or a set of rules. It is extremely important however, as an ideal to aim for, and a guide at every stage of planning, running and evaluating services (O'Brien, 1981).

Although this philosophy has gained widespread acceptance there are those who cannot reconcile it with their personal or professional approaches and practices. Work is still needed therefore, to share it with care professionals, planners and managers, members of authorities and the general public. It requires exposure to good practices, clear demonstration that theoretically humane approaches actually achieve better and more satisfying lifestyles for intellectually impaired people. It also needs demonstrating that they can be contained within reasonable costs for health and social services, and do not threaten improvements for other needful groups. The public health 'campaign' is still needed to promote positive attitudes to life and health in the widest sense, and the rights of individuals.

INTER-PROFESSIONAL CO-OPERATION AND CHANGING ROLES

There is a fundamental dilemma in implementing 'normalisation' in service delivery, in balancing integration at risk of neglect, with special provision at risk of alienation and stigma. The most important specialist roles therefore, are advocacy and negotiation, but these require a depth of experience not readily gained in generic services. The current scene is complex and confusing. The field characteristically attracts a multiplicity of professional involvement. For new styles of services new styles of work are required. Doctors have been by training and tradition weak on inter-disciplinary co-operation essential in this field. They can claim only partial knowledge, experience and skills which do not necessarily feature large in the total perspective of care. The influence of psychiatrists has diminished with loss of administrative power and shortage of satisfactory recruits. Paediatricians have become more involved and paediatric neurology is developing as a sub-speciality. Current management issues have required increasing involvement of Community Physicians, but shortage of experienced people with appropriate skills limits their current contribution. Clinical medical officers often have wide 'clinical' experience, but seldom assume managerial roles. The specialist medical contribution to the field is thus diverse and divided and some integration of roles might be more efficient and effective in serving clients (Tyne, 1981). There are overlapping roles with clinical psychologists who now feature prominently in assessment, therapy, evaluation, and promotion of community based care. Nursing in mental handicap has also been changing. Many already exercise a wide range of care, support and habilitation skills and welcome the opportunity to work in community based services, either in domestic style residential care settings or in providing domiciliary support. Others value their association with nursing traditions and some find it difficult to change. They constitute the greatest resource of manpower with experience and commitment but there has been relatively little progress towards training a new profession of care workers envisaged by the Jay Committee (DHSS, 1979) of which the nurses would form the principle constituent. There is progress however, in the development of community nursing, employment of nurses in social services facilities and establishment of joint-agency community mental handicap teams (Hall & Russell, 1980).

Social work in Britain largely abandoned mental health specialisms after the establishment of generic social work departments in 1971. This 'integrated' service however, diverted experienced personnel and provided little opportunity for new recruits to gain experience. Recently there has been a reversal of this process with reversion to specialist social workers in both mental illness and mental handicap.

Lessons could be drawn from the incorporation of special education into the general system also in 1971, where special facilities were retained within a generic agency, guaranteeing all learning disabled children similar standards of provision and staffing as others, plus special skills and special resources (Warnock Report, DHSS, 1978b). Further integration — into ordinary schools — is tentative in Britain, but progressing in a very personalised way (Gottlieb, 1981). There is also some progress towards using ordinary facilities in further education, training, and employment (Rowan, 1980). However, adult training centres remain the principle service and staff are generally aware of the need to improve quality and move towards more appropriate educational and occupational models (Whelan & Speake, 1977). They also need to work more closely with psychotherapists, occupational therapists, speech therapists and others contributing to the habilitation and re-habilitation of adults with intellectual impairment.

This plethora of professions, this diversity of interests, this richness of resources requires careful co-ordination if it is to be effective and efficient. Co-operation is not always easy and is hindered by separate training as well as separate structures. The new context in which professionals are being asked to work has profound implications for recruitment and training (Mittler, 1979). In particular all professions need to understand the wider context of colleagues with quite different orientations, how to work in teams, which is barely acknowledged in current curriculae, and how to work with parents (Mittler & McConachie, 1983).

The organisational structures in which people work together are very much the concern of community medicine and three levels of team-work are currently uneasily co-existing in this field.

At a senior level, Joint Care Planning Teams (JCPT) have made much progress since 1974 in co-ordinating health and social service plans, but the achievement of comprehensive community based care will require further development towards joint management teams. This is discussed in detail later.

Multiprofessional District Handicap Teams (DHT) were proposed in the Court Report (DHSS, 1976) in association with Child Development Centres to be concerned with assessment, co-ordination of treatment and guidance to parents and other professionals in respect of *all* disabled children. They have been established in some districts but their extensive brief for a whole district population affects their ability to provide personal support and comprehensive advice for everyone. 'Key workers' for specific families have not often been appointed (Plank, 1982).

The National Development Group proposed Community Mental Handicap Teams (CMHT) to work personally and locally with families or individuals needing a more substantial programme of help and support (Mittler & Simon, 1978). The core of the team being a community nurse and a social worker, the proposal came at an opportune time for both professions, and has probably avoided much of the inherent conflict of roles in domiciliary work. Many are now working, with other professional members varying. They generally cover much smaller populations than a whole district and might theoretically work several to a District Handicap Team, but this seldom happens. They may thus lack expertise in other problems also common amongst intellectually impaired people, and may lack the support of senior colleagues in either principle agency. Without this they may find it no less difficult to negotiate access to generic services than clients or parents sometimes experience with general medical and dental practitioners, hospital departments, social security, employment and housing agencies. Yet it is through direct personal contact of this sort that the personnel of generic services are likely to change restrictive attitudes and practices. Plank (1982) has reviewed both DHTs and CMHTs.

In general, currently, the picture is very messy and unsatisfactory. There is a wealth of ideas and genuine commitment, and team work skills are slowly being learned — usually by experience. But co-ordination of all these developments in each district is generally lacking in the absence of an overall structure for the district service. The promotion of inter-disciplinary and inter-agency teams and team-work skills, their co-ordination and support, and the creation of an organisational structure which can satisfactorily manage the district service, are primary objectives and essential challenges for community medicine. If community physicians do not respond, who will?

CHANGES IN SERVICE STRUCTURES

There are two linked major issues currently exercising the minds of service planners in the field of intellectual impairment: the 'run down' of the hospitals and the general transfer of responsibility for care from 'health' to 'social services'. The future of the old institutions has been discussed for decades. Twenty years ago some local authority health departments reviewed their own hospital residents and brought many out into hostels or other accommodation (Susser, 1968). Most were competent mildly impaired people who did a lot of the work and needed little care. Relatively few similar people were recruited to the hospital populations to replace them, leaving hospitals with mostly highly dependent residents requiring higher staffing levels. More recently many hospitals, local health authorities and social services departments have tried to relocate residents either in hostel type accommodation favoured by earlier policies, or small group accommodation of domestic scale and style more consistent with normalisation. The public scandal about conditions inside some hospitals have helped to promote improved standards of care and alternative provision, but there are still hospitals and districts where relatively little movement has taken place.

Gradual run down of the hospitals has been a matter of national policy for a long time, and strong directives have been issued to remove children (DHSS, 1971). 'Care in the Community' (DHSS, 1981b) proposals are backed by extra finance but the larger hospitals include many people with serious multiple disabilities but a considerable life expectancy, and the process may be very extended in the absence of comprehensive plans for relocation. Some have argued that the only guarantee is to put dates on the closure of each hospital and to plan accordingly. Very recently the Government has required from District Health Authorities plans for closure of hospitals and this is a new step in national policy adding political and bureaucratic pressure to humanitarian motivation to change the nature of the service. At least one Authority has scheduled the closure of its large hospital by June 1986 (Exeter, 1983).

There are, however, many problems in fulfilling these good intentions. The most important is simply the dearth of satisfactory alternatives which genuinely offer a better lifestyle and better standards of care, on the scale that is required. Some health and social service authorities do not yet appear committed to comprehensive local provision or the principles of normalisation. But the outstanding reason is one of finance. Hospital and revenue costs are tied up within centrally funded health service budgets but alternatives in the community based service should be mostly in locally funded social services budgets. Appointed Health Authorities are more subject to government policy, whim or interference; elected Local Authorities more subject to local political control. Transfer of funds from one to the other is immensely problematic but currently there are imaginative attempts to do it. Joint funding schemes have gained ground by which the health service fund projects under social services jurisdiction, especially since recent extension of the period before the latter must pick up the cost. In some cases it is now virtually permanent funding. The government discussion document 'Care in the Community' (DHSS, 1981) and subsequent responses and decisions have paved the way to more effective transfer, but senior staff on both sides vary in their willingness to make new mechanisms work. It may be necessary in some districts for the NHS to create the new-style service within its own resources, as a first step. There are other possibilities: several voluntary bodies are providing substitute homes, day care or even domiciliary support services. Funding from the NHS may be easier but co-ordination of overall planning, administration and evaluation may become even more difficult. Health Authorities may provide alternative homes in ordinary housing, preferably through housing associations or authorities, transferring staff and funds with each group of clients. In general avoidance of the NHS or Social Services *owning* the property gives more flexibility and fewer finance problems.

The larger hospitals still contain large numbers from many districts some outwith the region. Liaison problems are considerable, especially as each hospital is managed by a single district health authority. Relocation of residents must take account of those with no obvious community of origin, or who after years of establishing contacts with the local community, would choose to settle there. Accepting people in excess of original complements should be recognised in district allocation of resources and this argues for regional involvement in managing the run down of the big hospitals.

The numbers of people with severe intellectual impairment from each district are manageable in planning terms once information is available. The sticking point for many professionals and planners appears to be people with profound impairment and multiple disabilities, yet these are so few in any one district, they should pose no great problem. Some will already be with their parents at home. Certainly arguments about this extreme end of the spectrum of dependency should not inhibit or delay the general movement forward of the relocation programme.

Problems of practice and principle arise with older and ageing residents who have lived in the hospital for decades. Should we require them to change all they know and how do we make genuine choices available to them? Yet unless alternatives are provided for them, the hospitals, and their funds, will remain. One way is for such people to move out with staff they know.

The re-deployment of hospital staff is a general issue of importance, but nurses who wish to stay in hospital service will have a considerable future yet. Perhaps a more important problem is maintaining morale and improving quality of care in progressively diminishing institutions, whilst giving priority to developing a new service. Many other workers are also affected and local employment must be taken into account when seeking alternative uses for hospital sites.

One thing is clear: there are ways of accomplishing the desired end if the will and imagination are there. Community Medicine should see the difficulties as problems to be overcome, not reasons for delay.

DISTRICT MANAGEMENT OF COMMUNITY BASED SERVICES

Planning, implementation, monitoring and evaluation of district services for intellectually impaired people necessarily involve the District Health Authority and the Local Authority Department of Social Services. They also need local education, housing and employment agencies, parent and voluntary groups. Within the NHS their co-ordination is primarily a task for community medicine.

The goal of comprehensive community based services emphasises the complementary roles of each agency and the overlap of current provision. They share common interests in the promotion of good practice, avoiding waste and evaluating all forms of care. The enhanced potential of joint funding requires close working at a senior level, and the progressive transfer of primary (but not exclusive) responsibility for district services to Social Services must be done together.

Since the 1974 reorganisation of the NHS, Joint Care Planning Teams have gained in experience and confidence in this as in other fields. However, they have often been unable to handle major issues because of inadequate delegation within either authority, and because staff of sufficient seniority, particularly from Social Services, were not fully involved. The pressures towards a new style of service, new responsibilities and their fiscal implications, have forced district personnel to consider much more powerful unified management structures. Generally speaking, there are four main options. Firstly, the NHS might manage the whole service. The main advantages are the nature of NHS funding and the presence in the health service of the largest body of trained, experienced and committed care staff. The disadvantages are, perhaps, less concrete but more persuasive. The NHS cannot generally claim to perform very well in the fields of disability; it is happier with illness models than disability models. Responsibility for substitute homes rather than 'hospitals', domiciliary family support rather than 'nurses', and habilitation rather than 'treatment' would rest uneasily on the bureaucracy and would have to incorporate similar facilities and personnel already provided by local authorities and voluntary bodies. If we truly had a national 'health' service rather than almost exclusively a national 'illness' service, such problems might not arise, but the reality seems to be that hospital type institutions and psychiatric medicalisation of learning disability have tended to separate, alienate and stigmatise. Of course, it is also possible for any other specialist or segregated care to have the same effects.

The second option is for Social Services Departments to manage the service with health and others providing help to individuals as required. This is consistent with long term national policy and movements towards integration into generic services. It emphasises the community base and local involvement and control. Disadvantages are several. New developments are difficult to finance out of local revenue, and transfer of national funds with strings attached is not favoured by local politicians or officers. Those committed to developing a humanitarian and effective service for intellectually impaired people are understandably unwilling to leave it to local political whim. Experienced health personnel in this position do not necessarily trust social services personnel to have the same knowledge or commitment and the social services case often lacks weight because of the dearth of experienced specialist personnel, though this is now improving.

The third option is for an agreed division of clients into two groups: those with predominantly 'health' needs and those with merely 'care' needs. Few people with experience of intellectually impaired people themselves would consider this remotely tenable. It is not possible to categorise people in this way except for a very few extreme examples. The common needs of intellectually impaired people of all ages and types are for health, education, social and employment services at appropriate times and in appropriate ways.

The fourth option is some form of joint district management structure between health and social services, incorporating also other interested bodies such as education, housing, employment, voluntary bodies and parents. Although most districts have probably not yet decided on the option they prefer, there is some general feeling that this is virtually the only viable one, at least as an interim measure before local social services are able properly to accept full responsibility. Many different forms are possible, but its main disadvantage may well be that it requires skill, flexibility, courage and imagination in management, qualities not always evident. It should be a specific contribution of community medicine to devise, negotiate and establish new management structures to solve new problems (Eskin, 1981).

It is on this basis that Sheffield District Health Authority and Sheffield Metropolitan District Council have accepted the recommendations of a working party of their Joint Consultative Committee (JCC) to create a joint team of officers for an interim period of probably 10 years, with the strategic aim of creating a unified service at the earliest opportunity, ultimately to be administered by the Local Authority with an input of medical, nursing and other support services as appropriate by the Health Authority (Sheffield, 1981). They are currently implementing their plan to form immediately a joint management structure to plan a single, unified, comprehensive, district service. Sheffield's proposals are particularly important since they derive from a very special recent experience. The Sheffield Development Project was a major attempt to implement, test and demonstrate a new pattern of community based services informed by similar thinking to that behind the 1971 White Paper, 'Better Services for the Mentally Handicapped'. An Evaluation Research Group was established which produced a series of 13 reports commenting positively and negatively on specific facilities (ERG, 1977–1981). The overall evaluation was constructive but highly critical of management arrangements, reporting ultimately that Sheffield 'entered the 1980s without even a reasonably well co-ordinated service, let alone an integrated one', and 'even the necessity for both the special co-ordinating committee (at member level) and the special executive working group (at senior officer level) to ensure that development project funds were spent responsibly, did not lead in Sheffield to a satisfactory delivery system, as we have seen. This was not a truly joint structure and the two separate systems were left almost completely free to go their separate ways.' They concluded that a single service was 'an absolute prerequisite for any significant improvement in services' (Heron, 1982; Heron & Myers, 1983).

A unified service is no new idea. There were strong movements towards it in a few Local Authority health departments 10 years before NHS re-organisation (Susser, 1968). In 1959 Denmark (with a population similar to a NHS Region!) had established a 'national mental handicap service' with a central authority concerned with all aspects of care. It proved an effective strategy for concentrating resources and effort into developing new services over a 20 year period. Concern about separateness led to devolution in 1980 to generic local authorities but with national and regional advisory bodies (see Heron & Myers, 1983). In the United States in 1970, local co-operation between parents and professionals led to a single service through the Eastern Nebraska Community Office of Retardation (ENCOR). After a decade of development, and in spite of many difficulties, ENCOR continues to gain respect and influence developments elsewhere (Thomas et al, 1978; Wing, 1982).

In the last few years several districts in Britain have formulated proposals for some variety of co-operative or joint planning and management. Newcastle (1980) proposed a 'management partnership'. Guys District (1981) sees a limited life for a joint structure, probably 10 years, and has therefore framed its proposals as a 'project', managed by a project team, not unlike Cardiff's NIMROD on a smaller scale

(Mathieson & Blunden, 1980). Staffed and financed from both health and social services, a team to be based in each social services department of the two Local Authorities concerned, would report to the district JCC. NIMROD has also influenced similar developments in joint management in the Isle of Wight. Wessex and North West Regional Health Authorities have published regional 'guidelines' which encourage districts to move towards joint management in one form or another, without imposing a single pattern, since local circumstances and personnel vary, and joint management structures can only work where those involved are committed to their success (Wessex, 1981; NWRHA, 1982). Relationships within a single management team must be negotiated and worked at in the context of firm commitments. The All Wales Working Party Report (1982) also eschewed a blueprint for planning and management arrangements at county level. Firmer guidance on structures might have helped, but it did propose that social service authorities should take the lead in preparing and submitting plans for comprehensive services. It also emphasised the 'exceptional managerial skill required' for developing the new service, implying some unification of service managements.

Many other districts are working along the same lines, facing conflicting demands and expectations and philosophies, varying degrees of ignorance and apathy, and problems of professional and personal relationships, all of which affect the degree to which co-operative management can be brought about. It is a considerable challenge to managerial, particularly interpersonal skills, and the special contribution of the Community Physician is crucial: understanding of organisations and social structures, knowledge of social as well as health services, responsibility for a whole population, concern with promotion of health, information skills. It is essential that community medicine takes the lead in devising local strategies and structures to achieve joint planning and management, and implement comprehensive community based care. The experience will not be without application to other services.

MEASURING PERFORMANCE: MANAGEMENT INFORMATION

Heron & Myers (1983) succinctly distinguish assessment, evaluation, monitoring and accountability. Assessment is best applied to abilities, skills and achievements of individuals. Descriptive, normative or formative evaluation is the measurement of effectiveness and efficiency of organisational methods of service delivery, to improve them. Monitoring generates information on the performance of a service system, in terms of its policies and objectives. Accountability is the broad concern with ensuring proper use of resources, including audit. Assessment has already been discussed in relation to measuring disability. The other three have specific community medicine connotations and in each there has been important developments in the field of intellectual impairment.

The most important example of descriptive evaluation of a district complex of services is the Sheffield study already alluded to. A brief summary was written up by Heron (1982) and the study set in a broader context by Heron & Myers (1983), but those concerned with planning district services should take the trouble to read the original reports, for the many practical details they comprehend (ERG, 1977–1981). There have been many other studies of services: (e.g. Heron et al, 1981), perhaps the best guide is an important review from the King's Fund, 'People First' (Ward, 1982).

Community Physicians should be able to offer new services the initiative, expertise and facilities for at least descriptive evaluation, but it is hoped that they may go considerably further. To help them, there have been several developments in normative evaluation. The All-Wales Working Party on Services for Mentally Handicapped People (1982) endorsed the 'check-list' approach following the lead of the National Development Group whose 'check-list of standards for improving the quality of services for intellectually impaired people' is thorough and comprehensive (DHSS, 1980b). These are not research instruments, but do require time and serious effort to apply properly.

Even more comprehensive and demanding is the package, 'Programme Analysis of Service Systems' (PASS), (Wolfensberger & Glenn, 1975). Its normative principles are derived from the philosophy of normalisation, and will raise staff awareness of standards and styles of care. For measuring service development it is not fully validated, but it has exciting possibilities for application in a British context (Kuh, 1978).

Community Physicians should ensure that evaluation procedures are built into any new plan. Descriptive and normative elements should ideally be complemented by formative elements in which principles, objectives and measures are agreed at the outset between personnel delivering the service and those evaluating it. The best known example in Britain is in the context of the NIMROD project, providing a comprehensive service to a population of 60 000 in Cardiff (Welsh Office, 1978; Mathieson & Blunden, 1980). Experience from NIMROD can help district plans elsewhere, but comparable procedures are needed in every district.

Evaluation overlaps with monitoring, and information systems have also seen important recent developments. A few 'mental handicap registers' have existed for many years. The Salford Register has collected data continuously for 23 years, the Wessex Register for slightly less and that in Sheffield from the early 1970s, as part of the Development Project. These Registers generally combine service monitoring and management information with research facilities. They have produced considerable literature relating to the epidemiology of intellectual impairment and the evaluation of services.

The movement towards comprehensive community based services has created a demand for accurate local information for planning and evaluation. It has been realised that data from national or other district sources are inappropriate to the style of planning required. It is insufficient to plan from the top, the provision of staff, systems and facilities. The planning process has to take account of a wide range of individual and changing needs, changing and merging professional roles, varying patterns of work, views and choices of clients, families and care staff, the need to negotiate inter-agency and inter-professional co-operation, and the need to build evaluation into any programme. Many social services departments and health districts want to know who is intellectually impaired in the district, where they are and what they are like, so that they can plan for particular people. They also wish to monitor the progress of service development and have seen registers as serving these needs comprehensively for a community-based service.

These registers are necessarily collaborative, and encompass data input and information output for both principle authorities. They can monitor the movement of people from the large institutions to alternative accommodation, and mostly incorporate some form of disability assessment. Quite a number use versions of the 'Kushlick form' (Kushlick et al, 1973; DHSS, 1978), the Wing DAS described earlier, or schedules of their own devising. Registers are generally intended to serve local care providers with immediate individual information, as well as managers with grouped information and this has favoured the use of micro-computers, and an interactive system. Several systems are being developed but the most advanced package is at the Westminster Hospital (Farmer & Rohde, 1982).

Few encompass research objectives or aetiological data from paediatric sources. They have sometimes lacked epidemiological oversight and have not used standard categories which facilitate comparison of statistical output. Some have been difficult to set up well, when the experience of others was not readily obtained. Other districts are contemplating setting up a Register and a recent publication attempts to guide them as to satisfactory conditions, data most likely to be collectable and of use, and the ways in which standardisation of procedures may facilitate their development and increase their value (Fryers, 1983). Research is now in progress (Cubbon, 1983) to evaluate registers themselves.

Accountability includes responsibility for best use of resources, but detailed costings of service elements are rarely available. Gross (1981) clarified some of the inherent difficulties, pointing out the varieties of cost reporting approaches which need to be specified to be understood. Cost benefit studies have appeared for some preventive programmes (e.g. Sardharwalla, 1979) and cost effectiveness studies for a few elements of care (e.g. Gross, 1977; Yates, 1977). Identifying units of care or service is problematic (Bowers & Bowers, 1976) but more studies like that of Vinni et al (1981) in Mental Illness would be a helpful start.

A recent report from the Department of the Environment Audit Inspectorate (1983) researched 'value for money in the care of mentally handicapped people by local authority Social Services Departments'. This will be a useful contribution, but it also reveals how difficult it is to avoid over-simplification and contentious or out-dated assumptions. It makes clear many gaps in financial information and the need for joint management to maximise cost efficiency. It comments on the wide disparity in local authority spending found also by Moores & Barrett (1976).

The Audit Inspectorate does not appear to have considered savings deriving from improved development of individuals to minimise future dependency. Conley (1973) looked also at the costs of ignoring this in the USA; Moores (1979) has commented 'If, as a society, we continue to ignore the latent ability of mentally handicapped individuals, they will continue in adulthood to represent, to an unnecessary degree, a financial burden to the community in terms of services required'. Better services need also to be seen as a positive investment.

REFERENCES

Akinsola H 1983 Severely mentally handicapped children in Manchester. Unpublished MSc Dissertation, University of Manchester
All Wales Working Party 1982 Report on services for mentally handicapped people. Welsh Office, Cardiff
Anglin B 1981 They never asked for help. Help the Aged and Metro Toronto Assoc. for the Mentally Retarded. Toronto.
Anon 1983 Alcohol and the foetus — is zero the only option? Lancet 26 March 682–683

Bernsen A H 1981 Handicaps, skills and behaviour of mentally retarded children: an epidemiological research method. In: Cooper B (ed) Assessing the handicaps and needs of mentally retarded children. Academic Press, London

Bowers G, Bowers M R 1976 The elusive unit of service. Project Share, Washington DC

Clark D 1974 Psychological assessment in mental subnormality. In: Clarke & Clarke (eds) Mental deficiency: the changing outlook. Methuen, London

Conley R 1973 The economics of mental retardation. Johns Hopkins University Press

Cooper B, Liepmann M C, Marker K R, Schieber P M 1979 Definition of severe mental retardation in school-age children: findings of an epidemiological study. Social Psychiatry 14: 197–205

Cooper B, Lackus B 1984 The social-class background of mentally retarded children. A study in Mannheim. Social Psychiatry 19: 3–12

Corbett J 1981 Prevention of mental retardation. In: Cooper B (ed) Assessing the handicaps and needs of mentally retarded children. Academic Press, London

Crawfurd M D'A 1982 Severe mental handicap: pathogenesis, treament and prevention. British Medical Journal 285: 762–766

Crawfurd M D'A, Gibbs D A, Watts R W E 1982 Advances in the treatment of inborn errors of metabolism. Wiley, London

Cubbon J 1983 Personal communication

Cunningham C, Sloper P 1984 Early intervention for the mentally handicapped child. In: Croft M (ed) Tredgold's mental retardation (13th edn). Baillière and Tindall, London

Cunningham M A 1981 A survey of mental handicap in Dumfries and Galloway: A study of needs. Dumfries and Galloway Health Board, Dumfries

Department of the Environment 1983 Social services: Care of mentally handicapped people. HMSO, London

DHSS 1971 Better services for the mentally handicapped. Cmnd. 4683. HMSO, London

DHSS 1976 Fit for the future. Report of the committee on child health services (Court Report). HMSO, London

DHSS 1978b The Warnock Report. Special Educational Needs. Report of the committee of enquiry into the education of handicapped children and young people. Cmnd. 7212. HMSO, London

DHSS 1978c Facilities and services of mental illness and mental handicap hospitals in England, 1975. HMSO, London

DHSS 1979 Report of the committee of enquiry into mental handicap nursing and care (Jay Committee). HMSO, London

DHSS 1980a Mental handicap: Progress, problems and priorities. HMSO, London

DHSS 1981a Pertussis Report. DHSS, London

DHSS 1981b Care in the Community. Consultative document. DHSS, London

Doll E A 1953 The measurement of social competence. A manual for the Vineland social maturity scale. Educational Publishers, Minneapolis

ERG 1977–1981 Reports 1–13 of the Sheffield development project evaluation research group. University of Sheffield

Eskin F 1981 (ed) Teamwork in the NHS. Occ. Papers 4. Unit for continuing education, Department of Community, University of Manchester

Evans H J 1977 Chromosome anomalies among live births. Journal of Medical Genetics 14: 309–312

Exeter 1983 New local services for mentally handicapped peoples: A plan for implementation by 1986: Exeter District Health Authority

Farmer R, Rohde J 1983 A register of mentally handicapped individuals using a micro-computer. Journal of Mental Deficiency Research 27(4): 255–274

Fryers T 1981 Measuring trends in the prevalence and distribution of severe mental retardation. In: Cooper B (ed) Assessing the handicaps and needs of mentally retarded children. Academic Press, London

Fryers T 1983 Altere schwer geistig behinderte Erwachsene: Die Grosse de Problems, in Alterwerden von Menschen mit geistiger Behinderung. Bericht des Internationalen Workshops 1981. Band 7. Grosse Schriftenreihe. Marburg/Lahn

Fryers T 1983 Standardisation of district mental handicap registers. Association of Professions for Mentally Handicapped People. King's Fund Centre, London

Fryers T 1984a Handicap due to intellectual impairment. In: Holland W, Detels R & Knox G (eds) Oxford Textbook of Public Health. Oxford University Press, London

Fryers T 1984b Epidemiology of severe intellectual impairment: Dynamics of prevalence. Academic Press, London

Fryers T, Mackay R I 1979a Down's Syndrome–a 17 year study: prevalence at birth, mortality and survival 1961–1977. Early Human Development 3: 29–41

Fryers T, Mackay R I 1979b The epidemiology of severe mental handicap. Early Human Development 3: 277–294

Gasser T H, Verleger R, Mocks J, Bacher P, Lederer W M 1981 The EEG Patterns of mildly retarded children: clinical and quantitative findings. In: Cooper B (ed) Assessing the handicaps and needs of mentally retarded children. Academic Press, London

Gottlieb J 1981 Mainstreaming: fulfilling the promises? American Journal of Mental Deficiency 86(2): 115–126

Gould J 1981 Psychometric tests – their uses and limitations. In: Cooper B (ed) Assessing the handicaps and needs of mentally retarded children. Academic Press, London

Gross A M 1977 The use of cost-effectiveness analysis in deciding on alternative living environments for the retarded. In: Mittler P (ed) Research to practice in mental retardation. UPP, Baltimore

Gross A M 1981 Determining the costs of alternative living environments for the mentally retarded: Can we afford deinstitutionalisation. In: Mittler P (ed) Frontiers of knowledge in mental retardation. UPP, Baltimore

Grossman H 1973 A manual on terminology and classification in mental retardation. Series 2. Washington DC, American Association on Mental Deficiency

Gunzburg H C 1974 The primary progress assessment chart of social developments. SEFA Publications, Birmingham

Gustavson K H 1981 The epidemiology of severe mental retardation in Sweden. International Journal of Mental Health 10. 1: 37–46

Guys Health District 1981 Development group for services for mentally handicapped people: Report to district management team

Hagberg B 1978 Severe mental retardation in Swedish children born 1959–1970: Epidemiological panorama and causative factors. In: Major mental handicap: methods and cost of prevention. Ciba Foundation Symposium 59, Amsterdam

Hagberg B 1979 Epidemiological and preventive aspects of cerebral palsy and severe mental retardation in Sweden. European Journal of Paediatrics. 130, 71–78

Hall V, Russell J A O 1980 A national survey of community nursing services for the mentally handicapped. Mental Health Studies Research Report. 10. Bristol University

Heron A 1982 Better services for the mentally handicapped? King's Fund Centre, London

Heron A, Kebbon L, Ericsson K, Blunden R 1981 Evaluation of services for mentally handicapped persons: Symposium on recent studies in Sweden and Britain. In: Mittler P (ed) Frontiers of Knowledge in Mental Retardation. UPP, Baltimore

Heron A, Myers M 1983 Intellectual impairment. The battle against handicap. Academic Press, London

Humphreys S, Lowe K, Blunden R 1981 The administrative prevalence of mental handicap in the city of Cardiff: an examination of geographical distribution. Research Report 11. Mental Handicap in Wales, Research Unit, Cardiff

Iivanainen M 1981 Neurological examination of the mentally retarded child: Evidence of central nervous system abnormality. In: Cooper B (ed) Assessing the handicaps and needs of mentally retarded children. Academic Press, London

Innes G, Johnston A W, Millar W M 1978 Mental subnormality in North-East Scotland: A multi-disciplinary study of a total population. HMSO, Edinburgh

King's Fund 1980 An ordinary life: Comprehensive locally-based services for mentally handicapped people. King's Fund Centre, London

Korner E 1983 (Chairperson) Reports of the committee on health services information. HMSO, London

Kuh D 1978 Review of the technique 'Program Analysis of Service Systems.' (PASS) Exeter, The University Institute of Biometry and Community Medicine

Kushlick A, Blunden R, Cox G 1973 A method of rating behaviour characteristics for use in large scale surveys of mental handicap. Psychology in Medicine 3: 466–478

Linna S L, Koivisto M, Herva R 1981 Chromosomal aetiology of mental retardation: a survey of 1000 mentally retarded patients. In: Mittler P (ed) Frontiers of Knowledge in Mental Retardation. UPP, Baltimore

Mackay R I 1976 Mental handicap in child health practice. Butterworth, London

Martindale A 1980 The distribution of the mentally handicapped between districts of a large city. British Journal of Mental Subnormality 26: 9–20

Martindale A 1983 Trends in the prevalence of mental handicap in Sheffield since 1975. Case register report. Ryegate Centre, Sheffield

Mathieson S, Blunden R 1980 NIMROD is piloting a course towards a community life. Health and Social Services Journal, 25th January, 122–124

Mittler P 1979 People not patients: Problems and policies in mental handicap. Methuen, London

Mittler P, McConachie 1983 Parents, professionals and mentally handicapped people — approaches to partnership. Croom Helm, London

Mittler P, Simon G 1978 Building support for the mentally handicapped and their families. Health and Social Services Journal 88: 541–542

Moores B 1979 Economics of retardation. In: Fryers & Whelan (eds) Current research in mental handicap. North West Regional Health Authority Publication, Manchester

Moores B, Barrett J 1976 Variations in local authority provision for mentally handicapped person. Health and Social Services Journal 86. 6: 258

Mulcahy M, O'Connor S, Reynolds A 1983 Census of the mentally handicapped in the Republic of Ireland, 1981 Irish Medical Journal 76: No.2: 71–75

Munro J, Fryers T 1984 Disability patterns in mentally handicapped adults. In preparation

National Development Group 1978a Helping mentally handicapped people in hospital. DHSS, London

National Development Group 1980 Improving the quality of services for mentally handicapped people: A checklist of standards. DHSS, London

Newcastle City Council, AHA (T) 1981 A blueprint for a local service. Newcastle CHC

North West Regional Health Authority 1982 A model district service. North West Regional Health Authority, Manchester

Nirje B 1970 The normalisation principle: implications and comments. British Journal of Mental Subnormality 16 (2)

O'Brien J 1981 The principle of normalisation. A foundation for effective services. Campaign for mentally handicapped people. London

Ort M, Liepmann M C 1981 The schedule of children's handicaps, behaviour and skills: Reliability and discrimination. In: Mittler P (ed) Frontiers of Knowledge in Mental Retardation. UPP, Baltimore

Plank M 1982 Teams for mentally handicapped people. Campaign for mentally handicapped people. London

Rowan P 1980 What sort of life? NFER Publication. Windsor, England

Russell J A O, Hall V 1980 Mental handicap studies. Research report No. 6. Department of Mental Health, Bristol

Sardharwalla I B 1979 Cost benefit of phenylketonuria screening. In: Fryers & Whelan (eds) Current research in mental handicap. North West Regional Health Authority Publication, Manchester

Sheffield Area Health Authority, Metropolitan District 1981 Strategic planning of services for the mentally handicapped

Snyder R D, Stovring J, Cushing A, Porter K 1981 Meningitis, the CT scan and neurological disabilities. In: Mittler P (ed) Frontiers of Knowledge in Mental Retardation. UPP, Baltimore

Steiner H, Neligan G A 1983 Perinatal morbidity and the quality of survivors. In: Barron S L and Thomson A M (eds) Obstetrical Epidemiology. Academic Press, London

Susser M W 1968 Community psychiatry: Epidemiologic and social themes. Random, New York

Sweeney D P, Wilson T Y 1979 Double jeopardy: The plight of aging and aged developmentally disabled persons in mid-America. Ann Arbor, Michigan

Thomas D, Firth H, Kendall A 1978 ENCOR — A way ahead. CMH Paper 6. Campaign for Mentally Handicapped People. London

Townsend P, Davidson N 1982 Inequalities in health. Pelican, London

Tyne A 1981 Who's consulted? CMH Enquiry Paper 8. Campaign for the Mentally Handicapped, London

Van Den Berghe H, Fryns J P, Pavloiv C, Deroover J, Kenlemans M 1981 Domestic causes of severe mental handicap. In: Mittler P (ed) Frontiers of Knowledge in Mental Retardation. UPP, Baltimore

Vinni K, Sillanpaa A, Anttinen E 1981 Cost study of mental health services. In: Stromgren E et al (eds) Epidemiological research as basis for the organisation of extra-mural psychiatry. Acta Psychiatria Scandinavica Supplement 62: 285

Ward L 1982 People first. Developing services in the community for people with mental handicaps: A review of recent literature. King's Fund Centre, London

Warren S A 1977 Using tests to assess intellectual functioning. In: Mittler P (ed) Research to practice in mental retardation. vol 11. Education and Training p. 3–11. UPP, Baltimore

Weatherall J A C 1982 A review of some effects of recent medical practices in reducing the numbers of children born with congenital abnormalities. Health Trends 14: 85–88

Welsh Office 1978 NIMROD: Report of a joint working party on the provision of a community-based Mental Handicap Service in South Glamorgan, Cardiff

Wessex Regional Health Authority 1981 Management proposals. Winchester

Whelan E, Speake B 1977 Adult training centres in England and Wales. Report of first national survey. HARU, University of Manchester

Whelan E, Speake B 1979 Learning to cope. Souvenir Press, London

WHO 1980 International classification of impairments, disabilities and handicaps. Geneva

Williams P, Shoultz B 1982 We can speak for ourselves. Souvenir Press, London

Wing L 1979a Comparison between Camberwell and Salford. In: Wing J K (ed) Recent Research in Psychiatry. Review of Scientific Work 1979. MRC Social Psychiatric Unit. Institute of Psychiatry, London

Wing L 1979b Prevalence of different patterns of impairment in immigrants. In: Wing J K (ed) Recent

Research in Social Psychiatry. Review of Scientific Work 1974–1979. MRC Social Psychiatric Unit. Institute of Psychiatry, London

Wing L 1981 Language, social and cognitive impairments in autism and severe mental retardation. Journal of Autism and Development Disorders

Wing L 1981 A schedule for deriving profiles of handicaps in mentally retarded children. In: Cooper B (ed. Assessing the handicaps and needs of mentally retarded children. Academic Press, London

Wing L 1982 Report on visit to ENCOR. Personal communication

Wing L 1983 Personal communication

Wolfensberger W 1972 The principle of normalisation in human services. National Institute for Mental Retardation, Toronto

Wolfensberger W, Glenn L 1975 Program analysis service systems (PASS 3). National Institute for Mental Retardation, Toronto

Wolfensberger W, Zanha H (eds) 1973 Citizen advocacy and protective services for the impaired and handicapped. National Institute for Mental Retardation, Toronto

Yates B T 1977 A cost-effectiveness analysis of a residential treatment program for behaviourally disturbed children. In: Mittler P (ed) Research to practice. UPP, Baltimore

Index

Intellectual impairment (*contd*)
  changes in prevalence, 286–289
  hypothesis, 289
  implication of change, 288
  incidence, 286
  social class gradient, 288
  terminology, 279, 281
Intelligence quotient (IQ) evaluation, 284
Interpreting evidence during investigation, 27
Inter-professional co-operation, patients with
    intellectual impariment, 290–294
Iodine
  deficiency, 159–160, 166–170
  disorders, terminology, 170
    see also Cretinism, endemic; Goitre, endemic
  supplementing, methods, 173–176
    evaluation, 176
    oil, 174–175
    others, 175–176
    salt, 173–174

Kaposi's sarcoma and human travel, 197–198
Karelia Heart Disease Prevention Project, 51
Korner Committee, 51

Lassa fever
  and human travel, 198–199
  transmission, 207
Lead
  impairment, 282
  and multiple sclerosis, 107
  poisoning, distribution, 96
Legionnaires' disease and human travel, 193–194
Leptospirosis control, 213–214
Liability, 30–31
Lifestyle conducive to health, WHO targets, 16
Listeriosis control, 208, 214–215
London Health Planning Consortium, 1981, 70

Marburg disease and human travel, 199
Malaria
  and human travel, 194–196
  prophylaxis for travel, 182
Mapping disease
  aim, 97–98
  collation studies, 101–102
  history, 93–97
  hospital and general practice statistics, contrast,
    109–110
  individual studies, 96
  infant mortality, 110–111
  methods, 97–98, 104–105
    aspects, 111–112
  migration and distortion, 98–99
    studies, 102–103
  multiple sclerosis, 105–108
  place of death or residence, 99
  population estimates, 100–101
  presentation, 101
  regional variation in survival, 99
  space-time clustering, 102–104
  validity, 98

Mapping disease (*contd*)
  validity of cause of death, 100
  water hardness and cardiovascular disease, 108–
    109
Maternal
  death, avoidable causes, 79
  mortality, 1881–1981, 224
Measles and human travel, 193
Medical profession
  disillusion with therapeutic progress, 79–80
  and growth of health consumerism, 80–82
  limiting power, 80
Mental handicap *see* Intellectual impairment
Methodology, 24–30
  implications, 24–25
  interpreting evidence, 27–29
  prescribing action, 29–30
  tacit assumptions, 26
Migration causing distortion of disease maps, 98–99
  studies, 102–103
Milk
  -borne infection, 212–213
    statutes controlling, 212–213
  consumption and multiple sclerosis, 107
Monkeypox virus, 207
Morbidity of the poor, 65–66
Mortality
  area, Registrar General, 94
  from cancer, and smoking, 66
  infant, mapping, 110–111
  maternal *see* Maternal mortality
  perinatal *see* Perinatal mortality
  principal causes 1980, 42
  rate 1980, 40
  and social class, 63–64
  standard ratios, 2
Multiple sclerosis, mapping, 105–108
  conclusions, 107–108
  environmental factors, 107
  genetic susceptibility, 106
  geographical variation, 106

Necessities, definition, 59
Nicotine dependence, 136–137

Obstetric care, criticisms and changes, 81
Office of Population Censuses and Surveys, 231–
  234
Old age, health in, 269–278
  efficiency, 275
  financial measurement not complete cost, 274–
    275
  fitness, loss, and disease, 270–272
  health care, planning for, 275–278
  identifying effective interventions, 273–274
  indicators, 274–275
  nature of challenge, 269–272
  objectives, 272–273
  patient's point of view, 275
  quality of life, 274
  self-care and informal care, 272
  social problems, 270